RURAL HEALTH NURSING
STORIES OF CREATIVITY, COMMITMENT, AND CONNECTEDNESS

Edited by
Patricia Winstead-Fry, PhD, RN
Julia Churchill Tiffany, EdD, RN
Raelene V. Shippee-Rice, PhD, RN

National League for Nursing Press • New York
Pub. No. 21-2408

ISBN 0-88737-524-3

The views expressed in this publication represent the views of the authors and do not necessarily reflect the official views of the National League for Nursing.

This book was set in Garamond and Palatino by Publications Development Company. The editor and designer was Rachel Schaperow. United Book Press was the printer and binder. The cover was designed by Lillian Welsh.

Printed in the United States of America

This book is dedicated to the Tri-State Rural Health Consortium which itself exemplifies the themes of creativity, commitment, and connectedness. The editors wish to thank the nurse administrators of the Universities of Vermont, New Hampshire, and Southern Maine for their encouragement and support. Their support enabled the editors to share equally in creating *Rural Health Nursing: Stories of Creativity, Commitment, and Connectedness.*

Preface

The purpose of *Rural Health Nursing: Stories of Creativity, Commitment, and Connectedness* is to introduce nurses and other health care providers to the issues, trends, and unique aspects of practice in the rural environment. The editors have included papers describing what is occurring in rural health and rural health nursing.

The idea for this book emerged from discussions among faculty from the Universities of Vermont, New Hampshire, and Southern Maine. These three northern New England states are characterized as rural. During discussions, the theme of rurality became a focus with which we could all identify. The concept was broad enough to allow a diversity of individual interests and yet give a coherence to our joint endeavors. On the basis of this common theme, the three universities formed the Tri-State Rural Health Consortium. For this book, we reached out to colleagues in other parts of the country who are also studying solutions to rural health problems.

Rural Health Nursing does not attempt to be exhaustive of the domain of rural health. It rather serves to highlight unique aspects of the rural health nursing experience. These chapters convey a feeling for the practice of nursing in communities where people know one another well and have often lived in close proximity for generations. Without denying the reality of the problems facing rural health care, this book offers a vision of how creativity, commitment, and connectedness can bring about positive effects.

By addressing rurality, this book advances the environmental aspect of the metaparadigm of nursing. It encourages scholars to explore other unique environments which shape nursing practice.

As the elements of person, nursing, and health are understood in an environmental context, the science of nursing will expand and raise new challenges for serving the health care needs of people.

The editors could not have accomplished this volume without the help of the many nurses who contributed their talents in writing and critiquing *Rural Health Nursing: Creativity, Commitment, and Connectedness.* We thank them for their participation in this work.

Patricia Winstead-Fry, PhD, RN
Julia Churchill Tiffany, EdD, RN
Raelene V. Shippee-Rice, PhD, RN

Contents

CONTRIBUTORS

Marilyn Barba, CNOR, RN
Graduate Student, Nursing Administration
University of New Hampshire
Surgical Supervisor
Huggins Hospital
Wolfeboro, New Hampshire

Mary Bayer, RNC
Co-owner and Consultant Administrator
Sandy River Health Alliance Nursing Care Centers of Maine
Portland, Maine

Beverly J. Chasse, MSEd, RNC
Nurse Counselor
Franklin Memorial Hospital
Farmington, Maine

Deborah A. Clark, MS, CS, RN
Behavior Specialist
School Administration District No. 47
Ashland, Maine

Lorraine M. Clarke, EdM, RN
Associate Professor
University of Vermont
School of Nursing
Burlington, Vermont

Judith A. Cohen, MS, RN
Associate Professor
University of Vermont
School of Nursing
Burlington, Vermont

Candace Corrigan, PhD, RN
Flagstaff, Arizona

Holly A. Cozzi-Burr, MSN, RN
Community Health Nurse
Bar Harbor Division of Community Health Services
Bar Harbor, Maine

Ruth Davis, MSN, CS, RN
Director of Behavioral Health Services
Franklin Memorial Hospital
Farmington, Maine

Carol Green-Hernandez, PhD, FNS, RNC
Associate Professor
Graduate Program in Nursing
University of Vermont
Burlington, Vermont

Brenda Pauline Hamel-Bissell, MS, EdD, RN
Associate Professor
School of Nursing
University of Vermont
Burlington, Vermont

Margaret Hourigan, EdD, RN
Senior Vice President, Clinical
Stevens Memorial Hospital
Norway, Maine

Karen R. Johnson, EdD, RN
Associate Professor of Nursing
University of New Hampshire
Durham, New Hampshire

Kathleen Ann Long, PhD, RNCS, FAAN
Dean and Professor
College of Nursing
Montana State University
Bozeman, Montana

Theresa A. B. Lyons, RNC
Nurses Diversified
Fairbanks, Alaska

Diane Feeney Mahoney, PhD, RNC
Coordinator, Graduate Program in Gerontological Nursing
College of Nursing
University of Massachusetts at Boston
Boston, Massachusetts

Dorothy Malone-Rising, MS, RNC
Gerontological Nurse Practitioner
Assistant Professor of Nursing
University of Vermont
Burlington, Vermont

Laurie Murray, DNS, RN
Assistant Professor
University of Vermont
School of Nursing
Burlington, Vermont

Mary Val Palumbo, MSN, RNC
Clinical Assistant Professor
University of Vermont
Burlington, Vermont

Raelene V. Shippee-Rice, PhD, RN
Director, Undergraduate Studies
University of New Hampshire
Department of Nursing
Durham, New Hampshire

Julia C. Tiffany, EdD, RN
Associate Professor
University of Southern Maine
School of Nursing
Portland, Maine

Lorraine Wargo, RN
Nursing Care Coordinator
Professional Nursing Service, Inc.
Burlington, Vermont

Clarann Weinert, PhD, SC, RN
Professor
College of Nursing
Montana State University
Bozeman, Montana

Patricia Winstead-Fry, PhD, RN
Professor
University of Vermont
School of Nursing
Burlington, Vermont

Diane York, CCRN, RN
Intensive Care Unit Head Nurse
Rumford Community Hospital
Rumford, Maine

Introduction

Rural America is a phrase that calls to mind cows, sheep, fields of grain, and the gentle people who live in this environment. This bucolic image is not the whole picture. To understand rural life today requires including images of poverty, economic problems, and under-served health care needs. *Rural Health Nursing: Stories of Creativity, Commitment, and Connectedness* focuses on the health care needs of rural people. This book contains material on unmet needs, but most of the chapters are stories of success—successful actions by consumers and providers of health care.

Scholarly inquiry into rural life is not new. Recent government actions, however, have highlighted the need for a focus on rural life. The Office of Rural Health Policy was created during the Reagan administration to promote projects and research germane to rural concerns. Congress has also begun to direct its attention to rural life. There are numerous proposals in committees addressing the needs of rural people.

One of the first difficulties a student of rural life encounters is that of definition. There is no generally agreed upon definition of rural. The lack of consensus reflects the diversity of rural populations. There are four generally used definitions. The first is by population density. "Frontier counties" are those with fewer than six people per square mile. Frontier counties are found in the West, but are not common in the rest of the country. A second way of defining rural is by population size. A town with a population of less than 2,500 is rural. The populations in the first two definitions may be either farm or non-farm communities. A third typology classifies counties as metropolitan or non-metropolitan. Counties with an urban population center of 50,000 or more are metropolitan. All other counties are non-metropolitan. The fourth way of classifying areas as rural is by distance from a health care facility. If a community is more than 60 minutes from a health care facility, it is rural.

The editors made no attempt to define rural in this book because there is no need to define rural from a nursing perspective. The eventual definition(s) that guide scholarly inquiry and discussion of rurality must be multidisciplinary because understanding and serving the needs of rural people is always an interconnected endeavor among many people. Instead of trying to achieve a definition, the editors asked contributors to either offer a definition for their chapter or to give a description of the rural area they were writing about.

Rural Health Nursing: Stories of Creativity, Commitment, and Connectedness makes no claim to be exhaustive of rural health issues and solutions. Rather, each chapter is a piece of a kaleidoscope that offers readers an insight into some aspect of rural nursing. In reading the chapters, the autonomy and creativity of the nurses and their colleagues will be impressive. The commitment of the nurses to their communities and the connectedness of people to one another and to health care organizations is equally impressive.

From the first chapter which introduces Irene Kent, a nurse who hung out a shingle and provided care to her neighbors for 30 years, to the last chapter in which Long and Weinert discuss appropriate theory for rural nursing, all of the chapters reflect aspects of creativity, connectedness, and commitment. The chapters are arranged to achieve a balance of theory and practice. Chapters one through 6 focus on the connectedness of families and caring. Chapters 7, 8, and 9 highlight the creativity and commitment of consumers and providers in meeting the support needs of people. Chapters 10, 11, and 12 exemplify the creativity in management that typifies some rural approaches to health care problems. Chapters 13 through 16 offer pieces on creative approaches to research, governance, and education in rural settings. Finally, Chapter 17 provides readers with a theoretical model of rural nursing into which they can transpose their pieces of the kaleidoscope to form a more complete set of ideas about rural health nursing.

Part I

Families and Caring

1

Nursing on Swans Island, Maine, 1938–1975

Holly A. Cozzi-Burr

Provision of nursing care to island communities is a service which people in these unique environments depend on greatly for support, for information, and for direct care. An island nurse is a person who has chosen to practice nursing in an environment where physical isolation, culture, and interpersonal relationships greatly affect one's practice.

A qualitative methodology was used during the research for this paper, as there is little known about the domain of island nursing and because this researcher attempted to describe the phenomenon from the "native's point of view," that is to say from the island nurse's interpretation of events in her domain.

Oral history was the qualitative approach used for this research. This method generates the type of rich description called for in the purpose of this research. Oral history is defined here as taped interviews with an island nurse about her recollections of nursing in the past. Unlike other histories of nursing, oral history enables the researcher to vicariously experience the past. That experience then combines with an intellectual ordering of past events and reasons for why events happened the way they happened (Sitton, 1986). Oral history as an approach to inquiry gives

3

the nurse an opportunity to describe her practice in the context of what was happening in the world, on the island, and in nursing.

The histories obtained for this paper give testimony to the fact that distance, travel, and isolation did not impede the ability of the island nurses to effectively serve their communities (FNS Quarterly, Summer 1987).

Mary Breckinridge, founder of the Frontier Nursing Service (FNS), recounts her experiences accompanying patients on wintertime trips via "ambulance" (FNS Quarterly, Autumn 1980, pp. 37–38). Breckinridge's experiences of emergency boat travel down the Middle Fork River (Kentucky) are not unlike the unexpected trips made by nurses and their patients on the Swans Island Ferry or the Sunbeam—the only ice breaker available in the early 1970s. Either vessel might depart Swans Island in a variety of unsavory weather conditions for a five-mile crossing of Blue Hill Bay to an awaiting vehicle in which the patient would be transported to Mount Desert Island Hospital 20 miles away.

A glimpse of the work of Swans Island nurses from 1938 to 1975 was found in old town reports at the island library. Data about island subsidies for nurses, expenses for telephone, drugs, and travel, and some indication of public health nurse involvement on the island were found in reports from 1938 through 1975. Data contained in these reports is useful in gaining an objective view of life and health care on Swans Island.

The town report for February 3, 1947, indicated that a sum of $1,800 was appropriated for nurse services and $125 for a dental clinic. A reprint of that agreement between Swans Island and the Sea Coast Mission, which provided the island with adjunctive health services and a stipend for nursing services, refers to employment of a public health nurse in 1946:

> . . . a salary of $1800 would be paid and $75 would be contributed for a dental clinic . . . . $50 would be raised to help pay off-island telephone calls made in the line of duty and not paid for by the sick person or family. Nurse charges .50 for a daytime call, $1.00 for an evening call, $2.00 to stay all night. Monies received will be turned in to the island treasury. The nurses will receive $35.00 per month car allowance, and charge .50 for use of her car

(Mission will make up the balance at the end of the month). Thus she will carry out preventive medicine and public health. . . .

A town report from 1966–1967 includes a Public Health Nursing Report outlining the services provided:

. . . visits to expectant mothers, infants, preschool children and adults. Special service clinics include orthopedic, pediatric, cardiac, mental retardation, cystic fibrosis, vision and hearing defects, x-ray, speech evaluation, and are available on physician request . . . . [Annual Report, 1966–1967]

The report also indicated that the Division of Public Health Nursing (PHN) administered DPT, DT, Small Pox, Salk vaccines, and Tine tests, and conferred with teachers about children. The appropriation for PHN was $80.00, and remained fairly constant through the early 1970s, although PHN expanded immunization schedules and service clinics to include treatment of epilepsy.

Monies received from the patients varied from $108 to $175 per year during the time of Irene Kent's nursing practice. The nurse's salary did not increase beyond $1,800 through the 1970s.

During the search for artifacts, biographical data about Irene Kent was found in a newspaper article written during the 1940s entitled "Island without a doctor: Three Maine nurses act in emergencies." A photo of the health care providers was captioned "Health Sentinels of Lonely Outpost." The data in the brief article sensitized the researcher to the appreciation islanders had for the three nurses who were living there at the time. The nurses, Irene Kent, RN; Leila Whitehill, RN; and Ann Cally, RN, were also housewives and mothers. While living on the island, however, they were likened to soldiers who "upon hearing call to arms, snap to attention and rush forth to join the fray" (Bernstorf, 1948).

ONE NURSE'S STORY

Irene Kent, RN, the primary respondent selected for the oral history, was a nurse on Swans Island for 17 years. Kent shared with this researcher a great deal about her life. Kent approaches longevity with an affirmative attitude and a clear-eyed view of reality. Although she had initial doubts and fears of not having "anything interesting" to offer, experience in the process satisfactorily cut through those qualms. Like a room full of books, Kent had a story to be revealed—finally someone ventured to ask.

Kent, an active, alert woman of 87 is not an island native. She came to the island in the 1940s and spent years traveling between her native New York and Swans Island before retiring to the island in 1972. In the time of her living on Swans Island, Kent provided nursing services to residents in their homes and from a clinic, which remains adjacent to her home. Pending her duties as an island nurse, the private realm of her life included homemaking, child rearing, and work in the public domain on the island Health Committee. Although "time-off" was her own, Irene's role on the island was characteristic of the barefoot doctors of China. For example, Kent's role and ability to handle medical problems while working at "non-health related work" was a significant force in the community, the family, and the social group (Denton, 1985, pp. 94–96).

Kent's description of her transition to an isolated island community is of an experience many would have found uncomfortable. It is in the breadth and depth of her description, however, that one reaps an appreciation of the characteristics which are necessary for a successful island nursing experience.

Upon arrival to Swans Island in 1946, Kent's impression was of "going back 100 years." The island lacked "facilities": several homes were without plumbing, electricity, heat, or phone. There were no autos or a passenger-carrying ferry until 1959. Yet these environmental circumstances did not inhibit her interest in living on the island or in getting to know members of the community.

The beauty of her surroundings and the invigorating salt air did not engender romantic notions about island nursing for Kent. Kent practiced on the island during a period when there were no pharmacy services on the island or readily accessible distributors of medical supplies. "Having to make do with whatever you had" was common in her practice. A mixture of Kaopectate and

Paregoric for abdominal cramping and adhesive taping in lieu of sutures were well used innovations.

The clinic as Kent remembers it was always simply appointed. A small waiting room at the end of a long entrance corridor contains the original furnishings; two chairs and a sofa. The examining room had an examining table, a sink, and a refrigerator. The house sits close to the road on one of the major island roads, approximately one mile from the ferry terminal. A small sign hung from the clinic entrance read "Irene Kent, RN—Clinic," indicating to the passerby or would-be patient that help in the form of professional nursing care was available in that beautiful, yet remote corner of the world.

A significant feature of her island practice was the kinship she developed with her advising physicians on the mainland. Although Kent had no preparation for island work, she enjoyed being away from the "structure" and routine of hospital work and being out on her own with physician backup.

Swans Islanders are independent and self-sufficient; these cultural norms influenced the type of nursing care that was needed and given. If Kent had an ethnocentric viewpoint, it was quickly discarded in favor of listening to what the islander thought was best for him or herself. Kent's story of learning about the island custom of applying salt pork to a wound, in lieu of traditional soaks, exemplifies her acceptance of the different practices, values, and attitudes of the islanders. Kent clearly understood that a nonjudgmental approach was essential in caring for a patient who was fearful of leaving the island to go to the hospital in Bar Harbor. Essentially, the island nurse learns to work with patients who have backgrounds different from her or his own. It is the nurse's relationship with people that made the work enjoyable.

Within the matrix of an independent practice are interrelationships and a reliance on community efforts in times of trouble. Kent recognized that without collective cooperation from islanders, good health and positive outcomes would be less likely to be enjoyed. The island's isolation dictated the need for interdependence and Kent's ability to think and act fast in an emergency. The skill for making appropriate decisions in a timely fashion has resulted in 40 years of her knowing that "no one ever died because they were on the island and couldn't get help." Kent learned to evaluate the patient data at hand and fully exercised her nursing abilities before medical intervention became accessible.

When referring to her role as island nurse, Kent speaks with a sense of assurance and adequacy and a satisfaction that addresses the privilege she has felt in being able to practice in this unique style.

The types of nursing duties performed by Kent were pragmatic and similar to lay nursing. Even though confined by the limits in technology inherent in nursing during the 1950s and 1960s, as well as by the strains of a remote work site, Kent was uninhibited in her ability to provide "general old-fashioned nursing." The care arrangements Kent could make included assessments, dressing changes, administration of immunizations, assisting with bed and baths, "sitting up with patients," and other care-oriented functions.

Kent remembered that "a great many times all I could do was just sit there and talk to them patients, tell them what I expected . . . they were glad to see a nurse . . . it took the responsibility off their shoulders—it was somebody they knew." She was quick to add that families did most of their own nursing and were pretty much "self-sufficient . . . while the nurse just came in like a doctor."

Kent married in 1933 and reduced her nursing activities to devote herself to her family. Familial obligation was commended at that time as "the most important institution in democratic society" and the caretaking function demanded one's full attention (Kalish, 1986, p. 121). The duties of wife and mother were obligated to husband and society. Kent was willing to give up her career for "the duty and glory of womanhood" (Gilman, 1970). Following the war effort, women who had previously worked in nontraditional roles returned to the function of making a happy home. The image of the postwar homemaker is a salient part of the bond between Kent the woman and Kent the nurse:

Adaptability and resourcefulness, the ability to improvise in emergencies are required when unpredictable events affect the household suddenly. Illness, accidents, financial

crises, and emotional shocks are the most serious. . . . If
she is inflexible or goes to pieces in a crisis, she aggravates
the situation. [Zapoleon, 1970]

Kent recalls herself as being "organized and in a routine" and
never having any problems balancing her duties as a homemaker
and as a nurse when she moved to the island. She was efficient and
eventually became the economic head of the household.

Kent was part of the work force in the 1950s through to the
1970s, working in various nursing roles. For the most part, nursing
during those years was the occupational equivalent of marriage.
The language of duty and obligation was relevant not only to
homemakers, but also characterized the historical ideology of
nursing and Kent's practice. In Kent's viewpoint, her care-giving
self was prominent in her life history; the self who became
"involved more closely with people than do nurses today."

RECOLLECTIONS OF OTHER ISLANDERS

The story of Swans Island illustrates the richness and challenges of
rural nursing. Willing informants, data found in historical records,
artifacts, and the clinic where Kent used to practice provided additional sources of information.

Author Perry Westbrook provides data showing island nursing (and doctoring) as a "challenge for those who were more
interested in doing a good job than in money" (1958, p. 179).
He also recognized that there was a significant reliance on "self-
doctoring . . . that goes back to the days of when one had to rely
on their own knowledge of herbs or sail to the mainland for professional help . . ." (p. 179).

Westbrook (1958) reveals a vivid sense of what the Swans
Island nurse of the past encountered when severe weather made it
impossible to get to the mainland. He describes a time during a
"nor'easter" when a Baptist minister suffering from acute appen-
dicitis was operated on right in the parsonage by the island physician. The nurse who was summoned by the physician was taken to
the parsonage by horse and sleigh on a network of interior logging

roads. By the light of oil lamps, reflectors, and flashlights, the surgery was successfully performed (p. 179).

Islander John Martin tells of home cures used when he was a youngster growing up on Swans Island:

> *Back then you didn't go to the doctor as often as you do now. People doctored themselves . . . they had Vicks Vapor Rub for colds. . . . I can remember flannel cloth and hen's grease . . . they take the hen's grease, melt it down and put it on flannel [to put on the chest] and give it to us to be taken internally. They had Carter's Liver Pills . . . Doan's Pills and Johnson's Back Plasters . . . today you can't buy them.*

Bernice Carlson, another island native, grew up using and still uses Father John's for colds if " . . . you get down so you ain't got much of an appetite." Whether a result of nostrums used by islanders or not, most enjoyed good health and died of old age (Westbrook, p. 179). Further data about the divergent life-styles, the provision of nursing care to the island community, and the health of the islanders was reflected in other interviews with selected respondents:

> *Anna Scott . . . she checked on me all the time. She would come right in day after day, check on me and tell me what to do. She would come to Johnny quite a lot, but if I wanted to know something I would call and ask her. Once she found out there was something wrong, you didn't have to call her. She would come and check on you. She was a good person, a very good person, she was a willing person . . . when she gave you advice it would be sound advice. If she said you should go see a doctor, then you should go see a doctor. She was one of them kind. I think it relaxes a lot of people, someone like her. She moved here and I think once she got acquainted some, she would go to people and they'd ask her this and that and I think it relaxed them, rather than saying, 'Well could you tell me what my problem is . . .' She would go find it out and ask them and I think it relaxed them to think that she was interested.*

Bernice Carlson illustrates the utilization of the island nurse many years ago:

Edith Spires was an RN that saved mama's life. There was no doctor available when sister was born. Mother had birthed at home and developed milk fever when the baby was born. The baby was born dead . . . mother had lost all of her hair and finger nails. Miss Spires administered hot baths and aspirin to mother who was out of her mind for a spell. When she improved she would no longer take aspirin having associated it with illness.

Eugene Norwood contributes his thoughts about needing emergency health care when living in isolation:

Esther McDuffy was smart, I thought. I remember she would come to me, I had this ulcer and you could look right in and see the bone and cords . . . and she would come every day to repack it. I walked on it for a long time before I did anything about it. That was one of the big problems on here, if you could run to a clinic you could get things done easy. I think if you live in Southwest Harbor or Ellsworth somewhere near a clinic, you can say, 'I don't feel good, I'm going in.' With a place like this, it's too much effort. My philosophy about staying well is just hope and pray, I guess.

The previous reminiscences contribute to a history of nursing duties and illuminate a way of life and tradition for Swans Islanders.

The characteristics of the subculture of island nurses as explored through the oral history of Irene Kent correlate with what the literature reveals about rural nursing. Although there is no consensus about what unique characteristics are essential to the successful performance of rural nurses, certain components have been described. Descriptions of the rural nurse which have been cited include: "generalists"; "flexible"; "versatile"; "adaptable"; "resourceful"; "culture conscious"; "self-reliant"; and "skilled in" obstetrics, maternity, intensive care, and emergency room nursing (Biegel, 1983; Bond, Bailey, Hansen, Wierda, 1984; Thobaden & Weingard, 1983). Certainly, the life of Irene Kent illustrates these characteristics.

REFERENCES

Annual Report of the Town Officers of the town of Swans Island, Maine (1966–1967). pp. 27–28.

Bernstorf, E. (1948). "Island without a doctor: Three Maine nurses act in emergencies," unreferenced newspaper article.

Biegel, A. (1983). Toward a definition of rural nursing. *Home Health-care Nurse, 1*(1), 45–46.

Bond, L., Bailey, S., Dommer, J., Hansen, M., Wierda, L. (1984). Rural nursing: Unique practice opportunity. *The Michigan Nurse,* 4–6.

Denton, J. A. (1985). Registered nurses: The barefoot doctors of the United States. *Nursing Forum, 21*(3), 94–96.

Frontier Nursing Service Quarterly Bulletin. (1980, Autumn). *56*(2), 32–38.

Gilman, C. P. (1970). The family relation. In A. F. Scott (Ed.), *Women in American life: Selected readings* (pp. 92–95). Boston: Houghton Mifflin.

Kalish, P. A., & Kalish, B. J. (1986). *The changing image of the nurse.* Menlo Park, California: Addison-Wesley.

Thobaden, M., & Weingard, M. (1983). Rural nursing. *Home Health-care Nurse, 1*(2), 9–13.

Westbrook, P. D. (1958). *Biography of an island.* New York: Thomas Yoseloff.

Zapoleon, M. (1970). Homemaking as a career. In A. F. Scott (Ed.), Women in American life: Selected readings (pp. 154–158). Boston: Houghton Mifflin.

2

On Fear and Courage: A First Encounter with AIDS in Rural Vermont

Laurie Murray
Lorraine Wargo

This chapter is a moving account of fear and courage. It is presented as a personal narrative to preserve the intense feelings that colored the activities in caring for a family with AIDS. To preserve the "story" of an early encounter with an uncommon, killer disease is of interest to students of the human spirit. Both authors were involved in the care of the family. For the sake of presenting a coherent account, however, the narrative is presented as Lorraine Wargo's remembrance of her work with the Campbell family, as they coped with AIDS. All names have been changed, except Wargo's.

To orient readers, the names given the Campbell family in this narrative are as follows:

Jane: the patient's mother

Dan: the patient's father

Margaret, "Meg": the adult AIDS patient

Greg: the patient's husband

Amy: the child AIDS patient, daughter of Greg and Margaret

Vicki: Amy's sister.

THE AREA

The town in which the events occurred is one of several in a valley. It is a ski area. Recreation is the main industry and farming is the second one. The valley population is between three and four thousand. It is a rural community. Because it is a resort area, it has many inns and restaurants. Most of the people who live in the town work there, but a number of people also commute out of town to work. The community itself is made up of Vermonters who have been there for several generations, of transients who come to the town during the ski season to work, and people who are transplants to Vermont. Transplant Vermonters are those people who visited the area, fell in love with the community, and decided to move there. Most transplants are from Massachusetts, New York, and New Jersey. The community is sort of a melting pot. The mix of old and new residents can cause some friction and tension, but basically it's a very caring community. People care about their neighbor, but also stay out of their neighbor's business. There is an incredible "communication system" that far exceeds Ma Bell. I wouldn't describe it as gossip. It's a real communication system, one that can be positive, as well as negative.

I am a traditional Vermonter, born and raised in Burlington. I am considered a real Vermonter. I left Vermont for ten years after college and went to Washington, D.C., to work and to get other nursing experience. My family and my roots remained in Vermont, and so we came back.

THE FIRST EXPERIENCE

I knew Jane because she lived in the area. I met her at the clinic where I worked. The health center is the only medical facility within a 30-minute drive.

I met Jane first in the community, bumping into her here and there. In February 1989, she came into the clinic obviously upset. Approaching the window, she asked to have her blood pressure checked right away, stating that she didn't feel well. I was walking by and took her into a room and checked her blood pressure. It was very high, and she was visibly upset. I asked her what was bothering her and commented that she looked stressed. She said she "couldn't talk about it right now." I accepted that and asked her to sit there for a while so I could monitor her blood pressure.

After a time, I decided to move her to a quieter room. I sat down just to be with her and to check her blood pressure. Finally, she said she had to talk to somebody; she felt she would "burst" if she didn't tell somebody what was going on. I encouraged her. She asked if I knew Margaret. Although, I hadn't met Margaret, I knew she was Jane's daughter.

She wanted me to promise that I wouldn't tell anybody her secret. I assured her that anything she said was confidential. She said she didn't want it written in her chart. I accepted that, but asked if I could tell Dr. Baker if it turned out to be something that might affect her medically. She agreed and then blurted out, "Margaret has AIDS." She started to cry. It was unbelievable. I sat there, held her hand, and let her cry. Then she added, "Even worse than that, the baby has AIDS too." She was in a state of disbelief—not wanting anybody to know—absolutely frightened that somebody would find out—knowing that in a small town, things get out. She worried about what the illness would do to the rest of her family as she had five other children. I knew some of her other kids. Some of them went to school with my kids. At this point she seemed to be responding to the stigma of having AIDS. What if people found out? What would happen to the rest of the family? What would happen to Margaret—to the dog—to Vicki? She raced on exhibiting totally out-of-control fear. We talked. Basically, I listened. I checked her blood pressure again. It was a little bit lower. I left her, found Dr. Baker, and told him. He went in and spent some time with her. That was how I came to know about Margaret.

Jane kept coming in, off and on. We would just talk. At that time, other than Jane and her husband, Margaret and her husband were the only ones who knew the true diagnosis. The rest of the family were told that Margaret had a blood disease, leukemia. The four were afraid to tell the family the truth. The fear of "it" getting out—not knowing how the community would react—the stigma of having this disease—all of these things left them in absolute terror of people finding the truth.

Dan worked for one of the biggest building companies in the valley, while Jane worked at a local store that sold fabric and novelties. Both were very active in their church. They were an extremely visible couple. Everyone knew them. People thought of Jane and Dan as positive, warm, loving people. Jane was the kind of person who said what she thought. Dan was a kind, Santa Claus-type person. They were afraid of being banished from the community. Greg had a parts and repair business in town. If word got out that his wife and daughter had AIDS, how would he support his family? There was a real financial as well as an emotional threat.

AIDS was a death sentence. People believed that AIDS didn't exist in Vermont. The feeling was, "We don't have that in rural Vermont, it is a city problem." We believed we were safe in rural Vermont. We came here to get away from the problems of the city. We didn't even lock our doors! I had a difficult time accepting that AIDS was in my home town, even though this was not my first encounter with it.

My first experience with AIDS was bad. A young man from San Francisco came to Vermont to vacation and decided to stay. While in Vermont, he started feeling badly. His friends noticed he was having memory problems. He came to the clinic with chest congestion and memory problems. I did a strep screen on him first, then took a history. We had an outbreak of strep at the time, so I figured he had strep, but the memory loss confused me. Dr. Brown and I checked him over, but we couldn't diagnose him. We started him on antibiotics. He didn't get better.

One day, as I was reading a magazine article about AIDS, I thought, "Gee, this guy sounds just like the people in this article." I had not seen AIDS yet, so the next day I talked with Dr. Baker. He thought I was crazy, but said, "Okay, let's check him for AIDS." The young man was positive.

I still remember the day Dr. Baker told him that he had AIDS. I've had other patients with AIDS since then, but this one was really traumatic for me. The fact that the man had AIDS wasn't a problem. To me it was just another disease and a patient who needed care. But that Vermonter part of me kept whispering, "This can't happen, not here in rural Vermont. Nothing bad happens to our families here in rural Vermont. We're protected out here in the country." You see, in Vermont we live with nature. We live with the environment, and the people care about the environment. Something like this just doesn't happen. On that day, the reality of the disease came crashing into my awareness.

The young man ended up leaving Vermont because he thought there was nobody there to help him. He was afraid that because he was a homosexual, he would be an outcast. He went back to San Francisco where he died alone. That was very hard!

Margaret's fears were just as real. She was just as scared, even though she was not a homosexual or an IV drug user. The fact that she had AIDS was just as scary to her as it was to this young man. Both of them were absolutely frightened of anybody finding out. The situation of secrecy stayed like this for over a year.

THE SITUATION BEGINS TO CHANGE

Eventually, Margaret came to the clinic because Amy had an ear infection. Margaret looked healthy and so did the child. No one mentioned AIDS. Indeed, when they left, Dr. Baker asked me if I was sure Jane was correct about them having AIDS.

Jane and I kept in touch. She would come into the clinic to have her blood pressure checked. I would see her and we would chat about how things were going.

In the fall of 1989, Margaret began to look a little sick—a little thinner. Although always thin, she started to look a bit more gaunt.

In February 1989, Jane started helping out in the home during the day, taking care of Amy and Margaret. Greg would come home at night and would take over the care. Sometimes Greg would stay up all night and go back to work in the morning. He maintained this pattern for a year and a half. Neither Jane nor Greg wanted to bother anybody. They wanted to keep it to themselves and take care of it themselves. They didn't seek any help. They were still afraid of the community's reaction.

Severe financial difficulty began because Greg was not able to handle working and taking care of his family. Everything started to crumble. They tried social welfare to get some assistance, but they had a house so they didn't qualify for any programs. Again, AIDS was not mentioned. They didn't tell the agency how much they were paying for drugs and other things. Greg had not tallied the costs. He just put the bills away in a box.

One of the ways Greg dealt with the stress was to occasionally drink alcohol. He avoided talking about AIDS with his friends. Margaret was involved with an AIDS support group at this point, but Greg did not join any support group, nor did he talk with his mother-in-law or father-in-law. He did reach out to his mother, but she was unable to deal with what was happening. He made a plea for help to her shortly before he committed suicide, but she thought he only wanted financial help. She didn't send him anything. He might have asked for help from his best friend, but he couldn't directly say, "I need you here."

In June, everything changed. Greg committed suicide. He had written his best friend a letter right before he died telling what a wonderful friend he had been. He also made a tape and wrote a letter for Vicki, his oldest daughter. In it, he explained that he couldn't cope and he thought they would be better off without him. He hoped that with him gone, they would qualify for social services.

Margaret was in the hospital for pneumonia when Greg committed suicide. Baby Amy was also in the hospital because she was not eating and was very thin. Amy had lost incredible ground quickly. The family was preparing themselves for Amy's death when Greg became extremely despondent and killed himself.

Margaret left the hospital to go to the memorial service and to help take care of the arrangements. Amy remained in the hospital. After the memorial service, Margaret went back to the hospital for continued treatment.

Not long before Greg committed suicide, some of the family members had begun to guess Margaret and Amy's real diagnosis. They had some raring, tearing fights because the family was upset that they weren't told, but had to guess. Nobody else in the community knew. No one even suspected AIDS. Margaret simply did not fit anyone's stereotype of an AIDS patient.

After Greg died, Margaret began to "go public." She applied and was qualified for the disabled children and home care program. It is a state program, Medicaid-funded, for any child with a medical need. Family income is not a criteria for participation. The child began to receive nursing care from Professional Nursing Service (PNS), the program I had moved to in April.

At the same time, Margaret was using the Visiting Nurse Association and another high-tech company to administer the IVs needed for her chemotherapy. Now she had to decide whether she wanted to continue working with different companies or choose one. She eventually decided it would be easier to work with PNS.

At a Bernie Seigel meeting, she stood up and told everybody that she had AIDS and received a big hug from Bernie Seigel. She also went to the Federated Church, and during the service, told everybody she and her daughter had AIDS. She wrote an open letter to the editor of the local paper, disclosing that she had AIDS and that that was one of the contributing factors to her husband's suicide. Margaret no longer wanted to live a lie. It became very important that she live and die with dignity. She also wanted to bring AIDS out of the closet and for people to realize that anyone can get it. She wanted people to know that it affected the whole family—that the entire family can die.

Margaret was due to leave the hospital on a Friday in the summer. It was a coordinator's nightmare! We stepped into a family situation that was already highly emotional. Greg had just committed suicide. Margaret and her daughter had AIDS, with Margaret going public. The family would have to deal with the community. I needed nurses who could walk into a situation where everybody is grieving and the whole family is in crisis.

As nurses, we must decide if we want to take care of a family that has AIDS, whether we will feel comfortable doing that. There were nurses who feared getting AIDS. They worried for their significant others and their children. Some of the husbands and lovers didn't want their nurse family member to take care of an AIDS client. People had to really look at what this illness meant to them. Nurses and their families had to come to grips with their value systems.

As the care coordinator, I spent most of my time educating the family and the nurses. Nurses caring for an AIDS patient in the home must draw blood, give medications, change dressings, insert nasogastric (NG) tubes, and clean up vomitus and diarrhea. They must bathe these people, touch them, and hug them.

Because the PNS nurses would live with Margaret for eight hours at a time, they might eat from her utensils and use her toilet. They feared they could get AIDS. What is played up is the fact that the patient can give the nurses AIDS. In actuality, that's not the problem. The problem is the AIDS patient's immune system is depressed and *we* are the ones who could kill the patient. I had to screen the nurses. They couldn't be sick. If their kids had chicken-pox, they couldn't work with this family.

We had three nurses who had experience with AIDS, and were comfortable with it. The majority, however, were uncomfortable and needed in-service education to go over universal precautions and discuss how AIDS is spread. Soon, most of the nurses began to feel comfortable with AIDS. For some nurses, the AIDS wasn't a problem, but the emotional aspects of the case were overwhelming.

Being in a rural area, we didn't have the experience with this type of case. We didn't have the support systems that are available in urban areas for nurses who work with AIDS patients. We were treading in virgin territory. We dreaded dealing with the insurance companies who also had little experience with this disease. Our organization had other AIDS clients, but the complexity of a mother and child having AIDS simultaneously and the complex family dynamics involved was new for all of us.

Despite all the problems, Margaret and Amy did come home. I was on call that weekend and decided to get in touch with them later that Friday evening to see how things were going. They got home around 5 o'clock. I received a phone call minutes later. It was an attack of Murphy's Law. Everything that could go wrong did go wrong. Amy pulled her NG tube out. Margaret realized this was the first time Amy had been home since her father's death. It was shocking for Amy to come home and not have her daddy greet her. This was also the first time Margaret was going to be there without Greg in the house.

I arrived to find Margaret in the bedroom, frustrated and upset. Amy was lying on the bed, and Vicki was walking around, sucking her thumb, clinging to everybody. Margaret was really trying to be in control. It was very important for Margaret to insert that NG tube tonight. So I helped her organize the equipment she needed. She said she couldn't do this, and at the same time said, "I have to do it. I have to do it. I want to be in control. I've got to carry my family on. I'm the only person who can really hold my family together." I walked her through putting the NG tube in. When she did it, she was incredibly proud of herself. Although, she never did it again by herself, she knew she could if it became necessary.

Margaret was convinced she could continue to take care of Amy through the night without any help. Jane was coming in during the days. The nurses were there during the day and we gradually increased our time to cover the evening also. The family planned to take care of the weekends. Those plans didn't last long. The family couldn't keep up such intense caretaking.

The challenge for me was to get more staff and to find the money to pay for it. Justifying the need for care became difficult because Amy was beginning to gain weight. The NG feeds were being successful. She was getting strong. Some of the nurses bonded particularly well with her. She was feeling comfortable with them, and they were challenging her. She started to walk. She was thriving, happy, and laughing. Margaret, on the other hand, was slowly deteriorating.

Margaret went back into the hospital about ten days later. One of the challenges in nursing the AIDS patient is the seesaw nature of the case. One day you come in and the patient can't get out of bed because of a fever of 103. The next day you come in, the patient is running around, feeling great, wanting to go shopping, do this, do that, drive the car. You never know what the needs will be. Trying to coordinate staffing is thus very difficult because in the country, you can't easily call a nurse in. There are not that many extra nurses available. At the same time, in spite of all of the problems, the goal is to allow the patient to be in control. Margaret wanted to help care for Amy, but she couldn't when she was sick.

During this time, the community rallied. The phone was ringing off the wall with people wanting to help. This was positive for Margaret. As the media gave her more coverage, she started getting letters, telegrams, and flowers from all over the country. On the negative side, all of these people calling did increase the demands on her. The nurses had to act as public relations personnel. We monitored phone calls and took messages. A few people wrote saying, "God is punishing you" and "You must have done something evil." While most were positive, and none of the negative ones were local, it was always hit or miss whether a letter would be positive or negative.

Margaret had to perform now, and that stressed her, as well as the family. The family, who was very, very private, had all of the sudden become very public. Newscasters from everywhere wanted interviews.

The nurses had to deal with all of this. It was not a case a nurse could be emotionally distant from. When the nurses walked through the door, whether they liked it or not, they were involved. As Margaret made more public appearances, it was a matter of whether the nurse could deal with all of this and work. Some nurses couldn't cope and had to leave.

It became a balancing act. The nurse had to have a good sense of herself to work there. Sometimes the nurse had to comfort somebody. Sometimes the nurse had to hug someone or to leave them alone in a corner so they could cry. Sometimes the nurse had to be the mediator of discussions, other times a fly on the wall because the family needed privacy. On top of all that, the nurses had to be aware of the feelings of the physicians and the representatives of the insurance company and Medicaid.

The sustaining goal was to keep Margaret at home because she wanted to die at home. She wanted to die with her family around her and she wanted to die with dignity. We wanted to make all those things happen for Margaret. The community was rallying. It developed fund-raisers, gave money, and provided meals. Their help relieved some of the demands on Margaret and her family.

A major nursing role was dealing with the family. Family members had no other support services. The nurses, therefore, became the ones to intervene in the family's burdens. For example, when Margaret's niece came to visit, she had no idea that her aunt was dying. The niece found out that Meg had AIDS only after Greg committed suicide. Her mother, denying how sick her sister was, only told the girl that Meg had AIDS and was sick. The niece came and saw her aunt looking like a skeleton and her cousin looking very sick. The visit stimulated questions about her uncle's suicide, about her aunt's and cousin's futures, and about whether they were going to live. The nurse facilitated a discussion between the niece and her grandparents. Because every member of the family went through phases of denial and then acceptance, the nurses went through the grieving process with each of them.

Providing emotional support to everyone became a major role for me. Family members would call me at home or I would get a phone call from Jane who would need support. The nurses who worked the case would call me to say they couldn't go there again. It was affecting their personal lives. I was sustained by knowing that this good family, with help, could make it through this terribly unjust situation. This case took an incredible amount of energy and time. I had to find time and support for myself because I couldn't constantly give out and not get replenished. I found support sometimes talking with other nurses. We developed a communication book in which we shared feelings and experiences with one another. The communication book was a wonderful tool for expressing caring. We left messages about having a tough shift or a good shift, notes to cheer one another, and offers to help if needed. We developed a strong sense of "we-ness" which grew stronger as Meg's condition declined.

During the last two weeks of Margaret's life, we became more involved with the family, as we tried to get them to come to grips with Meg's pending death. Each person would talk to us individually, asking, "Is Margaret dying? When is she going to die?" We supported each other and tried to spend a lot of time with the family also.

Margaret had promised me that she would call me when she knew death was close. On the Sunday before Labor Day, I got a phone call from the nurse who said Margaret wanted to see me right away. When I arrived, Margaret was in bed, shaking from head to toe. She looked up at me and shouted, "Lorraine, I don't know what to do. What do you want me to do? Maybe I should go to the hospital." She started making wild suggestions. I answered her, "Now wait a minute. The issue is not what I want, but what you really want." She just screamed at me, "I want to die. I'm done fighting. I have fought for so long I want to die. I am finished fighting and I hurt so badly. I hurt everywhere." I leaned over and said softly, "If you are ready to go, what do you want me to do?" She wanted me to call her parents because she needed to finish some business. I did that. Then she wanted me to help her sit on the edge of the bed so I could hold her. As I did that, I felt a tremendous sense of relief. She was ready to go, and she was in a good place. Now it was time to let death happen.

As I hugged her, she repeated, "Let me die, let me die." We sat for a while holding one another. Both of us were comfortable with her wish to die. Now the challenge was to prepare everybody else. I called her parents. It took a while for them to come because they were camping. When they came, I started to leave. They looked at me and said, "We're close, aren't we?" I said, "Yes." They were very upset and cried a bit.

Meg spent those last two days getting things straightened out. She assigned tasks to each person, gave away her belongings, and decided her sister would raise Vicki. She asked her mom to promise that the girls would not be separated, as long as Amy was alive. Our role as nurses during this time was to be supportive and to keep some distance.

Pain control became a big problem. It was a holiday weekend and there was no place to get morphine. I remembered that our local doctor kept demoral and phenergan in his office. I called him; I was desperate. He had his secretary meet me, and I took all the demoral, phenergan, needles, and syringes he had. We gave her demoral and phenergan IM, and increased her morphine by mouth. That combination controlled her pain and we continued that regimen for the entire holiday weekend. She experienced little pain, but she was definitely deteriorating.

Those last days were very intense emotionally. All the family started to come. They were grieving. Margaret seemed to be holding on because Tuesday was the day Vicki would begin school. When Tuesday arrived she was in bed. Although she was very weak and filling up with fluid, she wanted to see her Vicki off to school.

We wrapped her in a blanket and her brother carried her outside. As she saw her daughter get on the bus, she said softly, "I've seen everything now."

After we put her back to bed, she was fighting and so restless, we couldn't make her comfortable. We gave her massive doses of medication. In the evening, she finally quieted down and slept. The family went home to get some rest and so did I. Around 4 AM Margaret woke up and asked for everybody. The entire family came back. Her mother did not leave her side until she died that afternoon.

That morning on my way to work, I stopped in to see Margaret. I hadn't had a moment alone with her since Sunday. I sat with her and asked, "How're you doing?" She looked up at me and asked, "Lorraine, how are you doing?" "I'm okay," I responded. "I'm okay, too," she replied. That was the last personal moment we had together.

I came back about 2:30 that afternoon. She was gasping. It was very difficult for the family to see her like that. We couldn't figure out what to do to help her let go. She kept holding on and we couldn't figure out why. Her brother wanted to take her to the hospital. He couldn't stand this. I said, "We will not go to the hospital; we're not going to do anything. We've got to wait until she's ready to let go." I knew how strongly she felt about dying at home.

I walked away and went outside for a minute to compose myself, wondering what I could do to help. The idea came to me. Wash her! I got a basin of warm water, and walked into the bed-room. Everybody looked at me like I was crazy. I told the family and Margaret we were going to wash her. Everyone pitched in giving her a back-rub and changing her position. As we were turn-ing her, I said, "Margaret, you are clean now." She looked at me, took one breath, and smiled. I said to everyone, "Look at her face." Her mother beamed, "Oh my God, she's so beautiful. Look at her face." The smile faded slowly away, and she was gone. Margaret always had a "thing" about neatness. I guess she had to be clean before she could go. The whole family was in Margaret's room. Though they were very upset and crying, there was a great sense of peace and relief. Margaret had died as she wanted. It had been very difficult, but there was a sense of pride. I was happy with our part in the process that allowed this to happen.

I immediately withdrew with the other nurse. It was our role to become shadows. Our job with Margaret was finished. The pastor who had been waiting went into the family. It was time for his healing. We went to Amy. She was all alone and frightened. She knew something had happened to her mom. The family wanted to be with Amy also. Sensitivity to the family's needs at the time of death is a delicate balance. We were still responsible for Amy. A nurse must develop the skill to be there but not be there. We called the physician and everybody else.

The funeral director took Margaret out by the back door so the family didn't need to see that. Slowly the family left, until finally the caregiver, Amy, and I were the only ones left. The house was so quiet. The other nurse did not want to be alone. I stayed with her until quite late. We cleaned up. Finally, I went to call the caregivers who had asked to be called when Meg died.

Word got out immediately that Margaret was dead. It made all the newspapers and television stations. The next days were intense. Mobs of people came to the funeral. It was painful to see that, during this time, Amy was really losing ground. We kept hoping it was because she was grieving and that she would turn around.

AMY'S STORY

We moved Amy from her mother's home to her grandmother's home. After the first night, it became apparent she could not remain in that home. It was too filled with memories of her mom and dad. Being there alone with the nurse was too much to expect. Amy never rallied. She cried and was unhappy. There were a few times where she would be like her old self, but most of the time she wasn't.

Her gastric tube insertion site did not heal. It was becoming more and more of a problem. It wasn't infected, but she wasn't healing. Her body was deteriorating. She was in great pain. About three weeks later, she started oozing gastric secretions from around the G tube. We called the physician and he told us to bring her to the emergency room, though there was really nothing we could do for her. We decided to wait until the next day, when Dr. Yaeger, a specialist, could see her.

The following day, she was admitted to the hospital. She was covered with herpes lesions. No matter what we did, we couldn't make her comfortable. The family didn't want to lose her. They seemed to need her even more than she needed them. They made a very unselfish decision and Monday morning called a care conference. They asked the doctor, me, and the hospital nurses some tough questions. Dr. Yaeger suggested all kinds of things that could be tried, but said nothing would give her more than a month or two to live. The family decided they weren't going to put her through any more. Within an hour, we were on our way home, to care for her until she died.

The pressure was off to save her. She slowly deteriorated. I was going to Dallas to a medical convention for six days. Before I left, I asked Amy if she would wait for me to come back home. She didn't say anything. I really didn't expect her to survive, but when I got home on Friday, she was alive.

She died gradually over the next couple of weeks. A slow change in her respirations marked her decline. She died Sunday evening at 10:30. We were with her. Vicki cried that night. She had not cried much after her mother died, but that night she sobbed uncontrollably. It was tough to watch, but I think it was best for her to let it out.

Vicki continues to live with her grandmother. She has counseling on a weekly basis. She is not living with her aunt, although that was Margaret's wish, because she needs some stability. If she were to move to her aunt now, she would have to change schools again. That would be three schools in less than two months, and two major moves. It is working well. She is blossoming. She is gaining weight and looks wonderful.

I see her often because she goes to the same school as my son. She has real problems still, concerns about death and dying. They revolve more around her dad's death than the death of her sister and her mother. She can understand their deaths because they were sick. She goes to the cemetery quite frequently, and brings her papers to show to her parents. She gets nervous when either grandparent has to go to a doctor. They take her with them when they go to the doctors and show her it's a routine check-up.

The rest of the family is coping well. Jane is talking to people in the community and to reporters which I think is very therapeutic for her. The community and the health care providers learned a great deal from this experience. Because of it, we are better prepared for the next situation.

ORGANIZATIONAL LESSONS

PNS learned some valuable lessons from this first encounter with an AIDS patient. Currently we have an AIDS client who was referred from Boston. We became involved with him much earlier and provided early respite care to save the family resources.

A major problem with Margaret and Amy was providing continuity of care. We now have a core group of nurses who are skilled in dealing with AIDS. Working with Margaret and Amy helped nurses sort out their reactions to AIDS and to dying. Some nurses came to realize they cannot deal with the death of a youngster. Others are challenged by it. We now have nurses who know themselves and know how long they can deal with such an intense situation.

PNS has started a support group for nurses who work with dying clients. We learned that it is not enough to start such a group as the client is beginning to decline. It must be offered from the beginning. The communication book has become a standard aspect of care. In addition to the emotional support, the book contains what works and doesn't work with a client. Nurses feel supported by one another and feel that they can better support the patient and family.

We are much more sophisticated about pain management. Some of the nurses had trouble with the massive doses of analgesic we were giving Amy. The doses could have killed an adult, but Amy needed them to be comfortable. We are more knowledgeable in dealing with the physicians, some of whom don't think AIDS patients have pain. We also have access to medication on the weekends now. No one will have to go through a Labor Day weekend on less desirable medication.

RURAL CONSIDERATIONS

The degree of community support that Margaret experienced is perhaps unique to a rural area. On the negative side, the fear that characterized the early period of the diagnosis is also probably uniquely rural. Over time, we all learned that people do not get AIDS from casual contact and that protective measures can be taken.

Vermont continues to list only those AIDS patients who are diagnosed in the state in its statistics. This under-reports the number of cases and may decrease the services available. However, we are able to meet the needs of our clients.

Support groups for AIDS clients are not readily available in our area. People still have to go to Burlington, Hanover (New Hampshire), or Albany (New York) for them. They also have to go to these urban areas for many of their medical services. A plus of the rural setting is the degree of cooperation we were able to achieve among the physicians and with insurance companies. Everyone wanted what was best for this family, and people made it work, even though it was a first experience for most of them.

We need to do more with the legal and ethical issues around "no code." "No code, do not resuscitate," does not mean not helping the person or taking care of them. That was one of the stumbling blocks we had with the family and the physicians. They had to come to grips with the idea that no code is not a sign of defeat.

The opportunity to protect Margaret's dignity, which was so important to her, was probably more achievable in a rural area because we knew her and her family. Looking her best was also important to Margaret, and that was great. It became a two-edged sword though. She would pull herself together to look great during the physician's visit. A couple of hours later when she "crashed," we had to convince the same physician that she had a problem.

I remember one day when Margaret was going to do an interview with the Associated Press and I was in the home. The interviewers were on their way, and she was trying to pull herself together. She was wearing a wonderful outfit and her make-up and everything was perfect, but she was feeling very poorly. She went out onto the deck and looked out across the mountains. She just stood there and took a deep breath, soaking in strength. She came back in, and said, "I can do it now." She maintained her composure through four hours of intense interrogation. As soon as they left, she collapsed.

Courage is not a rural characteristic, but Margaret drew strength from the mountains, and we drew strength from her.

3

Being There and Caring: A Philosophical Analysis and Theoretical Model of Professional Nurse Caring in Rural Environments

Carol Green-Hernandez

Without being there for my patients, there's no basis for my nursing. I have to be there for them in order to give caring to them. If I don't let my patients know I'm there for them and really be there for them, I don't feel satisfied that I'm really giving nursing.

Clinical Supervisor

That caring is integral to nursing is no longer a subject for scholarly debate. Multiple analyses and studies now document that caring defines nursing practice, validating the long-held value that caring is central to professional action (Gaut, 1983; Hernandez, 1987, 1991a, 1991b; Leininger, 1977; Watson, 1989). Caring connects one human being with another (Mayeroff, 1971; Noddings, 1984). That human presence, or "being there," can support one's caring for another, even to the extent of aiding healing, is not a new idea (LeShan, 1966; Nygren, 1932). However, that nursing's therapeutic intent requires being there for the client-family as a caring presence that is holistic in its attendance has only recently begun to undergo scrutiny (Hernandez, 1987, 1991a, 1991b; Watson, 1989). This chapter explores the concept of being there, and traces from a philosophical inquiry both caring and being there as the basis for nursing.

APPLICATION OF THE THEORETICAL MODEL OF PROFESSIONAL NURSE CARING TO RURAL NURSING

Other chapters in this book present data relating to the special needs of rural clients who often live in isolated areas. The meaning of the nursing presence is especially significant to people living in rural regions because they are frequently underserved by other health care providers. Willits, Bealer, and Timbers (1990) explored the meaning of rurality in a survey of 1,241 residents of Pennsylvania. They found that respondents connected the word rural with more positive than negative images. Of relevance to this chapter's examination of the importance of being there to the nursing presence, however, was their discovery that both quality of life and quantity of services and opportunities were perceived as compromised in rural areas, as compared to mainstream America. This finding correlates with that of a report by the National Advisory Commission on Rural Poverty (1967) a generation earlier. The commission stated in part that

> . . . in educational facilities and opportunities, the rural poor have been shortchanged . . . public services . . . are grossly inadequate . . . [and] few resources [are available] with which to earn incomes adequate for a decent living and for revitalizing their communities [p. X].

Lack of needed social and educational service opportunities allies with the traditional hesitance of some rural residents to accept so-called assistance from outside immediate community or family social structures (Hernandez, 1984). Rural areas tend to encompass a large percentage of older individuals as well as a higher percentage of older individuals who also live in poverty (Bourg, 1975; Hernandez, 1984; Johansen & Fuguitt, 1984;

Willits et al., 1990). Resistance to accepting outside assistance may stem from the so-called independence and pride inherent in many older residents of rural areas (Hernandez, 1984; Moen, 1978). It is also possible that this resistance can be correlated to the greater discrimination rural residents traditionally demonstrate in developing and maintaining social affiliations, as compared to non-rural dwellers (Goudy, 1990). Within this context, then, the nurse's being there for the client-family in a rural culture must take on the essence of such an affiliation. The rural resident may more readily perceive professional nurse caring from a nurse whose therapeutic presence reflects the values of the rural community, whereby the nurse recognizes client need for controlling independence.

THEORETICAL MODEL OF
PROFESSIONAL NURSE CARING

The following definitions organize this author's theoretical model of professional nurse caring: *Natural caring* is a human process in which one assists another in growth and actualization. One can potentiate self-actualization through giving caring to another (Hernandez, 1987, 1991b; Mayeroff, 1971). *Professional nurse caring* operationally enfolds natural caring, and can only be taught to nurses following and/or concurrent with their living the experience of natural caring. Professional nurse caring is learned and is transmitted with therapeutic intent as a direct nursing intervention. The nurse intentionally uses professional caring as the *modus* or therapeutic means for meeting a client's assessed needs, in order to attain nursing and client health care goals. The energy for giving professional caring emerges from the nurse's relationship with the client-family. Within the context of this model, the client can be an individual, group (either related or not), or a population. The client is the co-participant in nursing care (Hernandez, 1989, 1991b).

Co-existent with the nurse's practice of client-centered professional caring, collegial caring can provide actualization to the nurse who otherwise may perceive either diminished or absent actualization in giving professional caring to clients. Such actualization can be fostered because the process of collegial caring includes the implication that the nurse will experience reciprocation of that caring. That is, a professional environment organized around this theoretical model is one in which caring given is also caring received (Hernandez, 1989, 1991b).

Nursing is the process of professional nurse caring, wherein the nurse co-participates with the client as a whole in implementing the nursing process. The primary focus of professional nurse caring is direct, intentional, and therapeutic involvement with the client. Every individual is a unique human being who interacts and interfaces as one with the environment. The individual communicates with, responds to, and has an impact on both self and others using the whole self, and within the context of all of creation. Human beings are but one explication of the environment. Cognizant of this environmental inclusivity and of each human's individuality, the nurse involves the client in using the nursing process to assess, plan, implement, and evaluate care directed toward meeting identified needs. Health is an ongoing process. Health's focus is positive. Nursing's health goal is one of making the client aware of health choices, helping the client to achieve optimum wellness, or helping the client to meet death with dignity.

Assumptions

Although a collegial caring environment is fundamental to the practice of professional nurse caring, a pre-nursing natural caring experiential grounding must underpin the nurse's practice of professional caring. This lived experience can also be provided and/or supplemented during the education process in nursing. Three basic assumptions thus frame this theoretical model:

1. the capacity to give and receive caring is a natural ability;
2. the nurse's ability to practice professional caring is predicated upon one's achieving the lived experience of natural caring;
3. the nurse cares for and respects one's own self.

Propositions

Five propositions organize this theoretical model. They reflect the philosophic as well as research perspectives which contributed to the model's development and refinement (Gustafson, 1981; Hernandez, 1987, 1988, 1989; Ingle, 1987, 1988; Rosenthal & Bourgeois, 1983). These propositions suggest that the nurse:

1. participate in collegial caring activities, e.g. staff meetings and formal/informal support groups, in order to facilitate self-actualization;
2. believe in the value of professional nurse caring;
3. have the desire to act;
4. know that one will intentionally act;
5. recognize that professional nurse caring is a process that can be directly and intentionally communicated.

Requirements

The natural caring experience grounds the nurse's practice of professional caring. Successful practice of professional nurse caring is based on meeting three conditions:

1. *learning* both how and how best to give professional nurse caring through formal and informal exposure to and practice of caring;
2. achieving psycho-motor technical *competence,* which leads to feeling professionally competent. Collegial validation of this competence empowers the nurse, supporting self-actualization;
3. achieving professional *confidence,* which is closely allied to learning as well as feeling technically competent. This confidence is achieved through the give and take of professional experience as well as collegial and client validation of nursing skills.

These conditions need not be met in any particular order. Meeting these conditions helps nurses to develop unique ways of working with clients and families, while enabling them to practice professional caring that is both therapeutic and unself-conscious. A heuristic for these conditions serves to illustrate their function in professional nurse caring:

$$\text{Learning} + \text{Competence} + \text{Confidence} = \text{Caring}$$

Learning how to practice professional nurse caring as well as gaining technical competence and professional confidence facilitate the development of a caring repertoire.

The Theoretical Model of Professional Nurse Caring is guided by seven concepts. Figure 3–1 presents a schematic of these concepts.

The nurse, by *being there* for the client, provides comfort and security. This support can be both verbally and nonverbally expressed, but is dependent upon the nurse's demonstrated, predictable, and nonjudgmental presence for the client. In this way, the nurse transmits *support* through providing nurturance, advocacy via reliable alliance, and health information access. Such involvement requires that the nurse have empathy for the client. *Empathy* derives from life experience and as such enables the nurse to understand and accept the client—in other words, to enter into the client's reality—without attempting to influence or change the client.

Professional nurse caring is transmitted to others through interpersonal *communication*. This communication can be verbal or nonverbal. Touching can be a powerful method of communicating professional nurse caring. Through being there for the client, while using the empathic self to communicate one's support, the nurse can effectively help the client to attain health and/or care delivery goals. *Helping* others requires that the nurse perceive that *time* is available to practice caring. Within this model, the practice of professional nursing is holistic. Lack of time can reduce nursing's practice to delivery of technical tasks, thus negating nursing's holistic practice.

In order to maintain and/or re-charge one's caring capacity, the nurse must feel that one's practice of professional caring with clients as well as colleagues is reciprocated. *Reciprocity* of caring is fundamental to the nurse's practice of professional caring

Figure 3–1
The Seven Concepts of Professional Nurse Caring

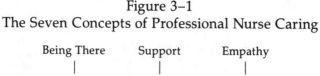

because it is through caring's reciprocation that the nurse can achieve self-actualization. Client reciprocation of caring may not always occur. In addition, client caring may not always lead the nurse to experience the self-actualization needed to gain and/or maintain the psychic energy required to continue to give professional caring. The nurse can also achieve actualization through giving and receiving professional caring from colleagues. If a nurse is not perceived by one's colleagues as both technically competent and professionally confident, however, professional caring's reciprocation may be compromised. In other words, through providing for professional self-actualization, collegially experienced professional nurse caring can both validate one's nursing practice as well as provide the psychic energy necessary to the nurse's continued ability to transmit professional caring to clients. This is especially true in those scenarios where the nurse is unable to engender client acknowledgment that caring was either received and/or valued.

Collegial participation in professional nurse caring is more than a benefit of practicing nursing using this model. That is, the nurse's fundamental ability to practice professional caring with the client depends upon the experience of professional caring with colleagues. (Such caring can be expressed, for example, in the respect of one colleague for another.) As an adjunct to natural caring the nurse might experience in personal life, professional caring practiced with colleagues can facilitate that self-actualization which is necessary to the caring process.

Figure 3–2 illustrates the foregoing conceptual model in only one dimension. It is not technically feasible to present the model

Figure 3–2
Schema of the Theoretical Model of Professional Nurse Caring

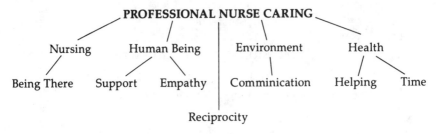

as a hologram. The reader is, therefore, asked to creatively visualize this schema as a holistic, multidimensional reality.

In the final analysis, caring cannot occur if one is not present for another. Integral to the caring process and definitive of the caring moment, being there connects one human being with another. Being there to give caring to another is a powerful metaphor for standing witness to one's own humanity.

UTILIZATION OF THE THEORETICAL MODEL IN ADMINISTRATION, PRACTICE, AND EDUCATION

The following discussion presents data excerpted from a study undertaken to provide validation for the model and the concept of being there. The author conducted open, unstructured interviews with a sample of 13 nurses whose professional practice is guided by the theoretical model, and who work in administration, practice, and education in nursing in rural northern New England. The author asked: "Tell me about your practice within the Theoretical Model of Professional Nurse Caring and, specifically, of your practice of being there. Explain as fully as possible." Data were audio-recorded and transcribed. Participants' rights were protected.

Administration

The model forms an administrative practice framework for both a busy nurse administrator overseeing a large outpatient department, as well as the department head of an upper division baccalaureate nursing program. The first administrator stated: "One of my strongest values is my need to nurture my staff. The model enables me to put this [value] into perspective." She added that through practicing being there:

> *I communicate in a variety of ways that I am there for my staff. For me, it's [providing] mentoring in my work with staff. By being available, by giving them information and helping them process it and apply it, I guide them in managing themselves.*

The second administrator echoed the above, adding that her management style is guided by the model because:

> *I care about my faculty as people. I look for people's strengths to give [them] the confidence to try other things that they may not otherwise like as well or feel confident about doing.*

She added that, for her, being there means that ". . . you start from the perspective of the consumer [whether student or faculty] and what she thinks she'll need, and then build on that with her."

Practice

The words of a nurse working in critical care at a regional medical center serving rural clients validate the importance of being there to the practice of professional nurse caring:

> *I can't just give technical care — I have to give biopsychosocial — and spiritual — care. If I don't do this, I don't feel that I'm giving my patients nursing in my ICU. Oftentimes my patients and their families are so scared and I have to help them through that fear.*

This nurse added that, through being there:

> *. . . I'm sure about the parameters of my practice. I let my patients know that I'm there for them, and I come back to check on them both when I say I will and in between. Being*

there is also about being a therapeutic listener. The Profes-
sional Nurse Caring Model supports me in validating my
nursing.

Another critical care nurse asserted:

The model frames how I plan and carry out my nursing.
Using professional nurse caring validates my nursing prac-
tice because it [the model] says what I value in nursing,
and also helps me to explain what I do in my nursing.

She went on to state that:

Being there just supports all this, because being there for
my patient and his family supports me in doing my techni-
cal stuff and the bio-psycho-social-spiritual things—and
following through on all this with them.

Education

The Theoretical Model of Professional Nurse Caring is being tested
at Vermont College of Norwich University in Montpelier. Adopted
as the school's conceptual framework in 1989, the model forms
the basis for the upper division baccalaureate curriculum for registered nurses (Vermont College of Norwich University, 1990). The
Vermont College faculty's teaching experience with the model
illustrates how the framework is used by both faculty and students,
offering further validation of the importance of being there in
professional nurse caring.

Faculty. One educator teaching within the model stated the following:

In teaching community health nursing, I find that the sys-
tem focuses on the patient [only], not the caregiver. I teach
that the client and the family have to be cared for as a
whole. Using the concept of being there, the student focuses
on the family as a whole, teaching the caregiver as well as
the patient, and letting them know that she is there to
provide comfort and listen. So the client and the family

develop a security that the student will deliver because the student repeatedly comes through and is there with [health] literature and answers to questions. So they can begin to develop trust with the student. There's an intangible relationship; the client can rely on "his" nurse. The model validates my teaching philosophy.

A second professor described how she creates a learning environment that is centered on the model's concept of being there:

I see being there as primary to my teaching of therapeutic communication. Being there is active listening. If you aren't fully attentive to what the person is saying and his affect and what he's doing, if you're not really there to that degree, you're missing a great deal of the communication process. Being there is essential to any communication. I don't think you can really be there and not care, or care and not be there. I think if you don't care, you're just physically there. Being there is more than "I'll sit here"—it's "I value what you have to say even if I don't agree." I value this process [of being there]. Being there is being aware that this process is happening and encouraging it to happen, and that's a responsibility I have as a group leader and as a teacher.

Students. One experienced nurse described her learning within the Theoretical Model of Professional Nurse Caring as:

. . . making me sensitive to my clients as human beings with full lives. My own nursing [practice] is less fragmented [since] using the model.

She further related that her use of being there:

. . . means I'm able to connect [my patients] to services they need because I've been there for them and seen and talked with them about what they'll need, as well as options they might have. I verbally express being there to my patients and demonstrate it in the way I communicate with them, [and] in how I can help them. For me, being there is connecting with the patient and his family.

Yet another student explained that her exposure to and learning based on the model's concepts meant that:

> . . . *my consciousness was raised about caring as a value. The model legitimized caring for me, allowing me to practice as a professional in a more meaningful way.*

She further describes that, as a student and also as an experienced upper management administrator:

> *I'm using more than my technical skills for a patient or my staff when I practice being there. I strive to empower the person to achieve his potential—and I can't do that if I'm not really there for them.*

The preceding assertions were echoed by a student who entered the upper division program as an inexperienced recent graduate of an associate degree program. She stated that her education within the model meant that "I learned how important it is not to confuse my values with my patient's." She believes her student testing of being there means:

> . . . *the clients I have know I'll find a way for them, to help them get what they need and that, because I'm not judging them, I feel I can develop a trusting relationship with them that we might not otherwise have had. And that's great— that's why I became a nurse and that's why I'm here to stay.*

Nursing students enrolled in Vermont College's baccalaureate program test out the model's concepts in their own nursing practice and give credence to its applicability to real-world nursing. As one student described:

> *Before I was exposed to the model and especially to [its concept of] being there, I thought that nurses had it [caring] or they didn't. My experience supported that. But I've seen that caring can be learned. And for me, being there for the patient is really caring in a nutshell because when I'm*

really *there for him, listening and checking on him fre-*
quently and all that—then I'm practicing nursing. And
that makes me feel good about me and what I'm doing.

Student-Nurse as Patient. What is the salience of the model's
concepts as perceived by the nurse whose baccalaureate education
and subsequent nursing practice are based on professional nurse
caring, and who is now living the experience of patient? The nurse
whose experiences and feelings are recounted below was critically
injured in an automobile accident and required extensive hospitalization and subsequent rehabilitation:

> *As a nurse, I've seen a lot of nurses who emphasize their*
> *technical skills in their practice. Certainly that's been my*
> *experience [in working with colleagues] as a nurse in CCU*
> *[Cardiac Care Unit]. But since being a patient for this past*
> *year, I find myself thinking about the nurses I've had. The*
> *one who was most helpful—and healing—was the one who*
> *would check in on me during the day and be supportive.*
> *When she said she would be there physically, she was, so I*
> *began to have confidence and trust. Her calmness helped*
> *me through embarrassing things like enemas and bedpans.*
> *She was always there and available, for me, physically and*
> *emotionally.*

This same nurse clearly believed that the nurse's nonverbal behavior had an impact on whether she felt the nurse's being there:

> *Another of my nurses was always letting me know that she*
> *was too busy to be there for me. She just acted harried. I felt*
> *like I would be putting her out if I asked for anything so I*
> *found myself not asking her for help, or prn's [pain medica-*
> *tion], or anything.*

That a nurse's caring nonverbal behavior does not totally comprise
this patient-nurse's perception of being there is suggested by this
assertion:

> *I had a new graduate for a nurse who was very caring but I*
> *remember her being very nervous when I started having*

*[muscle] spasms and told her what I needed and she just got
so nervous she brought another nurse in. So she was someone I viewed as emotionally able to be there but not technically able to be.*

This nurse also contrasted the importance of emotional caring and
support with technical competence in being there, describing a
primary nurse who was:

*. . . technically competent but he couldn't be there for me.
[For example], when I told him I was feeling sick—it was
like he didn't believe me, because when I did throw up, he
said "Oh, I guess you were sick." . . . So when I didn't
need his technical expertise any more I found I didn't want
him as my nurse—I mean I really didn't want him—
because he wasn't emotionally there for me.*

CARING AND BEING THERE:
THE ONTOLOGICAL PRESENCE

This section of the chapter will present a philosophical analysis
that will demonstrate the primacy of caring and being there as the
essence of professional nursing. The questions to be explored are:

- What is the meaning of being there in nursing?
- Does the presence of being there connote caring?
- What is the relationship between caring and being there in
  professional nursing?
- Does the ontology of being there in caring give meaning to the
  lived experience of day-to-day nursing?

To begin to answer these questions, the meaning of caring must
first be explored.

The Language of Caring: Entological, Theological, and
Philosophical Antecedents

Both the Greek *kara* or *karon* and the Old English *carian* contain
the rudimentary meaning of the modern word "care" as well as of

"caring." *The Oxford English Dictionary* (1933) notes that in about 1000 AD, caring was used prepositionally—as to charge one's mind with concern, heed, or attention. By the late 14th century this meaning was extended to include not only "attending to with care," but also to "care for" something. This meaning persists into the present. "Care" as a noun derives from *karn* or *caren,* which translates as mourn, trouble, or sorrow (*The Oxford English Dictionary,* 1933, p. 115). This meaning persists, in somewhat altered form, to mean that cares are sorrows.

As a verb, "caring" can also be used as "cared" and as "cares," and derives from *carian, carien,* and *cearian* (*Oxford English Dictionary,* 1933). Used in this way, the word means to have concern for; to feel an interest in; to look after or provide for; to have a liking, inclination, or regard. Thus one is inclined or disposed to have regard for, as in fondness or attachment for someone or something. The following discussion will demonstrate that caring's linguistic meaning is integral to understanding caring's conceptual meaning.

For persons raised in the Judeo-Christian heritage, there is a theological perspective to caring. Yahweh, in the Old Testament, has a "loving concern" for Israel (Williams, 1968, p. 33). In the New Testament, the caring of Jesus for humanity represents selfless interpersonal caring (Whitehead, 1933).

Because the New Testament was written in Greek, the Greek "agape" was used to connote the fellowship of love in Christ. Agape is inclusive of God's love for humankind, of humankind's love for God, and of human love for fellow humans (Nygren, 1932). The essence of agape's fellowship love is contrasted by that of eros' passionate love (Richardson, 1951). Conversely, however, eros can also connote the spiritual. Both Plato and Aristotle used eros to connote the upward movement of the soul toward God (Nygren, 1932).

The caring of God for people and of people for each other are both facets of the same ethic of agape (Nygren, 1932). St. Thomas Aquinas (translated by Goodwin, 1977) asserts that such human caring, in the spirit of agape, is "perfect charity." Perfect charity "totally bind[s people] to God" (p. 36). The goal of such perfect charity, or agape, is ". . . helping men to reach full self-affirmation, to attain the courage to be" (Tillich, 1952, p. 78).

Tillich's (1952) goal of "helping men to . . . attain the courage to be" is a powerful view of caring (p. 78). Mayeroff (1971) rendered this view an intelligible philosophy. Echoing Aquinas's notion of perfect charity, Mayeroff (1971) asserts that caring gives life its meaning. The orderliness of that life is derived from this meaning. He further describes caring as ". . . a human activity [and] a process that involves helping another grow and actualize himself" (p. 463). Thus, according to Mayeroff, ". . . caring is the antithesis of simply using the other person to satisfy one's own needs [because] . . . in the most significant sense . . . [caring means] to help [another] grow and actualize himself" (p. 1). As such, he continues, caring ". . . is a process, a way of relating to someone that involves *development*" (emphasis Mayeroff's, p. 11). It is this notion of caring, in which one individual facilitates another's developmental growth and self-actualization, that most compellingly describes caring as a process.

Through the caring process, the carer participates in the reality of the other. The carer sees the other as having potentialities which are expressed through the other's need to grow. The caring process is at once an extension of, yet separate from, the carer. In this way the other is not dependent on the carer, for the other is a participant in that caring. Mayeroff (1971) asserts that this process exhibits eight major components. These are: knowing, alternating rhythms, patience, honesty, trust, humility, hope, and courage.

The carer must know the other before one can render caring. Knowing the other enables the carer to help that person to grow (Mayeroff, 1971). Once the carer knows the other, both immediate and long-term needs are examined. This is the process of alternating rhythms. It is characterized by backward and forward movement. This movement occurs across both in a narrow, or short-term, and a wide, or long-term, framework. The carer must use past experiences in order to determine which framework best fits the other's need at a given point in time. Mayeroff determines that such a framework requires patience if ". . . the other [is] to grow in its own time and in its own way" (p. 12). As an active process, patience requires the carer to appropriately interpret the need for caring.

Caring as action is not apparent unless the assessment indicates that that action is both appropriate and meaningful. This process requires that those who care are honest in openly confronting their motives for caring. Honesty facilitates genuineness in those who care. Honesty is a prerequisite to trust. Such trust enables those who care to allow care recipients to grow toward independence in their own way and time. Trust that the cared for will achieve self-actualization nurtures those who care. Those who care are aware of—and trust—their personal caring capability. Thus, those who care experience growth in caring ability (Mayeroff, 1971).

The carer is genuinely humble. Humility facilitates one's willingness to learn more about self and other. The carer is not afraid to admit to and learn from personal mistakes. In a broader sense, the carer's humility prevents one's seeing others as existing merely to satisfy the needs of the carer. The carer focuses on the other rather than the self (Mayeroff, 1971).

The carer possesses hope. This hope realistically encompasses what is, yet can envision what could be as well. That the carer possesses hope enables one to have courage. The carer must have the courage to trust the other. The carer does not know whether the caring relationship will endure, or grow in a positive direction, or have a happy course. The carer must have the courage to care nonetheless. Such courage is not naive, as it is a logical outgrowth of past experience (Mayeroff, 1971).

Mayeroff's (1971) notion of caring is not that of a casual or transitory interest in another. Rather, caring is the use of self in order to help another to grow toward self-actualization. The carer inevitably is helped to grow toward self-actualization. It is the caring process rather than its action that bestows self-meaning and, hence, gives meaning to one's life.

May (1969) asserts that the meaning of one's life is related to the world in which one lives. The concept of care provides one's meaning in that ". . . in care one must [be] involve[d] with the objective fact. [One must] do something about the situation" (p. 18). Care is a necessary part of humanness. May's notion of care is one of action. This notion essentially mirrors Mayeroff's (1971) view of caring as process. Whether viewed as action or as process, care does not exist unless and until it is enacted. Care as both action and process brings love and will together. Love and will enable one to care for or about another. Such care is definitive of humanness. Care is thus ". . . ontological in that it constitutes man as man . . ." (p. 288). The New Testament agape of selfless, loving fellowship is enhanced by May's notion that care is human-centered. Further, May's belief that ". . . care brings love and will together . . ." connotes the essence of agape (p. 288). Thus, care is natural to and definitive of humankind.

Buber (1970) and Marcel (1964) take a subject-object view of caring in the human relationship. Each sees the "I-You" relationship as not dialectical but, rather, dialogical. This view is definitive of the concept of empathy (Halpern & Lessor, 1960). Empathy occurs only as a between-people phenomenon in the presence of genuine dialogue. This dialogue requires that a degree of openness exist between self and other. Marcel (1964, p. 89) describes this as a process of one's "making room" within the self in order to communicate empathetically with another. In other words, the carer must penetrate the other's reality, becoming a co-presence with that other. Thus the I-Thou encounter is transformed into a transcendent co-presence of carer and recipient (Marcel, 1964).

Buber (1970) essentially concurs with this view. He asserts that co-transcendent communication requires that one both see and experience the other from one's own as well as from the other's perspective. This notion moves beyond empathy, wherein one experiences the other's reality as the other experiences it. Co-transcendence requires that the self experiences something from both one's own as well as the other's reality. Such an experience is a concretization of the notion of genuinely being there for another.

This view of caring is one that is essentially selfless. Such caring is consistent with the selfless fellowship of agape, ". . . convey[ing] feelings that you are there to support [another], to contribute to his development, because you value him for what he is" (Buber, 1970, p. 16). This notion is, in essence, care. As such, care is the action whereby May's (1969) love and will are united. Its process is kinetic. Heidegger (1975, translated by Hofstader, 1984) sees this kinesis as *Umschlag,* which he describes as motion indivisible from that which is moving. This notion of *Umschlag* characterizes both the moment and process of caring. The interpersonal interchange of the caring moment can be expressed by the carer's actual or implied being there in both space and time for the other. Such being there is the expression of one's essential humanity at its most basic, caring level. What, then, is the ontic of this expression?

Being There: The Moral Commitment of Caring

The foregoing discussion supports the premise that caring requires that the carer be there for the other. In order to understand this assertion, however, the nature of being there must first be probed within the ontology of Dasein (wherein one contemplates the self) and its reflection of personal being. When considered within the caring definitional framework, the examination of being is a quest for self in relation to others. Indeed, Aristotle's scrutiny of *logikos,* the what-it-was-to-be, indicates that each person's being is unique such that one is what one is by virtue of oneself alone (Heidegger, 1976, translated by Sheehan, 1976; Lewis, 1984). This "what is" of being-as-human is akin to the divinity of Yahweh's I-Am-Who-Am. The uniqueness of this human beingness is explicated through one's living and being in the world. When taken within the context of human experience, living and being connect Aristotle's *logikos* with the image of one's humanity. Being is thus intelligible as human, connoting one's humanity (Levinas, 1989). Within this perspective, being there is a human process wherein one is present as a whole person for another. The caring definitional framework denotes this presence as one that is interpersonal and, hence, mandates sharing of self with other (Hernandez, 1987, 1989, 1991b). In examining the nature of this interpersonal presence, however, one must ask whether being there is the sharing of Dasein. It is important to know of what is this being there comprised, and to identify its ontic, if the phenomenon of being there is to be made explicit in professional caring.

The Ontic of Being There

Heidegger generally asserts that Dasein focuses on the being of self (1962, translated by Macquarrie & Robinson, 1967). Nevertheless,

Heidegger implies that Dasein is also other-focused when he states that "Dasein is essentially for the sake of others" (1962, cited in Bernasconi, 1988). Certainly the ontic of a being that focuses on others as well as self is very different from a being that primarily contemplates only self. This other-focus underpins the being there of caring and, as such, elevates the notion of Dasein (wherein one contemplates self) to involvement with another wherein one commits the self to being there for the other.

Levinas (1989) believes that human involvement of one with the other ". . . is the dramatic event of being in the world" (p. 122). This writer would add that, when one intentionally seeks such involvement, or being there for the other, one must accept responsibility for that involvement and its consequences beyond those of the caring moment itself. The other also shares in that involvement and, hence, in its consequences. This relationship with another through being there is intimately tied to the caring moment, for to be there for another, one must put aside the concerns of self, at least for that moment in time. Being there thus expresses the moral commitment inherent in caring, for to be there for another is to be in relationship with that other, who also embodies the being of Dasein. Therein lies the kernel of a moral commitment, for being's involvement with the other is merely the opposite of commitment to self. The nature of this commitment best emerges from a theoretical conceptualization of caring.

REFERENCES

Aquinas, St. T. (1977). In R. P. Goodwin (Trans.), *Selected writings of St. Thomas Aquinas.* Indianapolis: Bobbs-Merrill Educational Publishing.

Bernasconi, R. (1988). "The double concept of philosophy" and the place of ethics in Being and time. *Research in Phenomenology, 18,* 41–57.

Bourg, C. J. (1975). Differentiation, centrality and solidarity in rural environments. In R. Atchley (Ed.), *Rural environment and aging.* Washington, D.C.: The Gerontological Society of America.

Buber, M. (1970). *I and thou* (W. Kaufman, Trans.). New York: Charles Scribner's Sons.

Gaut, D. A. (1983). Development of a theoretically adequate description of caring. *Western Journal of Nursing Research, 5*(4), 313–324.

Goudy, W. J. (1990). Community attachment in a rural region. *Rural Sociology, 55*(2), 178–198.

Gustafson, D. (1981). Passivity and activity in intentional actions. *Mind, 90,* 41–60.

Halpern, H. M., & Lessor, L. N. (1960). Empathy in infants, adults, and psychotherapists. *Psychological Review, 47*(3), 32–42.

Heidegger, M. (1967). *Being and time* (J. Macquarrie & J. Robinson, Trans.). Oxford: Blackwell. (Original published in 1962).

Heidegger, M. (1976). On the being and conception of Aristotle's *Physics B,1.* In T. Sheehan (Trans.), *Man and world.* Bloomington: University of Indiana Press.

Heidegger, M. (1984). *The basic problems of phenomenology* (A. Hofstader, Trans.). Bloomington: Indiana University Press. (Original published in 1975).

Hernandez, C. M. G. (1984). Hunger and the rural elderly: An examination and proposal for nursing and legislative action. In F. Smalkowski (Ed.), *Readings in public policy and health care.* New York: Adelphi University Press.

Hernandez, C. M. G. (1987). *A phenomenologic investigation of the concept of the lived experience of caring in professional nurses.* Unpublished doctoral dissertation, Adelphi University.

Hernandez, C. M. G. (1988). *A phenomenologic investigation of the lived experience of caring in technical nurses.* Unpublished research.

Hernandez, C. G. (1989). Caring as a paradigm for nursing. *Conference Proceedings: International Council of Nurses, 19th Quadrennial Seoul Congress.* Seoul, Korea; *and Conference Proceedings: Advances in International Nursing Scholarship, Sigma Theta Tau International Research Congress.* Taipei, Taiwan.

Hernandez, C. G. (1991a). A phenomenological investigation of caring as a lived experience in nurses. In P. Chinn (Ed.), *An anthology on caring* (pp. 111–131). New York: National League for Nursing.

Hernandez, C. G. (1991b). Professional nurse caring: A conceptual model for nursing. In R. M. Neil & R. Watts (Eds.), *Caring and nursing: Explorations in feminist perspectives.* New York: National League for Nursing.

Ingle, J. (1987). *Utilization in nursing practice of Hernandez's conceptual model of caring.* Unpublished doctoral research, The School of Nursing in the Graduate School, The University of Alabama at Birmingham.

Ingle, J. (1988). *The business of caring: The perspective of men in nursing.* Unpublished doctoral dissertation, The School of Nursing in the Graduate School, the University of Alabama at Birmingham.

Johansen, H. E., & Fuguitt, G. V. (1984). *The changing rural village in America: Demographic and economic trends since 1950.* Cambridge, MA: Ballinger Publishing.

Leininger, M. M. (1977). The phenomenon of caring: The essence and central focus of nursing. *American Nurses Foundation* (Nursing Research Report), *12*(1), 2, 14.

LeShan, L. (1966). *The medium, the mystic, and the physicist.* New York: Viking Press.

Levinas, E. (1989). Is ontology fundamental? *Philosophy Today,* (2), 121–129.

Lewis, F. (1984). New essays on Aristotle. *Canadian Journal of Philosophy, 10,* 127–130.

Marcel, G. (1964). *Creative fidelity* (translated by R. Rosthal). New York: The Monday Press.

May, R. (1969). *Love and will.* New York: W. W. Norton.

Mayeroff, M. (1971). *On caring.* New York: Harper and Row.

Moen, E. (1978). The reluctance of the elderly to accept help. *Social Problems, 25*(2), 293–303.

National Advisory Commission on Rural Poverty. (1967). *The people left behind.* Washington, D.C.: U.S. Government Printing Office.

Noddings, N. (1984). *Caring: A feminine approach to ethics and moral education.* Berkeley: University of California Press.

Nygren, A. (1932). *Agape and eros* (Vols. 1–3). London: S. P. C. K. *Oxford English dictionary.* (1933). London: Oxford University Press.

Richardson, A. (Ed.) (1951). *A theological word book of the bible.* New York: Macmillan.

Rosenthal, S. B., & Bourgeois, P. I. (1983). Lewis, Heidegger and ontological presence. *Philosophy Today, 27*(4), 290–296.

Tillich, P. (1952). *The courage to be.* New Haven: Yale University Press.

Vermont College of Norwich University. (1990). National League for Nursing reaccreditation report. Montpelier, VT.

Watson, J. (1989). *Nursing: Human science and human care. New York: National League for Nursing.*

Whitehead, A. N. (1926). *Religion in the making.* New York: Macmillan.

Whitehead, A. N. (1933). *Adventures of ideas.* New York: Macmillan.

Williams, D. D. (1968). *The spirit and the forms of love.* New York: Harper and Row.

Willits, F. K., Bealer, R. C., & Timbers, V. L. (1990). Popular images of "rurality": Data from a Pennsylvania survey. *Rural Sociology, 55*(4), 559–578.

4

Mental Health and Illness Nursing in Rural Vermont: Case Illustration of a Farm Family

Brenda Pauline Hamel-Bissell

HISTORY OF FARM FAMILIES AND MENTAL HEALTH AND ILLNESS CARE

In passing through a lunatic asylum the visitor is some-times surprised to learn that the most numerous class of unfortunates are from the farm . . . [T]he key to the so frequent cases of insanity and suicide among farmers [is that] their subjects of thought are too few; their life is a ruinous routine. There is a sameness and a tameness about it[,] a paucity of subjects for contemplation most danger-ous to mental integrity.

> *Isaac Newton*
> *U.S. Commissioner of Agriculture*
> *1862* Annual Report

Our understanding of farmers and farming is largely mythic. Two dominant myths exist about farmers. The first is that the coun-try or rural setting as opposed to the city is a place of healthy home and upright, sober, contemplative, and moral people. The corollary

55

to this myth is a view of the city as a breeder of luxury, ambition, and corruption. The second dominant myth about farmers is antithetical to the first. In this view, the country or rural setting is seen as a place where nothing happens except for the routine of back-breaking, mindless work—a life untouched by culture or resources. This myth defines the rural setting as home to the hayseed and cloddish boor. As Newton's comments indicate, it was true that 19th-century insane asylums were packed with farmers. This situation was partly an accident of demographics since at that time the majority of Americans lived on farms. City people have long replaced farmers in today's mental illness care facilities (Pistorius, 1990).

Most health care professionals lack an in-depth understanding of the health care desires and needs of farm families. Health care professionals in general believe the same two dominant myths about farmers and learn about farmers primarily from today's 30-second television news spots that highlight only problems related to the present farm crisis. Several questions remain unaddressed. What are the desired health care needs of farmers? What services do and would they use? Are farmers still different (if they ever were) from other people? Do health care professionals need special knowledge and skills to care for farm families experiencing a member's mental illness?

Existing literature on the topic of mental health and illness care delivery to rural Americans is admittedly in the formative years in addressing these issues and questions. Many authors advocate the need to complete more research on the topic and to develop theoretical frameworks for conceptualizing farm families' needs as well as appropriate interventions for health care professionals. Various authors who have examined the delivery and use of rural mental health services conclude that the quality of life is lower for rural people and that rural residents receive poorer services than urban dwellers. They point out, however, that their conclusions are made from the urban health care professional's eyeview. Thus, the needs of rural people have been most often assessed using urban people's standards. The literature itself is tainted by the two previously described myths about country people and farmers. Some authors argue that successful health care practice in small towns and rural communities requires a unique set of skills and knowledge or at least a reordering of these skills within those sets. Most authors agree that effective mental health practice is sensitive to the social environment and culture of the people served. Health care delivery needs to be consistent with the realities of life in rural societies. Mental health practitioners need to be able to work with the distinctive features of rural environments and the people who live in those environments.

This chapter identifies some features of rural communities that have an impact on the delivery of mental health services in those environments. The identification of these features is meant to advance our understanding and appreciation of the diversity and pluralism of rural America.

RURAL MENTAL HEALTH AND ILLNESS CARE

Delivery Issues and Needs of Farm Families

Most of the literature that addresses the issues surrounding rural mental health care and needs of farm families comes from the fields of sociology, psychology, and agriculture. There is no one theory of mental health delivery for rural residents. As Long and Weinert (1989) note, the development of a theoretical base for nursing practice in rural settings is in its infancy. Although limited and difficult to compare, most research regarding rural health has focused on identifying the unique characteristics, attitudes, and values of rural individuals; the distinctive features of rural physical environments; the skills needed by health care professionals serving these populations; and finally, the way these features affect delivery of mental health and illness care. Drawing on contributions made by earlier researchers (Bachrach, 1981; Flax, Wagenfeld, Ivens, & Weiss, 1979; Jackson, 1982; Martinez-Brawley & Munson, 1980), Coward, DeWeaver, Schmidt, and Jackson in 1983 designed the first comprehensive framework for mental health practice which incorporated many of the distinctive features of rural environments, rural clients, and rural health care providers. Coward et al.'s (1983) frame of reference for mental health practice is compatible with and includes many of the features described by Long and Weinert (1989) in their design of a theory base for rural nursing. The collective conclusion found by our survey of existing research is that indeed rural clients in the form of farm families differ from their urban counterparts and, thus, mental health services will work best if they are altered and modified to incorporate these distinctive features.

Features of Rural and Farm Family Populations

Certain demographic differences persist about rural residents. There is a notable difference in the age composition of rural and urban environments. Rural communities tend to have a larger proportion of the very young and the very old. Compared to the number of individuals in all other age categories, there are more people over 65 or under 18 years of age. These two periods of life are times when dependence on others and need for community services is often the greatest (Flax et al., 1979).

Rural families are changing and reflect many of the trends that have been witnessed already in urban families. The age at marriage has risen. Fertility has declined. Household size has diminished. The divorce rate has increased. The rate of labor force participation by women has grown. Rural couples, however, continue to marry earlier, have more children, seek divorce less often, and live in larger households than do urban couples (Brown, 1981).

Traditional wisdom has characterized rural people as more politically conservative, independent, self-reliant, distrustful of outsiders, fundamentally religious, and less committed to social welfare. Coward et al. (1983), in their review of national and local surveys, found moderate support for many of these stereotypes. On the other hand, extensive and comprehensive reviews of these attitudes by Glenn and Hill (1977) and Larson (1978) caution that many of these generalizations are due to limitations in the research methodology. This area of research remains controversial (Keller & Murray, 1982).

Rural individuals consistently attain lower levels of education than do their urban counterparts. Rural farm men who are 25 years and older have generally completed an average of 11 years of education in comparison with 12.5 years of education completed by urban men. Rural women are even more disadvantaged in the educational arena. The dropout rates of rural high schools are also higher. The more rural the area, the larger the percentage of 16- and 17-year-olds not enrolled in school. This pattern continues with regard to college education. People from urban areas are almost twice as likely to graduate from college as compared with those from rural areas (Keller & Murray, 1982).

One in six rural residents lives below the poverty line (National Rural Center, 1981). Rural poverty is often associated with chronically depressed areas and can thus affect several generations of the same family. Furthermore, minorities in rural America continue to experience greater deprivation and a higher incidence of poverty than their urban counterparts (Carlson, Lassey, & Lassey, 1980; Falcone & Rosenthal, 1981).

Earning a livelihood in Vermont's back country farms has always been a struggle. Unable to compete with the large mechanized farms of the West, small-scale farming has been declining in Vermont since the 19th century. In 1945, Vermont had 26,490 operating farms. Today, there are fewer than 5,000 (Duffy, 1985). This number continues to decline. Comstock (1987) concludes that the family farm is beyond salvation, practically speaking. The forces of the modern market and international competition seem to dictate that it will soon be impossible for a farmer to support a family on a farm grossing under two hundred thousand dollars a year and working fewer than two thousand acres.

Because of this decline in family farming, the diversity of rural occupations has sharply increased. At earlier points in history, "rural" was synonymous with "agriculture" but this is no longer a valid characterization in the United States. In 1979, only 10 percent of the rural population lived on farms (Bescher-Donnelly & Smith, 1981). Today, seven out of every ten rural workers are employed in either service, manufacturing, or retail trade (U.S. Department of Commerce, Bureau of the Census, 1978). In addition, the rate of out-of-home employment of rural women has risen at an astounding rate. It had been characteristic for rural women to remain in the home and assist with the farming. Now, it is more characteristic for the rural woman to seek employment outside the home in order to help support the family farm (Pistorius, 1990).

Physical and Mental Health Status of Rural and Farm Families

Because of the mind-body interaction and the impact that physical illnesses have on emotions, it is important to know what illnesses plague rural residents. Overall, the physical health of rural residents appears to differ from that of their urban counterparts. In some areas of health, rural people appear to be advantaged. They have fewer reported days of restricted activity, fewer days of bed disability, fewer days lost from work and school, less frequent limitations of activities due to chronic conditions, and fewer acute conditions (Hassinger, 1982). On the other hand, rural people report higher rates of infant deaths, more motor vehicle accident deaths, and much higher rates of injuries at work (often on farm machinery). "Farmer's lung," an allergic reaction to small dust particles and mold spores breathed in while working with hay and silage, is a threat to every farmer. It can become untreatable (Pistorius, 1990). These health conditions, whatever their magnitude, are compounded and escalated because there are fewer physicians and health care facilities in rural areas (Rosenblatt & Moscovice, 1982). Patrick Leahy, U.S. senator from Vermont, points out that for many small towns and rural communities, the development and delivery of effective, accessible, and affordable health services remains an elusive and unmet goal (Committee on Agriculture, Nutrition, and Forestry, 1984).

Great controversy exists over the incidence of mental illness in rural America. In a comprehensive review and critique of the literature, Wagenfeld (1982) found research that demonstrated a higher frequency of mental illness while other data suggested a lower rate. Huessy (1972) argues that psychiatric problems encountered in rural areas differ from those found in urban districts. Balacki (1988) notes difficulty in comparing results of various studies on the mental health needs of rural communities. She proposes, however, that in spite of methodology problems, literature over the past few years has dispelled some long-held myths about rural populations. According to Balacki, the notion that rural areas provide low stress environments for the inhabitants and that there is a decreased need for mental health services is inaccurate. There is a deficit of mental health services in rural areas. This underservice is due both to a lack of programs and an underutilization of existing programs. Many rural residents underutilize mental health services because they lack knowledge of and hold negative attitudes toward such services. There are also problems related to the accessibility of these services. In addition, rural residents can have an exceptionally high degree of tolerance toward the mentally ill. Except for suicidal, hallucinating, and delusional behaviors, rural residents tend to seek help for psychiatric problems from family practitioners rather than from mental health professionals. Family and church groups provide much of the crisis support in rural areas. The social network is a strong influence in rural communities (Flaskerud & Kvitz, 1982, 1983).

Chung-Chou, Sallach, and Klein's (1986) study of 275 rural and urban schizophrenics in Missouri indicates that there is a marked difference in symptomatology and social adjustment. Overall, rural patients have a better adjustment to home living. According to their views and those of their relatives, rural schizophrenics had a higher level of expectations and performance of social activities and more participation in free-time activities. Davies, Bromet, Schulz, Dunn, and Margenstern (1989), in a similar study with a different population of 124 urban and rural schizophrenics, support the above findings. They further note that chronic schizophrenic outpatients who live in nonfamily settings in an urban community function more poorly and encounter worse environmental conditions than do patients who live in a rural community. The exception is the physical condition of the dwelling, which was not directly associated with patients' levels of functioning.

Rosenblatt and Anderson (1981) present evidence that certain rural occupations, such as farming, are particularly stressful. Krach (1990) and Hendricks and Turner (1988) note that depression, suicide, and chemical dependency have risen dramatically in this population. The problems facing farmers have become so severe in Vermont that the Vermont Department of Mental Health and the Department of Agriculture have begun to work together so that services specific to the needs of farm families can be integrated into community mental health services (Dalton, 1989).

Rosenblatt (1990), in testimony gathered from 42 adults in 24 Minnesota farm couples, describes the concerns of farm families caught in the present economic crisis. Many farmers feel grief. Hope, money, effort, hardship, concern, love, dreams, and time are invested in a farm. As a result of the farm's economic troubles, all of this time, effort, and dreaming has come to count for nothing or might come to count for nothing in the near future. Families spend a great deal of time seeking advice from county extension agents, relatives, friends, farm publications, attorneys, bankers, extension and government hot lines, and government offices. All of these activities require energy and attention that take time away from family members and farm work. Some family decisions that are based on family relationships, history, loyalties, rules, obligations, rituals, expectations, feelings, and shared experiences can hurt the enterprise. On the other hand, the economically sound decision may not fit family loyalties or vision of the family's future. Feelings experienced by farm families over lost investments are those of devastating loss, loss of life's goals and meaning, loss of security.

Freidberger (1988) views the present farm crisis as a situation that farmers commonly faced in the past. The problems of the modern farm family, forced to sacrifice the farm which is home, livelihood, and legacy to their children, are the same as those experienced by farmers since the time the land was first settled. Even so, the present economic downturn has made both the community and the families highly vulnerable.

Manolis (1987) points out that even though rural mental health professionals are busier with farm crisis related problems, they are seeing only a limited number of individuals in need of services. This is due to the characteristic reluctance of farm and rural populations to use services available to them. Many farmers talk to no one and suffer in silence. This characteristic stems from traditional values such as stoicism, independence, and pride in self-sufficiency that become instilled in one's personality. These values prompt a vulnerability to depression that is based on guilt and shame, particularly when an individual is faced with losing a farm that has been in his or her family for generations.

In summary, mental illness does exist in rural areas. Effective utilization of available care services is not occurring. Delivery of services, however, may not be implemented in conventional terms given the paucity of trained mental health professionals and the personal characteristics of rural residents. Certainly, the image of the stress-free, trouble-free rural life-style is inaccurate for contemporary rural America.

Features of the Rural and Physical Environment

Scientists in social ecology and environmental psychology have found that the physical and social environments of rural communities impose unique conditions on the delivery of rural mental health services. They posit that the interactive relationship between social forces and the physical environment have a collective synergetic effect on individual behavior. Research findings support that physical terrain does influence social organization and interaction. For example, Heller, Quesada, Harvey, and Warner (1981) suggest that extended-kin-oriented familism is more characteristic of rural Virginia respondents, whereas primary-kin-oriented familism is more representative of the Nevada sample. Similarly, the plantation-orientated economy which characterizes the rural sections of flat coastal areas in Southeastern states has been contrasted with the yeoman farming villages of rural New England (Carlson, Lassey, & Lassey, 1980).

In her study of 296 midwestern farm families, Krach (1990) found that during this time of financial strain, farmers find emotional and physical support through kin relationships. Farmers have frequent, satisfying contacts with aged family members. Filial responsibility remains strong even when financial resources decrease. Krach points out that health interventions are dependent on an understanding of rural kinship patterns. Her study indicates that filial responsibility and affectional bonds are pervasive in rural families. While the threat or fear of losing a farm can tear away at individuals and destroy the entire family unit, health professionals can be at the forefront of preventing this by helping children, young parents, and aged parents become more resourceful.

Americans perceive rural landscapes as quality places to live. Rural people value access to the outdoors and open spaces and conclude that a rural location is superior for raising children. People report more preferences for rural residence. They are seeking a better quality of life. For example, only four out of ten urban residents are content in the city but nine out of ten rural residents wish to remain just where they are (Dillman & Tremblay, 1977; Fuguitt & Zuiches, 1975; Watts & Free, 1973).

Unfortunately, this higher quality of life and higher sense of well being is mostly just in the eyes of rural residents. Water system contamination, coal slag slides, forest fires, and the boom town development which accompanies new mineral extraction have all been shown to disrupt rural health and life (Clark, 1990; Erikson, 1976). Despite the pristine images of enormous white farmhouses in immaculate condition, housing is substandard for more than half of rural residents. Two-thirds of the houses in rural areas lack adequate plumbing (Bird & Kampe, 1977; Mikesell, 1977; National Demonstration Water Project, 1978). The inhabitants of the worst housing are often those that suffer multiple disadvantages of poverty, old age, minority status, and rurality (U.S. Senate Hearings, 1984).

The structure and operating procedures of rural communities are distinctive and tend toward the traditional. These structures have evolved as a function of the smaller scale, more personalized interaction, and local values and traditions of each rural community. These distinctive features are manifested in both the rural political structure with its yearly town meeting and in the economic structure which is now in decline because of the difficulties in agribusiness (Bryan, 1981; Vogeler, 1981). The general consensus is that small towns and rural communities conduct their business in styles that are different, not better or worse, than large urban centers.

Much has been written about the status and inadequacies of the educational, health, and human services that exist in rural communities. Such services have been shown to be fewer in number and less accessible, more narrow in their program scope and function, poorly financed because of smaller tax revenue bases, paying lower salaries for professionals, and serving large geographic areas that are sparsely populated and sometimes contain difficult terrain (Ahearn, 1980; DeWeaver, 1982; Nelson, 1980; Wodarski, 1983).

A local author, Peter Miller (1990), eloquently summarizes the attitude and state of affairs that many Vermonters face in relation to their physical and rural environment:

> *The Green Mountains, Vermont's backbone, are old and worn; they roll and dip, folding the country into pockets and peaks. What these mountains do is give to Vermont patches of geographical privacy; the paradox is that this privacy often is annotated by the breadth and openness of a mountainside view.*
>
> *Those who settled here overcame the severe winters and tamed the rock-embedded soil; they stamped their heritage on Vermont as they turned forests into mowings. It's difficult to say whether it was the temper of the people that made them Vermonters, or whether it was the roughness of the land and climate that forged these newcomers into such distinct personalities.*
>
> *Many of us have taken for granted our hills and valleys, our serpentine roads that skirt cornfields and slice through prim villages and narrow, forested valleys. Innumerable books extol the beauty of Vermont. Tourists come to see this bucolic anachronism that exists within fifteen hours; driving distance of fifty million people.*
>
> *And that is Vermont's problem. It is so accessible to metropolitan areas that many wish to have a second home here—for skiing, for a weekend, for a summer, or just as a social cachet. Others want to move here permanently. As demand increases, developments are created from farms and wooded hills. As our highways become better, the isolated pockets are no longer isolated. Real estate prices escalate. Farmers and townspeople sell their houses for what they think are ridiculously high prices; then, in a few years, wish they hadn't sold out.*

Vermont is losing its privacy, and some of its beauty is being tarnished as development steadily moves north. Our state, in the last decade of this century, is being gentrified. It is becoming more like the name it was first called in the eighteenth century: New Connecticut.

The biggest loss with this change is its people; the Vermonters we have known are unique. They love their state for its beauty, but they revere it more for the freedom it has given them. Most of the Vermonters carved out their own existence as farmers, woodsmen, craftspeople. They are a self-reliant bunch, independent as all get out. They don't need much, so they don't have to make much. If they don't have enough money, they paint the front of the house and not the back—if they are inclined to paint at all. Not so long ago each town took care of its poor, and country store owners gave credit to those who needed it during slack times.

Yet these Vermonters are more liberal than most New Englanders in their attitudes towards their neighbors; it's okay to be a bit different, to do things your own way. Vermonters never did like too many rules, written by government or unwritten by society. Vermonters are social, but social according to their own whims. They have learned to live happily in solitude. They would be aghast at how some downstaters exist within a corporate structure.

That's the anachronism of Vermont—it and its people just don't fit under a corporate, or social, structure; it's not their style. So, as Vermont slowly succumbs to a suburban culture, to development, to stringent state and federal regulations, its hard-core residents—the independent Vermonters—are retreating. Their homes and communities are changing hands and real Vermont neighborhoods are restricted to isolated villages and regions where farming is strong or roads are poor. [p. ii–iii]

Vermont deputy secretary of state, Paul Gillies (1991), echoes Miller's view and the view of many Vermonters:

Somehow, over time, Vermont got itself a reputation as a place where a combination of climate and geography produced a character that was conservative in fiscal matters and liberal on social issues; that was mildly xenophobic,

*but still unusually tolerant of different ways of thinking
and living; with a dry wit and a wry acknowledgement of
reality. Why harness a cow to a plow? To teach her life ain't
all romance.*

*The world thinks of Vermont as a place to retreat to, a
place to find a spiritual center that may have been lost in
the whirl of urban life, a place where nature remains un-
spoiled. Its image, real or not, has been photographed
and filmed and written about, almost to the point of self-
parody. [p. 5]*

CASE ILLUSTRATION OF A VERMONT FARM FAMILY

The family in this case study has given the author permission to use
pseudonyms and change some events and circumstances in order
to protect their confidentiality and anonymity.

The Laframboises are a family of ten. Stanley and Irene married when they were 18 and 17 years old. Both grew up in French-
Canadian farming families from the northern Vermont region and
both could boast of 12 to 15 siblings each if they counted those
who died in early childhood. After working as hired hands for
various established farmers, Stanley and Irene were finally able to
purchase their own dairy farm of 200 acres. This acreage consists
of several large hay producing fields, pasture, and woodlands. The
view north is a scenic vista of the northern Green Mountains and
the view south is of a large lake known for its clear waters and
fishing. The Laframboises have been able to consistently keep a
milking herd of forty jerseys in the barn which was built around
the turn of the century. The farmhouse is large and includes sheds
and enough bedrooms for their eight children in addition to a
spacious kitchen and living room. The nearest village, grocery,
and farm supply stores are ten miles away by dirt roads. Trips to the
village are mainly for a weekly Roman Catholic church service on
Sunday and occasionally for food or equipment supplies. The
Laframboises grow much of their own food in a garden, are supplied by eggs and chicken meat from their chicken flock, and, of
course, with milk and beef from their dairy herd. Stanley's view is
that this is not only cheaper, but better because fresh vegetables

such as corn on the cob and raspberries from the cane just cannot be gotten at the market.

Irene maintains the household. She does weekly laundry, which she hangs outdoors, and sees to the three meals per day. She does much of her own preserving and canning, often bakes her own bread, and ensures that the family has homemade pies and cookies to offer friends and regularly visiting relatives. The family enjoys breakfasts of eggs, milk, and bread; midday dinners of meat, potato, vegetables, and dessert; and a supper of soup, sandwich, or midday leftovers. Irene's outside work includes weeding and maintaining the garden and raising the young livestock. Stanley's routine consists of early morning and evening milking of the cows and midday cleaning of the barn. Summer haying from June to August includes these routines in addition to 12 hours a day spent preparing the hay in the fields. The children assist with the running of the household and farm. They are also busy with school. In addition to the morning and evening milking and three meals per day routines, there are seasonal mandates. Summer is occupied with haying so that the dairy herd will have food for winter. Spring is fence preparation and repair time so that the herd can be contained during summer grazing. Fall is field preparation time so that the land is replenished with fertilizers and nutrients for the next growing season and crops. Much of what the Laframboises earn is returned to their farm and the cycle repeats itself. They enjoy their lives and, although they do not have much in the way of stylish clothing and furniture, feel rich with the quality of their family. They are able to get through each day having their own place, generating their own food, and maintaining their family. Stanley and Irene describe this way of life as their reason for existence. "This was what we were brought up to do . . . raise a large family and make our way as farmers with our own spot of land."

The psychiatric nurse from the area mental health clinic met Irene and Stanley while they were in their middle 50s. They had incorporated their ten-year-old niece, Jeannette, into their family after Stanley's sister died in the state mental hospital. All except one daughter, 12-year-old Mary, had left Irene and Stanley's home by that time. Stanley describes his sister as having been "nervous" for years. "My parents watched over her until their deaths a few years ago. She became worse and had to be sent away since she broke down the screen door one day and could not be reasoned with." He feels he can give his niece a good home and that his sister would have wanted as much. Mary will be a great stepsister for Jeannette. "It is the least that we can do for our sister. It would be irresponsible and selfish of the family to allow Jeannette to be taken into a foster care home. It would just not be right. Yes, Jeannette is a bit nervous too but we believe this is the best place for her, among family."

For the next five years the Laframboises' lives continue with the usual farming routines. Jeannette is doing fine. It is accepted that she is a bit more highly tempered than Mary, is big for her age, and has moody spells. Irene takes Jeannette to their family physician in the town ten miles away for her yearly check-up. Stanley has recently been diagnosed with diabetes so their trips to town are more frequent. Stanley has steadily gained weight and is now on a weight reduction diet. "I guess Irene's pies have been too much for me," he says.

The next year Jeannette has a fight at school that continues as a group of her peers pick on her about her temper. Jeannette's grades worsen and she appears worried and preoccupied much of the time. She reports a visitation from Mary, Mother of God. The school counselor talks with the Laframboises about Jeannette and the family decides to consult with their family physician. The family physician prescribes a small dosage of Stelazine to be taken at bedtime. Irene is worried about her and notes that tensions are worse at home too. Stanley has not been feeling well for the past year and is finding the farm work and financial concerns at age 60 a bit too much for him. Also, he and Jeannette seem to get on one another's nerves and argue with each other which in turn makes everyone more nervous.

The family physician refers the family to the mental health clinic. The psychiatric nurse is unable to get the family to come to the clinic for an interview so she visits them at their house. When asked about future appointments at the clinic, Irene and Stanley relay that 30 miles is too far away to travel in view of all the chores on the farm. Also, they believe that their family physician knows them best and they feel more comfortable with him.

"We go a long way back," Stanley says. "Irene's mother acted as a midwife for our doctor's father who was the only physician in town when we were growing up. All of us kids were born at home back then. Irene's mother knew a lot about herbs and old-time remedies. Thorough-wort, sulphur, and molasses were good for the blood. We no longer take these remedies, but the cows sure do better on a little molasses on their hay during the winter months." When asked what concerned them most about recent events and what they needed help with, they shared their belief "that God helps those who help themselves." They would appreciate having information about the medication Jeannette was taking. They felt she was too doped up because she often fell asleep in the daytime and no longer had energy to do much. She was also gaining weight and complained of a dry mouth. They worried about not being available for Jeannette when she became an adult. "We are getting on in years and Stanley may have to sell out and retire," Irene said. "If we do not have the farm, we worry about whether we will have the space to keep her. We believe she does best here with us with the routines, fresh food, and outdoors that she has become used to and come to enjoy."

The nurse continues to see the Laframboise family in their home and discovers that the local Catholic priest, Father Tremblay, is also a frequent visitor and guest during the Sunday noon meal. The Laframboises share and discuss with him all their reactions, trials, and tribulations. The priest helps them explore their concerns, encourages them to seek resolutions, and praises them for what they have accomplished thus far.

In addition to their concern about Jeannette's health, the Laframboises are also concerned about the possible loss of their farm. The Laframboises have two sons who are in the armed services and who, according to Stanley and Irene, "never were much interested in continuing in their father's footsteps." Their daughters all remain in the area but are married and obligated to their husbands' occupations. No one else in the family is interested in the farm. Their daughters, grandchildren, and cousins are frequent visitors. Many discussions are held around the kitchen table as the family's concerns and options are debated. Stanley and Irene agonize about what is best to do. . . . The mental health nurse encourages these discussions; venting of feelings; and use of priest, family physician, and relatives for support during this time.

Stanley receives an offer from a summer tourist from the nearby lake to buy just the farmhouse and barn with ten acres. Stanley makes it clear that he would rather have the farm remain in the family or second best to sell the entire farm to another farmer. "I am against breaking up my place into little pieces. These new people come in and with them comes the loss of farming. Most of them go to Town Meeting and know how to change things, so they run the town and with them come higher taxes. I can't understand them. They buy a place like the Goddard's in good condition and tear out every partition and pretty near wreck it. Then they start over and build it again. God, they seem to need to spend money. I think they could do better with less." Finally, a nephew offers to work as the Laframboises's hired man in exchange for room and board only. This helps Stanley and Irene to temporarily solve one of their problems.

This case study of a Vermont farm family illustrates some of the issues facing nurses who practice mental health and illness care in this setting. Health care must fit with the population's priorities and desires. The distinctive features of these rural environments and populations are used by the mental health nurse to shape and determine specific actions, interventions, and programs.

FEATURES OF PROVIDING
RURAL MENTAL HEALTH CARE

A host of practitioners and researchers insist that it is different to be a service provider in a rural versus an urban setting. They propose a set of features that are necessary for health care providers to have in order to be successful in delivering rural health care. These features consist of educational preparation and training, knowledge and skills, and attributes and values.

Psychologists and social workers have debated the need for rural health care professionals to be generalists who are able to deal with a wide range of problems (Ginsberg, 1982). Some argue that the generalist model has been an obstacle to the development and delivery of rural services. Irey (1980) proposes a compromise by advocating that the rural health care professional should be a generalist who has specialized skills. Using an ecological perspective, she suggests that the rural worker should be educated to deal with the interaction between the person and the environment since these transactions may be the source of problems. More agreement exists on the knowledge and skills providers will need regardless of formal education. This knowledge is not a unique set of skills but requires a different ordering of these skills for professionals who practice in a rural environment. Rural practitioners need a broader mixture of knowledge and skills because fewer service options are available in their communities. The practitioner must be able to work with other disciplines, analyze the rural community, tap existing resources, and create new resources. Skills in management and community organization, and a willingness to change treatment styles (e.g., emphasis on more short-term, problem-oriented therapy), are necessities. Practitioners must be able to work independently or autonomously while they act as advocates for their rural clients and communities (Dengerink & Cross, 1981; Munson, 1980; Wodarski, 1983).

Some personal attributes and values have proven to be of greater success than others in rural practice. Ginsberg (1982) notes that a higher level of emotional maturity and a great desire for autonomy is helpful for rural workers. A conventional appearance also aids the worker in most rural communities. The appearance needs to fit the convention of the community. Bridging the cultural gap between provider and client is always a challenge. A great many mental health workers who now practice in rural communities are either urban-raised, urban-educated, or both. The myths and stereotypes about rural life they hold may need to be purged. Care delivery models must be culturally compatible with the social class, region, race, and ethnic group of the clients (Coward & Smith, 1982; Wagenfeld & Wagenfeld, 1981).

Certain demands of the rural environment can affect one's job performance and satisfaction. If the mental health care professional has formerly practiced in an urban setting, the process of adjustment to rural practice is critical. The number of professional helpers is smaller in rural areas. There are difficulties associated with recruitment, retention, isolation, lack of peer support, low renumeration, and excessive caseloads (Ozarin, 1981). Some rural providers have difficulty with the relative absence of privacy and anonymity that is due to the social visibility of their actions. This social visibility must be considered as a peculiar characteristic of rural practice by workers who want to be effective practitioners as well as active community members. Finally, the opportunity for supervision and consultation are lower in rural areas; hence the provider must be able to discover alternative methods to obtain necessary collegial feedback.

Work and the various routines of the family farm are of great importance in the rural area. Health care must fit in with these routines. These families cannot afford traveling and time away from farm work. These families are more likely not to utilize and seek out mental health professionals. Their pride, independence, and self-reliance dictate that they will decide for themselves what is best.

Nurses who work in rural communities will need to allow time for extended trust development with rural populations. Visibility and participation in community activities, organizations, and religious groups may help the nurse to become known and accepted as a person in that community. Time must be taken to learn about the various cultural values and beliefs. Careful listening to families' expressed needs will be most useful to the nurse.

The lower formal educational levels of rural populations indicate that the highly verbal and sophisticated communication styles commonly ascribed to mental health service providers may need to be modified. The patterns and forms of communication between client and agency or individual therapist will work best if they vary in accord with local reading levels, cultural compatibility, and language abilities. The more direct, concrete, and locally relevant methods of intervention may better serve these populations than the longer term introspective types of modalities.

Time and distance will also be major factors for the mental health service provider. Typical rural intervention strategies such as satellite service centers or circuit-riders may become cost prohibitive. One consequence of these physical circumstances may be a shift from a primarily ameliorative and intervention style to a more preventive, educational orientation. The provider may choose to rely more heavily on locally based resources, such as family physicians or clergy members, who have easier and greater access to clients even though they may not be trained in mental health. Lastly, rural mental health nurses may decide to place a greater emphasis on collaboration and cooperation with community leaders and/or natural helping networks.

REFERENCES

Ahearn, M. C. (1980). Health services are needed for rural children. *Rural Development Perspectives, 3*, 26.

Bachrach, L. L. (1981). *Human services in rural areas: An analytical review.* Rockville, Maryland: Project SHARE, A National Clearinghouse for Improving the Management of Human Services.

Balacki, M. F. (1988). Assessing mental health needs in the rural community. A critique of assessment approaches. *Issues in Mental Health Nursing, 9,* 299–315.

Beale, C. L. (1981). *Rural and small town population change: 1970–1980.* Washington, D.C.: U.S. Department of Agriculture, Economics and Statistics Service, ESS-5.

Bescher-Donnelly, L., & Smith, L. W. (1981). The changing roles and status of rural women. In R. T. Coward & W. M. Smith, Jr. (Eds.), *The Family in Rural Society.* Boulder, CO: Westview Press.

Bird, R., & Kampe, R. (1977). *25 years of housing progress in rural America.* Washington, D.C.: U.S. Department of Agriculture.

Brown, D. L. (1981). A quarter of a century of trends and changes in the demographic structure of American families. In R. T. Coward and W. M. Smith, Jr. (Eds.), *The family in rural society.* Boulder, CO: Westview Press.

Bryan, F. M. (1981). *Politics in rural America: People, parties and policy.* Boulder, CO: Westview Press.

Carlson, J. E., Lassey, M. L., & Lassey, W. R. (1980). *Rural society and environment in America.* New York: McGraw-Hill Book Company.

Carlson, L. R. (1984). No peers in my sphere. *Kansas Nurse,* 10–11.

Chung-Chou, C., Sallach, H. S., Klein, H. E. (1986). Differences in symptomatology and social adjustment between urban and rural schizophrenics. *Social Psychiatry, 21,* 10–14.

Clark, E. (1990). Troubled waters. *Yankee, 54*(4), 80–90.

Committee on Agriculture, Nutrition, and Forestry. United States Senate (1984). *Emerging issues in the delivery of rural health services.* Washington: U.S. Government Printing Office, 38-977-0.

Comstock, G. (1987). *Is there a moral obligation to save the family farm?* Ames: Iowa State University Press.

Coward, R. T., & Smith, W. M., Jr. (1982). Families in rural society. In D. A. Dillman & D. J. Hobbs (Eds.), *Rural Society in the U.S.: Issues for the 1980's.* Boulder, CO: Westview Press.

Coward, R. T., DeWeaver, K. L., Schmidt, F. E., & Jackson, R. W. (1983). Distinctive features of rural environments: A frame of reference for mental health practice. Burlington, VT: University of Vermont Center for Rural Studies.

Dalton, W. A. (1989). The State of Vermont Department of Mental Health Fiscal Year 1989 Statistical Report. Waterbury, VT: Department of Mental Health.

Davies, M. A., Bromet, E. J., Schulz, C., Dunn, L. O., & Margenstern, M. (1989). Community adjustment of chronic schizophrenic patients in urban and rural settings. *Hospital and Community Psychiatry, 40*(8), 824–830.

Dengerink, H. A., & Cross, H. J. (1981). *Training professionals for rural mental health.* Lincoln and London: University of Nebraska Press.

DeWeaver, K. L. (1982). Delivering rural services for developmentally disabled individuals and their families: Changing scenes. In R. T. Coward and W. M. Smith, Jr. (Eds.), *Serving families in contemporary rural America: Issues and opportunities.* Lincoln, NE: University of Nebraska Press.

Dillman, D. A., & Tremblay, K. R., Jr. (1977). The quality of life in rural America. *Annals of the American Academy of Political and Social Science, 429,* 115.

Duffy, J. (1985). *Vermont: An illustrated history.* Northridge, CA: Windsor Publications, Inc.

Erikson, K. T. (1976). *Everything in its path.* New York: Simon and Schuster.

Falcone, A. M., & Rosenthal, T. L. (1981). *Delivery of rural mental health services*. Cleveland, OH: Synapse Inc.

Fenton, M. V., Rounds, L., & Iha, S. (1988). The nursing center in a rural community: The promotion of family and community health. *Family Community Health, 11*(2), 14–24.

Flaskerud, J. H., & Kviz, F. J. (1982). Resources rural consumers indicate they would use for mental health problems. *Community Mental Health Journal, 18*(2), 107–118.

Flaskerud, J. H., & Kviz, F. J. (1983). Rural attitudes toward and knowledge of mental illness and treatment resources. *Hospital and Community Psychiatry, 34*(3), 229–233.

Flax, J. W., Wagenfeld, M. O., Ivens, R. E., & Weiss, R. J. (1979). *Mental health in rural America: An overview and annotated bibliography*. Washington, D.C.: National Institute of Mental Health (DHEW) Publication (ADM 78-753) U.S. Government Printing Office.

Freidberger, M. (1988). *Farm families & change in twentieth-century America*. Lexington, KY: University Press of Kentucky.

Fuguitt, G. V., & Zuiches, J. J. (1975). Residential preferences and population distribution. *Demography, 12,* 491.

Gillies, P. (1991, Jan 23). What Vermont has done for the United States. *The Chronicle & The Weekly News, 5,* Barton, VT.

Ginsberg, L. H. (1982). Social work in rural communities with an emphasis on mental health practice. In P. A. Keller & J. D. Murray (Eds.), *Handbook of rural community mental health*. New York: Human Science Press.

Glenn, N. O., & Hill, L. (1977). Rural-urban differences in attitudes and behavior in the United States. *The Annals of the American Academy of Political and Social Science, 429,* 36.

Hassinger, E. W. (1982). *Rural health organization: Social networks and Regionalization*. Ames, IA: State University Press.

Heller, P. L., Quesada, G. M., Harvey, D. L., & Warner, L. G. (1981). Rural familism: Interregional analysis. In R. T. Coward and W. M. Smith, Jr. (Eds.), *The family in rural society*. Boulder CO: Westview Press.

Hendricks, J., & Turner, H. B. (1988). Social dimensions of mental illness among rural elderly populations. *International Journal of Aging and Human Development, 26*(3), 169–189.

Huessey, H. R. (1972). Rural models. In H. D. Barten & L. Bellak, (Eds.), *Progress in community mental health,* 2. NY: Grune & Stratton.

Irey, K. V. (1980). The social work generalist in a rural context: An ecological perspective. *Journal of Education for Social Work, 16*(3), 36.

Jackson, R. W. (1982). Delivering services to families in rural America: An analysis of the logistics and uniqueness. In R. T. Coward & W. M. Smith, Jr. (Eds.), *Family services: Issues and opportunities in contemporary rural America* (pp. 69–86). Lincoln, NE: The University of Nebraska Press.

Keller, P. A., & Murray, J. D. (1982). *Handbook of rural community mental health.* New York: Human Sciences Press, Inc.

Krach, P. (1990). Filial responsibility and financial strain: The impact on farm families: *Journal of Gerontological Nursing, 16*(7), 38–41.

Larson, O. F. (1978). Values and beliefs of rural people. In T. R. Ford (Ed.), *Rural USA: Persistence and change.* Ames, Iowa: Iowa State University Press, 91.

Long, K. A., & Weinert, C. (1989). Rural nursing: Developing the theory base. *Scholarly Inquiry for Nursing Practice:* An International Journal, *3*(2), 113–127.

Manolis, D. C. (1987). Diffusing the crisis in rural mental health care. *Minnesota Medicine, 70,* 14–15.

Martinez-Brawley, E. E., & Munson, C. (1982). Systemic characteristics of the rural milieu: A review of social work related research. *Arete, 6*(4), 23.

Mikesell, J. J. (1977). *Population change and metro-nonmetro housing quality differences.* Washington, D.C.: U.S. Department of Agriculture.

Miller, P. (1990). *Vermont people.* Waterbury, VT: Vermont People Project.

Munson, C. E. (1980). Urban-rural differences: Implications for education and training. *Journal of Education for Social Work, 16*(3), 43.

National Demonstration Water Project (1978). *Drinking water supplies in rural America.* Washington, D.C.

National Rural Center (1981). *Rural Poverty.* Washington, D.C.: National Rural Center, 1828 L Street, N.W., Washington, D.C.

Nelson, G. (1980). Social services to the urban and rural aged: The experience of area agencies on aging. *The Gerontologist, 20*(2), 200.

Outlaw, C. H. (1983). Community mental health nursing in a rural setting. *Free Associated Press, 10*(3), 12–13.

Ozarin, L. D. (1981). Rural mental health programs and the federal government. In M. O. Wagenfeld (Ed.), *Perspectives on rural mental health* (pp. 93–97). San Francisco, CA: Jossey-Bass, Inc.

Pistorius, A. (1990). *Cutting Hill: A chronicle of a family farm.* NY: Alfred A. Knopf.

Rosenblatt, R. A., & Moscovice, I. S. (1982). *Rural health care.* NY: John Wiley and Sons.

Rosenblatt, P. C., & Anderson, R. M. (1981). Interaction in farm families: Tension and stress. In R. T. Coward & W. M. Smith, Jr. (Eds.), *The family in rural society* (pp. 147–166). Boulder, CO: Westview Press.

Rosenblatt, P. C. (1990). *Farming is in our blood.* Ames: Iowa State University Press.

U.S. Senate (1971). *Hearings before the Senates' special committee on aging (Part II).* Washington, D.C.: U.S. Government Printing Office.

U.S. Department of Commerce, Bureau of the Census (1978). *Social and economic characteristics of the metropolitan and non-metropolitan population: 1977 and 1970.* Current Population Reports: Special Studies 25, No. 75 Washington, D.C.: U.S. Government Printing Office.

Vogeler, I. (1981). *The myth of the family farm: Agribusiness dominance of U.S. Agriculture.* Boulder, CO: Westview Press.

Wagenfeld, M. O., & Wagenfeld, J. K. (1981). Values, culture and delivery of mental health services. In M. O. Wagenfeld (Ed.), *Perspectives on rural mental health* (pp. 1–12). San Francisco, CA: Jossey-Bass, Inc.

Wagenfeld, M. O. (1982). Psychopathology in rural areas: Issues and evidence. In P. A. Keller & J. D. Murray (Eds.), *Handbook of rural community mental health* (pp. 30–44). New York: Human Sciences Press.

Watts, R., & Free L. (Eds.). (1973). *State of the nation.* New York: Universe Books.

Wodarski, J. S. (1983). *Rural community mental health practice.* Baltimore: University Park Press.

5

Training Family Caregivers
of Rural Elderly

Raelene V. Shippee-Rice
Diane Feeney Mahoney

INTRODUCTION

Older adults, 65 years of age and over, constitute approximately 13 percent of the U.S. population. In 1986, for the first time in history, there were more persons over the age of 65 in the United States than children under the age of 18. By the year 2010, older Americans are expected to account for 20 percent of the country's total population. Although demographic projections may be altered to some extent by unanticipated changes in the birth rate and immigration patterns, there is no disputing that the total number of older adults will continue to increase. The greatest demographic increase is occurring in the category of those 85 years of age and over. In 1980 there were 13,000 adults over 100 years of age; by the year 2000 there will be over 100,000; by the middle of the 21st century, one million people will be over 100 years of age (Brody, 1990).

79

The Rural Elderly

The distribution of older Americans, however, is not consistent across the country. In 1980, the percentage of older adults in individual counties ranged from −16.5 to +13.5 percent, with a disproportionate number living in rural areas (Bohland & Rowles, 1988; Cutler & Coward, 1988; Lancaster, 1988; Patton, 1989). Rural residents comprise about 25 percent of the U.S. population, but they constitute over one-third of the nation's elderly population (Van Hook, 1987). Cutler and Coward (1988) suggest that place of residence is a critical variable in assessing needs of older Americans.

Older adults living in rural areas include those who have lived there all their lives as well as those who have migrated to rural areas in search of safety, lower taxes, and new life-styles. Those who have lived in rural areas for much of their lives are considered to be "aging in place." These older adults have more chronic health problems requiring more physician visits, enter hospitals twice as often, and stay hospitalized twice as long as those living in non-rural areas (Cutler & Coward, 1988; Lancaster, 1988; Patton, 1989). Older adults living in rural, non-farm areas are those with the poorest health (Cutler & Coward, 1988). They are also the least likely to have or take advantage of preventive health care (Talbot, 1985).

Rural older adults aging in place have few economic resources such as savings, private pensions, or health insurance (Nelson, 1980). They also have lower rates of education (Lancaster, 1988). Housing and transportation are two pressing needs of rural older adults (Krout, 1983; Lancaster, 1988; Montgomery, Stubbs, & Day, 1980; Nelson, 1980; Patton, 1989). Transportation, a key factor in access to health care, is hampered by geographic distances, difficult terrain, inadequate or non-existent public transportation systems, and poor roads (Hersh & Van Hook, 1989). When illness occurs, older adults may delay seeking medical care because of these transportation difficulties or because of the distance to health care providers (Lancaster, 1988). Such delays in seeking treatment may result in a severity of illness that requires hospital admission for treatment.

Rural Health Services

Older adults living in rural areas have fewer health care services available to them (Talbot, 1985). Of the 81 community hospitals that closed in 1990, 43 were in rural areas. At the present rate, another 600 may close in the next few years (AACN, 1989). Rural communities developing home health services encounter difficulty trying to provide services because of the great distances between home care beneficiaries and between beneficiaries and providers' offices. A nurse may have to devote the greater part of a single day to one client when the client lives several hours from the health care agency and the care required is extensive (personal communication, J. Tiffany, September 25, 1990).

A major hurdle to quality care in rural areas is the recruitment and retention of nurses (Ermann, 1990; Fickenscher, 1990; Thobaden & Weingard, 1983). There was a 9 percent decrease in the number of rural hospital beds in 1988 because of a shortage of registered nurses (Secretary's Commission on Nursing, 1988). Factors contributing to this shortage of nurses include, "Inadequate and inequitable salaries, fear of professional isolation, lack of modern facilities and inability for spouses to find acceptable employment . . ." (AACN, 1989). In addition, the knowledge and skills required to be effective in rural health nursing differ from those required in more metropolitan settings. Rural nurses make more decisions without input from colleagues and physicians, assume responsibilities for a wide variety of skills and procedures normally performed by physicians or allied health professionals in urban areas, and become more involved in their patients' lives because they live in the same small community (Mossefin, 1987). Few nurses are educationally prepared for these differences (Hassinger, 1982; Lassiter, 1985).

Thus, rural elders experience several health disadvantages: they have more health problems as a result of economic and housing conditions, have few health care resources available to them, and are restricted in their access to the resources that are available (Lancaster, 1988).

The implementation of prospective payment through Diagnostic Related Groupings (DRGs) has resulted in older adults being discharged from the hospital "sicker and quicker." It is not uncommon for older adults discharged from the hospital to home to require extensive assistance with personal care. This need for assistance places a concomitant demand on family members and formal care providers to provide this care (Fischer & Eustis, 1988; Shaughnessy & Kramer, 1990).

Rural Family Relationships

Rural families consider primary groups and social networks to be highly important and influential in their daily lives (Hassinger, 1982). Rural older adults use few formal services either because of lack of information about their availability or because of hostility toward government programs (Auerbach, 1976; Krout, 1983; Stoller & Earl, 1983). Hayslip et al. (1980) found that rural elders feared interference from agencies and viewed the use of home care agencies as the first step toward institutionalization. Bremer (1989) reports that rural older adults are reluctant to accept home nursing services unless they have severe symptoms. This reluctance is a major barrier to nursing involvement in home care. In a study of rural elderly poor, Scott and Roberto (1985) found that when children live in close proximity, older adults use few or no formal services. Thus older adults living in rural areas rely heavily on family and other informal networks for their home health care.

Nursing Implications

Although the family's role in providing home care to older adults has been a major research focus in the gerontological literature, nursing literature on this subject is sparse. According to Phillips (1989), "An appreciation for the importance of this work [preparing family] and a realization of its implications for nursing practice, however, have been slow to emerge." Schirm (1989) reflected a similar opinion when she reported that there is only limited nursing research on the functionally impaired older adult. When added together, the characteristics of rural elderly, functionally impaired and reliant on family caregivers, paint a portrait of a population that can benefit from nursing expertise.

Nurses caring for older adults must respond to the challenge of helping families to 1) become effective caregivers of their impaired older members; 2) carry out their caregiving responsibilities with minimal strain to themselves and to older care recipients; and 3) experience positive aspects of the caretaking experience whenever possible. The Seacoast Caregivers Project described later in this chapter was a pilot project that developed and tested a curriculum to train family caregivers in basic caregiving skills. The curriculum was published under the title of *Training Family Caregivers: A Manual for Group Leaders* (Mahoney, Shippee-Rice, & Pillemer, 1988). This chapter will present an overview of the curriculum and describe the testing of the curriculum with three groups of caregivers in New Hampshire and Maine. Before describing the curriculum and the pilot project, we will review the literature relevant to 1) characteristics of family caregivers and care recipients; 2) caregiving activities; 3) caregiver stress and burden; 4) caregiver satisfaction; and 5) group work with family caregivers. A discussion of the relevance of this project for rural health nursing and implications for nursing research will conclude the chapter.

LITERATURE REVIEW

Most of the studies on family caregiving use non-rural populations for study participants. This is not surprising given that most researchers are located in non-rural areas and the availability of subjects is much greater in larger population centers. Thus there have been few studies specifically addressing the long-term care needs and patterns of family caregiving among rural older adults and their families. What the literature does indicate is that many older rural adults have little use for formal services and depend primarily upon their spouses and their children for help and support (Scott & Roberto, 1985; Shanas et al., 1968). Although the following literature review may not be generalizable to the rural population, it is helpful as a background from which to begin nursing assessment and the application of interventions.

Family Caregivers

Caring is an affective aspect of family relationships; caregiving is the behavioral representation of that caring (Pearlin, Mullan, Semple, & Skaff, 1990). Consequently, caregiving is an integral part of family life. Traditionally caregiving has been associated with parenting and the nurturing and rearing of children (Brown & Kelly, 1987; Giele, 1982). As the population ages, caregiving for impaired spouses, parents, and other older family members consumes an increasing proportion of family time. "Having a dependent elderly parent [has become] a normative experience for individuals and families" (Brody, 1985).

Although not part of the normal aging process, chronic health problems are highly correlated with increasing age. Over 40 percent of those over 65 and 60 percent of those over 85 have one or more chronic health conditions. Most chronic health problems are associated with alterations in functional status such as difficulties in sleeping, eating, working, moving about, and thinking clearly (Dennis, 1990). Chronic illness is marked by periods of exacerbation and quiescence (Zola, 1990). With each exacerbation or as the number of chronic health problems increases, the ability of older adults to independently perform activities of daily living (ADLs) such as toileting, bathing, and moving about (Katz et al., 1963) and instrumental activities of daily living (IADLs) such as medication management, grocery shopping, and meal preparation (Lawton & Brody, 1969) may become impaired. When older adults are unable to perform the normal activities of daily living, families become the first line of support and assistance (Shanas, 1979; Weeks & Cueller, 1981). Over 80 percent of the care presently given to older adults living in the community is done by family caregivers (Brody, 1979; Shanas, 1979; Cantor, 1983; Mutschler, 1985; Stone, Cafferata, & Sangl, 1987; Rivlin & Wiener, 1988). Seventy-five percent of that care is provided without any help from social or health care agencies (Frankfather, Smith, & Caro, 1981; Rivlin & Wiener, 1988; Stoller & Earl, 1983). When professionals are involved in managing care of chronically ill older adults, families are often confused about who is responsible for which aspect of care, who the primary coordinator of care is, or who should be contacted when specific problems arise. The patient and the members of the family often have a better understanding of the illness and how to manage it than do health care professionals (Dennis, 1990).

Thus, the presence of an effective family unit is a crucial factor in maintaining the growing number of frail older adults in the community and preventing or delaying institutionalization (Toseland & Rossiter, 1989). The family is a valuable and important resource in the life and care of older adults; so, too, is it a critical resource to society in meeting the needs of its older members. The centrality of this caregiving role played by the family led Linda K. George (1990), a noted gerontologist, nurse, and policy analyst to write, ". . . [family] caregiving has generated more interest among gerontologists than any other topic."

Caregiver Characteristics

Family caregiver is a generic term. Researchers use the term family caregiver when discussing either or both primary and secondary caregivers; that is, those who assume the majority of caregiving responsibility (primary caregivers) and those that assume an assistive role (secondary caregivers) to the primary caregiver. Family caregiver as used in the research literature may refer to any member of the family providing care to an older adult or may be limited to specific relatives such as daughters, sons, spouses, or other kin. For example, in a study of 111 family caregivers, 37 were spouses (gender not indicated), 40 were children (gender not indicated), 21 were other relatives, and 13 were friends/neighbors (Cantor, 1983). The dynamics between the care provider and the older adult care recipient differ depending upon the familial relationship. Spouses, children and, to some extent, children-in-law are the dominant informal caregivers to older adults (Stone & Kemper, 1989). The spouse is usually the first line of responsibility for primary caregiving. If there is no spouse present, caregiving responsibilities fall to the adult children, usually a daughter; if no daughters are available to assume the role of primary caregiver, sons will assume caregiving responsibilities. However, the son's spouse will very often assume the hands-on direct care tasks (Horowitz, 1985; Johnson & Catalano, 1983). Overall, women supply significantly more care to impaired older adults (Brody, 1985; Cantor, 1980; Horowitz, 1985; Johnson & Catalano, 1983; Shanas, 1979; Stone & Kemper, 1989). As the majority of caregiving is provided by a spouse, daughter, or son, this section of the literature review will focus on the characteristics of spouses, daughters, and sons.

Spousal Caregivers

> . . . *spouses are willing to do almost anything . . . to prevent the nursing home admission of their lifelong companion. [Hess & Soldo, 1985, p. 79]*

The caregiver in an elderly couple is most likely to be the wife (Stoller, 1990). Women live an average of seven years longer than their husbands and are often younger than their husbands. Married older women are more apt to be institutionalized than are married older men, suggesting that wives may provide care longer for more severely impaired spouses than do husbands (Stoller, 1990). Husband and wives caring for impaired spouses are usually themselves over 65, suffer from one or more chronic health problems, and have limitations in activities of daily living (Barusch, 1988; Fengler & Goodrich, 1979; Mutschler, 1985). These caregivers may require some level of assistance for themselves (Hess & Soldo, 1985). In a sample of 89 spouses, Barusch (1988) found that 53 percent of the husbands and 70 percent of the wives experienced physical difficulty performing some care related tasks needed by their spouses.

Daughters as Caregivers

> *[Caregivers] are daughters and daughters-in-law who come from a range of economic, social, and ethnic backgrounds and have different combinations of personal circumstances. They may be 30 or 50 or 70 years old. Some are*

married; others are widowed, divorced, or have never married. Some are homemakers, some have worked all of their adult lives, and others are part of the huge number who have recently entered or plan to enter the labor force. Whatever their individual situations, what they have in common is that they are taking care of disabled older people in their families, have many other roles and responsibilities, and are feeling the pressure and strains. [Brody, 1985, p. x]

Most spousal caregivers live with the disabled older adult, but most daughters and sons live in separate households. When a parent does live in the same household with a child, it is most often daughters with whom they live. In the 1982 Long-Term Care Survey, the mean age of daughters providing care to a parent was 52.5 years (Brody, 1990). Twenty-five percent were under 45 and almost 15 percent were over 65.

More than half of spouses and children acting as caregivers work full time (Stone & Kemper, 1989). Brody (1990) reports that 11.6 percent of daughter caregivers were forced to terminate their employment because of caregiving demands, while another 30 percent had to reduce the number of working hours or take time off from their jobs without pay.

In addition to primary caregiving responsibilities, family members may assume secondary caregiving responsibilities. When the spouse is the primary caregiver, children provide social and emotional support as well as assistance with some of the activities and instrumental activities of daily living. In a study of daughter primary caregivers, daughters' husbands provided approximately 4 to 6 percent of instrumental (hands-on) care and 11 percent of other types of assistance as secondary caregivers. Siblings, children, and other family members were secondary caregivers providing approximately 20 percent of the assistance (Brody, 1990). Brothers as secondary caregivers supply significantly less support to sibling primary caregivers than do sisters (Brody et al., 1989).

Sons as Caregivers

Sons tend to be under-represented in caregiving research because 1) they are less apt to participate in survey research, 2) may be less personally involved in the caregiving role and thus less apt to participate in research studying that role, and 3) men who are at the age to be involved with caring for aged parents are more apt to have been socially and culturally conditioned to be less expressive and thus less likely to engage in interviews about their personal feelings and reactions to caregiving (Horowitz, 1985). Current literature on sons as caregivers indicates that sons become primary caregivers by default. It is only when the son is an only child or when no daughter or other female family member is available (Horowitz, 1985; Johnson & Catalano, 1983; Shanas, 1979) that sons assume final responsibility for parent care. Horowitz (1985), in a study of 131 adult children caregivers, found that sons who were caregivers had more education, with 41 percent having college degrees compared with 17 percent of daughters. Men were more likely to be employed full time. The reduction in family size as a demographic trend suggests that sons may be increasingly called upon to serve as caregivers to their older parents (Horowitz, 1985).

If married, sons' usually involve their wives in sharing the caregiving responsibilities. Sons assume responsibility for financial management or advising and decision making. Men who are primary caregivers experience some of the same dilemmas, share the same pains, and achieve the same sense of satisfaction as female caregivers (Stafford, 1988).

Care Recipient Characteristics

In a review of the literature on group interventions, Toseland and Rossiter (1989) report that 72 percent of caregivers in the studies cited provided care for a parent or relative with some form of mental impairment. The remaining 28 percent provided care to older adults with unspecified impairments. Barer and Johnson (1990), in their critique of the caregiving literature, identify the lack of specificity regarding the caregiving needs and characteristics of the care recipients as a major weakness. Although half the articles they reviewed focus on caregiving of mentally impaired adults, they state that, "Other recipients of care are simply described as being disabled, impaired or frail" (p. 27). Citing mental impairment, however, is as limiting in its specificity of the type of care required as does "being disabled, impaired or frail."

Given the constraints of the caregiving literature, we can nonetheless, make some assumptions about the characteristics of older adults who require assistance from families or friends. These assumptions are based primarily on reported results of national surveys. In a review of the 1984 National Long-Term Care Survey, Stone and Murtaugh (1990) report that 15 percent of all older community residents aged 65 and older who had been disabled for at least three months required assistance with at least one ADL or IADL. Most care recipients required assistance with bathing followed by help with toileting, dressing, getting in or out of bed, and eating. Grocery shopping, money management, laundry, and getting around outside were the instrumental activities of daily living for which help was needed. The most common daily IADLs with which older adults required assistance were meal preparation and taking medications.

Troll (1988), in discussing "new thoughts on old families," suggests that "rarely is the parents' perspective considered" in the gerontological family literature. The same could be said about the family caregiving literature: rarely is the affect, impact, issues of family caregiving on the care recipient addressed.

Caregiving Activities

Families providing care to older adults face the prospect of increasing responsibility as the impaired family member grows older, chronic illnesses progress, and functional abilities decline. This is a distinctive difference from child care in which the caregiver expects the child to grow up and the caretaking demands to decrease (Worcester, 1990).

The characteristics of the care recipient are major determinants of the types of caretaking tasks and processes family members provide. The caregiving needs of older adults living in the community are not dissimilar to those required by older adults in long-term care institutions. The response to the caregiving tasks is the result of caregiver characteristics rather than those of the care recipient. Caregiving spans a diverse array of tasks and levels of responsibility, involvement, skills, and activities. A critical variable in determining caregiving activities and responsibilities is the physical and mental health of the older adult and the severity of impairment. Activities range from driving the older adult for physician visits to complete bed side care. The time involved in carrying out caretaking responsibilities may range from a few hours on an occasional basis to around-the-clock care. Marks (1987) estimated that families providing physical hands-on care to older family members spend up to 120 hours a week in caregiving tasks. Caregiving may be given to older adults living in the same household with the caregiver, to those living in separate households within driving distance of thirty minutes or less or to those living hundreds to thousands of miles away. Each of these caregiving relationships creates similar as well as distinct demands.

Caregiving activities can be described or categorized in several different ways. Stone and Kemper (1987) categorize caregiving responsibilities according to the needs of the care recipients: those who have cognitive or other mental health impairment but do not need hands-on help, those who need help for conditions that are not chronic such as post-hospital care, and those who require assistance with ADLs (eating, toileting, dressing) and/or IADLs (preparing meals, taking medication, shopping for groceries). Older adults may require only financial or emotional support or assistance with home maintenance and care including light or heavy housework, laundry, and so forth (Stone & Kemper, 1989).

Bowers (1987) divides caregiving into five categories based on processes of caregiving. She describes the processes as instrumental (hands-on caregiving behavior or tasks); anticipatory (behaviors or decisions based on anticipated, possible needs of a parent); preventive (activities carried out for the purpose of preventing illness, injury, complications, and physical and mental deterioration); supervisory (an active and direct involvement in arranging for, checking up, making sure, setting up, and checking out parents' care); and protective (protecting the parent from the consequences of that which was not or could not be prevented).

Archbold (1980) describes the role demands of caregiving as preventing medical crises, controlling symptoms, carrying out treatment regimes, preventing social isolation, adjusting to disease course, attempting to normalize the living situation, and finding necessary resources and money for care.

Rew et al. (1987) suggest that providing care to older family members includes intervening on patient's behalf, listening, administering medication and treatments, providing comfort measures, and ensuring the safety of the care receiver.

Thus, caregiving requires different levels of caregiver involvement, skills, and activities. Miller, McFall, and Montgomery (1991) report that care given to older adults with greater functional limitations or to those impaired in a number of ADLs and IADLs requires significantly more caregiver involvement because of the increased number of tasks to be done and the extra hours required to do them.

Caretaking activities carried out by adult children fall along traditional gender lines. Daughters are more likely to help with hands-on assistance such as personal care, transportation, and household chores. Sons are more apt to be involved in helping with financial management, advice giving, and decision making. However, both daughters and sons engage in fulfilling family affective functions and see them as a part of the common caregiving role (Brody, 1990; Horowitz, 1985; Stafford, 1988; Stoller, 1990).

Caregiving has the potential to bring family members closer together, allowing new understanding between parent and child (children) or between husband and wife to develop. Maynard provides a description of this phenomenon in sharing her reactions to caring for her dying mother.

> *She had always fed and cared for me . . . It seemed fitting that now I should be cooking and caring for her. . . . We talked about many things over those meals . . . talked about her bitter struggles with her mother, and mine with her. . . . We talked about death and the relative merits of butter vs. vegetable shortening in piecrust. . . . when my mother lay asleep I thought a lot about mothers and daughters and the way we tend to pass on from one generation to the next a legacy of family patterns, good and bad . . . the way to live life, have a marriage, raise healthy and strong children. [Maynard, 1990, p. 104]*

The costs of caring, however, cannot be overlooked for they are not insignificant. Providing care to older family members places demands on a family's physical, emotional, psychological, and financial resources that involve not only the direct costs on family resources but also generate indirect or opportunity costs; the costs of not doing something else with their resources other than assigning them to the care of the older adults.

It is not unusual for family members to undergo emotional, physical and even financial strain as a result of providing care to their older family members. The strains they experience emanate from the perceived stresses and burdens associated with caregiving responsibilities and activities (Cantor, 1983; Zarit et al., 1980). Emotional strains are more frequently reported than are physical or financial ones.

Caregiver Stress and Burden

The gerontological literature is replete with research on the stresses, strains, and burdens associated with caregiving and the factors that correlate with them. Webster defines strain as "to tax to the utmost." Stress is defined as "a mentally or emotionally disruptive or disquieting influence" (Webster's Dictionary, 1986). Using concept analysis and role theory, Ward (1986) defines role strain as "an undesirable state perceived by the individual within a role arising from the stress associated with the role." She defines role stress as "a social structural condition in which role obligations are vague, irritating, difficult, conflicting, or impossible to meet." Although the words strain and stress are referred to in almost all articles on family caregiving, they are more often defined by scores subjects obtain on standardized measures rather than semantically. However, an analysis of the implicit meanings of the terms stress and strain as used in the gerontological caregiving literature indicates the definitions of Ward are the most applicable.

Burden can be conceptualized as composed of objective and subjective experiences. Montgomery and Borgatta (1989) define objective burden as the extent of disruptions or changes in various aspects of the caregiver's life and household. Subjective burden is defined as the caregiver's stress and nervousness related to the situation and the extent to which the caregiver feels manipulated by the demands of the care recipient.

More attention has been given to the negative effects of caretaking. Policymakers, health economists, and professional care providers are acutely interested in identifying those factors that contribute to strain and subsequent feelings of stress and burden. Families who experience negative reactions to caretaking may become "burned out" and develop health problems, provide poor care, and possibly mistreat the older adult (Fulmer & O'Malley, 1987). Families may have to rely heavily on community services or be forced to institutionalize the older adult. These responses to caregiving have the potential to increase public expenditures. However, if the sources of strain and the resultant stress and burden can be identified, interventions can be developed that will minimize the negative aspects of caregiving. By increasing family coping strategies and decreasing the strains of caregiving or the feelings of stress and burden, caregivers will feel empowered to carry out their caregiving responsibilities with positive feelings of regard for themselves and for the older care recipient.

Factors correlated with increased feelings of stress and burden are restrictions on caregivers' time and freedom, isolation from friends and relatives, conflict from competing role demands, and feelings of insecurity and incompetence in their ability to provide adequate care (Brody, 1990; Clark & Rakowski, 1983; Frankfather, 1981; Hirschfeld, 1983). The level of impairment of the care recipient seems minimally related to the level of stress experienced by the caregiver (Hawranik, 1985; Gubrium, 1988; Zarit et al., 1980). However, care recipients with psychological and behavioral impairments create more stress for family caregivers than do medical or physical impairments (Hirshfeld, 1983; Poulshock & Deimling, 1984; Worcester & Quayhagen, 1983).

Some caregivers respond to feelings of burden by providing inadequate care of institutionalizing the older adult. Other reactions include anger, anxiety, guilt, and depression (Brody, 1985; Drinka, Smith, & Drinka, 1987; Gallagher et al., 1989; George & Gwyther, 1986; Poulshock & Deimling, 1984). Physical responses of caregivers include fatigue, back problems, illness, and exacerbation of chronic health problems. Between 15 and 30 percent of adult children experience health problems in response to caregiving demands.

The type of care required by the care recipient, especially heavy physical care, and watching the health changes experienced by the older adult and the losses they experience create strain in the caregiver. Other factors include disruptive behavior, personality clashes, and negative interactions between parent and child. Miller, McFall, and Montgomery (1991) suggest that it may be the level of involvement of the family caregiver rather than the caregiving activities themselves that is significant in the generation of caregiver stress.

Spouses appear to have a "higher tolerance threshold than other caregivers" (Hess & Soldo, 1985). This conclusion is based on an analysis of a model proposed by Mindel and Wright and described by Hess and Soldo. The model examines the interactions between dependency needs of the care receiver, characteristics of the caregiver and the context in which care is given. Although spouses care for more impaired persons, experience more functional health limitations, and have fewer resources to relieve the burdens of caregiving, they provide care longer than do adult children and experience lower levels of distress (Hawranik, 1985; Jones & Vetter, 1984; Worcester & Quayhagen, 1983). It is unclear, however, whether it is the familial relationship that explains the difference or whether it is the number of role demands experienced by the older and younger caregivers. Several researchers suggest that the caregiving literature supports the hypothesis that it is the relationship of the caregiver to the older adult that is the most critical variable (Gubrium, 1988; Gwyther & George, 1986).

Caregiver Satisfaction

Several factors contribute to feelings of satisfaction with the caregiving experience or mediate the level of burden and stress experienced by the caregiver. These factors include availability of familial support and contact (Zarit et al., 1980), gratification in the relationship with the impaired older adult (Hirschfeld, 1983), and availability of formal supports (Jones & Vetter, 1984; Worcester & Quayhagen, 1983). Phillips and Rempusheski (1986) report several aspects as important in the development of a caregiver's perception that the relationship with the older care recipient is a good one or a negative one. These aspects include: reconciliation of past and present images of the elder, the degree to which the caregivers' standards and values of what it means to be in a caregiving situation are realized, caregivers' perception of history of events and of the elder and his or her behavior, the caregivers' role beliefs and normative expectations for the elders, and the caregivers' management strategies.

Families who experience higher levels of satisfaction are less apt to institutionalize the impaired family member. Thus, nurses must be as sensitive to promoting and reinforcing the factors that enhance the caregiving experience as they are to developing strategies to relieve factors that contribute negatively.

In addition to identifying factors correlated with caregiver strain, stress, and burden, researchers have been equally interested in finding ways caregivers adapt and cope with caregiving demands. Johnson and Catalano (1983) describe two broad categories of adaptive mechanisms: distancing techniques and enmeshing techniques.

Distancing techniques include physical and psychological behaviors which allow the caregiver to remove him or herself from the caregiving situation as the elder's physical and/or mental status deteriorates and caregiving demands increase. Some caregivers distance themselves by enlarging the family network to include others. In a poignant description of his experiences as the primary caregiver for his mother, Klaybor (1988) provides us with an example of distancing as an adaptive response:

> . . . *I needed to break away. . . . my plan to leave the scene required that Mom's other children cooperate to arrange for her care, and thus my brothers and sisters had a greater opportunity to help. . . . Mom became closer to Marsha, her own sister Alice, neighbors, and other relatives. With me away, there was more room for other people to share in her care. [Klaybor, 1988, p. 176–177]*

In enmeshing techniques, the relationship between the caregiver and care recipient intensifies to the exclusion of other relationships. This is common especially among older married couples. Role entrenchment is another enmeshing technique in which caregiving becomes accepted as a role that takes precedence over other social roles. In *Women in the Middle,* Brody provides us with verbatim descriptions of women's caregiving experiences with their parents. Even though Brody does use the concept of role entrenchment, an excerpt from one of the women, Mrs. Gordon, presents us with an experience that represents the concept of role entrenchment as a successful adaptive mechanism:

> . . . *I'm content. I'm doing a noble thing. . . . Mother complains when I'm not here. I am her security blanket. It's not an obligation. I'm glad to do it. It's my job. . . . She says she used to feel stressed and that she was giving things up, but no longer. [Brody, 1990, pp. 163–164]*

Group Work with Family Caregivers

Health and social service providers have responded to the stress experienced by caregivers by initiating groups wherein caregivers can explore their feelings about caregiving, receive emotional and psychological support, discuss their problems, and gain information. The caregiving literature is replete with descriptions of such programs and research evaluating their effectiveness. The major goal in using group strategies is to help family members increase their coping abilities and decrease feelings of overburden and stress. Most of the strategies reported involve the use of support groups, and to a more limited extent, educational groups.

Toseland and Rossiter (1989) reviewed and analyzed 29 caregiving groups reported in the gerontological literature between 1969 and 1987. They identified six themes prevalent among support groups for family caregivers: information about care receiver's situation, use of the group as a support system, emotional impact of caregiving, [caregiver's] self-care, problematic interpersonal relationships, and development and use of support systems outside the group. A seventh theme, included in only a few groups, was the improvement of home care skills. Most group programs lasted six to eight weeks with weekly sessions lasting one to two hours. Participants were predominately white middle class women aged 40 to 65 years who were wives or daughters of the care recipients (Toseland & Rossiter, 1989). Most (72 percent) were caring for adults with some form of mental impairment, usually Alzheimer's disease. Methods of program evaluation ranged from reliance on informal anecdotal information with little emphasis on data collection, to more formal methods that included standardized tests and measurements (Toseland & Rossiter, 1989). The research design most commonly used was the pre- and post-test. Post-tests were conducted immediately post-intervention, with some studies conducting a follow-up evaluation usually six months after the program (Toseland & Rossiter, 1989). The findings of Toseland and Rossiter are similar to those found in a review of the caregiving literature conducted in 1983 by Clark and Rakowski. In addition to these general reviews, several authors have written critiques of the caregiving literature (Barer & Johnson, 1990; Pearlin et al., 1990).

Major criticisms cited in the above critiques include 1) the lack of adequate description and specificity of the objectives and content included in the program; 2) focus of groups on middle class, white caregivers; 3) lack of operationalizing the term caregiver; 4) infrequency with which the type of care needed by care recipients is considered in the analysis, and 5) minimal attention to difficulties encountered in program implementation (Barer & Johnson, 1990; Clark & Rakowski, 1983).

In their review of the caregiving literature, Clark and Rakowski (1983) categorized caregiving tasks described by caregivers participating in educational and socio-emotional support groups. Several of the tasks that were reported as being particularly stressful for caregivers were performing basic ADLs for care recipient; gaining knowledge about the disease/condition; resolving disappointment or feelings of guilt over one's performance; avoiding severe drain on physical strength/health; and interacting with medical, health, and social service professionals. Yet few of the group interventions reported in the reviews by Clark and Rakowski (1983) and Toseland and Rossiter (1989) included teaching skills associated with physical caregiving.

Greene and Monahan (1989) report on a study that specifically identified the teaching of physical caregiving skills as an important goal of the program. The program consisted of eight two-hour weekly sessions. Each session included three components: an affective component articulating and sharing difficult and painful experiences; an educational component focusing on physical skills training, social skills development, processes of aging, and of course of diseases; and a third component focusing on relaxation training. Groups were led by a team composed of a social worker and a community health nurse. The purpose of the group intervention was to reduce stress and burden among family caregivers as measured by standardized instruments. Results suggest that the support group did help caregivers with high levels of stress to better cope with their caregiving responsibilities.

Where do families learn how to provide physical care to their members? As noted earlier, older adults are now discharged from the hospital while still needing assistance with their ADLs. Few families feel adequately prepared to assume the necessary caretaking activities (Baines, 1984; Clark & Rakowski, 1983; Rew et al., 1987). Families expecting the birth or adoption of a baby are offered numerous educational opportunities to help them prepare for their new role as parents or grandparents (Brown & Kelley, 1987). Parenthood is recognized as an important role transition, one that benefits from educational preparation. Community agencies sponsor programs in which parents-to-be learn how to care for their newborn's physical needs, while receiving emotional support to ease their transition into parenthood.

Caregivers of frail elders also experience role transition, yet there are few opportunities to learn the role of caregiver for the frail elderly (Rew et al., 1987). As noted in the literature review, the majority of caregiver programs described in the gerontological literature emphasize social support and information sharing. Although no one model of group support can meet the diverse needs of family caregivers, there is a demonstrated need for programs that will help family caregivers develop competence in meeting the demands of caregiving. If caregivers feel competent and comfortable performing physical caregiving activities; applying knowledge specific to the health and care needs of the care recipient; and using effective problem-solving, decision-making, and assertiveness skills, they may experience less strain and more satisfaction.

The Seacoast Caregiving Project was initiated to develop and test a curriculum to train family caregivers. The curriculum is designed specifically for nurses to use as a tool for teaching family members more effective methods of providing care to older adults. The curriculum was tested with three groups of caregivers. In the next section the curriculum, the pilot program to test the curriculum and its effectiveness with family members, and the evaluation of the program are described. The project was funded by the Foundation for Seacoast Health of Portsmouth, New Hampshire. This organization was established to provide financial support for programs and projects promoting the health and well-being of those living within its target area, coastal New Hampshire and the southwest tip of Maine.

THE FAMILY CAREGIVER TRAINING CURRICULUM

The curriculum developed by Mahoney et al. for the training of family caregivers is based on the rationale that providing informal caregivers with an opportunity to develop technical skills and knowledge in a supportive group environment will increase caregiver competence and lead to feelings of security and empowerment. As a result, family caregivers will experience more self-control and less physical and emotional strain. Caregivers will also feel more competent in interacting with the formal caregiving system and professional care providers.

The curriculum is based on three assumptions:

1. families want to provide safe, effective, and quality care for their aged family members;
2. traditional educational and socio-emotional support groups do not provide knowledge and skills relevant to hands-on caregiving required by elders with impaired ability to perform their activities of daily living; and
3. nurses are the most appropriate health care professionals to teach families caregiving skills.

Program Goals and Objectives

The goal of the program is to assist caregivers to meet their care-taking responsibilities with greater skill and knowledge and with less physical and emotional strain on themselves and their elderly care recipients.

The program focuses on helping family members to meet the following objectives:

1. increase their knowledge of personal care techniques and adaptations;
2. distinguish between normal changes associated with aging and pathological processes;
3. perform caregiving services in a more efficient manner;
4. expand their range of caregiving skills;
5. identify the meaning of the caregiver role to themselves and the care recipient; and
6. develop assertiveness techniques for use in both the family system as well as the formal caregiving system.

Conceptual Model

The program, as designed by Mahoney et al., is a partnership model between the nurse as facilitator and the caregiver. In this model, the caregivers identify the knowledge areas they think they need. The nurse's responsibility is to share professional information, promote skill development, and identify resources that will help caregivers to gain competence in the areas they identified. The agenda is consumer-driven yet professionally mediated in response to common as well as unique problems of caregiving. The group approach facilitates information exchange and enhances learning. The nurse-facilitator strives to

1. develop a collegial caregiver relationship by avoiding professional dominance;
2. encourage an interactive process of caregiver learning;
3. respond to unique needs of the caregiver/care recipient dyad;

4. help caregivers to feel empowered through the sharing of specialized knowledge and skills;
5. teach advocacy skills using an activated consumer approach;
6. affirm the value of caregivers' efforts; and
7. promote caregivers' self-esteem.

The conceptual model of the program is depicted in Figures 5–1 and 5–2. Figure 5–1 shows a caregiving system in which the negative aspects of caregiving outweigh the positive. In this diagram, whatever positive aspects present in the system are outweighed by the negative burden created by the demands on the caregiver. Figure 5–2 depicts the differences expected to occur as a result of participation in the caregiver training program. The nurse-facilitator encourages and promotes adaptations to optimize the care recipient's functioning and introduces caregiving skills and knowledge to minimize caregiver burden. The nurse-facilitator seeks to strengthen and support the existing positive aspects in the family system. Nursing efforts are directed at promoting family adjustment and supporting the caregiver.

Curriculum Outline

The training program is designed to be completed in seven sessions. Each week, one of the following key topics is offered: taking vital signs, managing elimination problems, confusion and sensory losses, using medications wisely, lifting and moving, hygiene, feeding, and oral health care. The order and emphasis of the sessions, however, vary according to the needs of the group.

Keeping with the program philosophy, the needs of the caregivers, not a pre-established agenda, drive the course. In the first session participants rate the issues that most concern them using an agenda setting tool (Appendix 5–A). The nurse-facilitator tabulates the aggregate results and reviews them with the group. Participants immediately see the areas of concern they have in common and realize how their individual needs will be met within the group setting. The overall program is sequenced according to the topics that received the highest interest rating by the group.

Figure 5–1
Negative Caregiving Situation

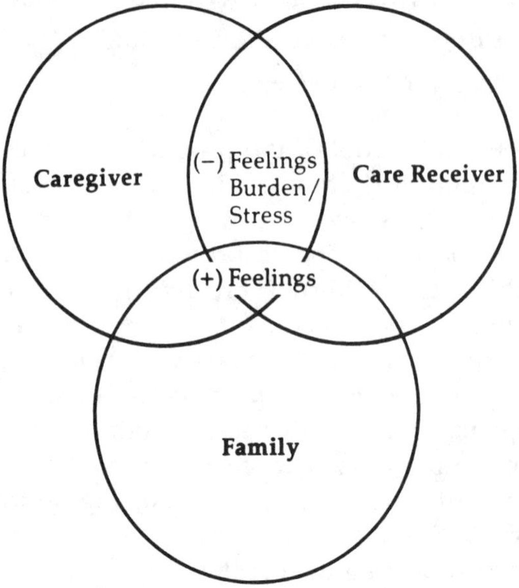

Consequently, each of the three groups had slightly different sequences in the program outline and topic emphasis (Exhibits 5–1 and 5–2).

Structure, not rigidity, is provided by having each session follow a similar core framework. During the opening segment, the nurse-facilitator encourages caregivers' questions about issues related to the topic for that session. Didactic information about the topic is presented for 15 to 20 minutes. The nurse demonstrates the technical skill(s) related to the session topic. A refreshment break in the middle of the session allows for informal contacts among the members and the facilitator. Information on local and national resources pertinent to the topic of the week is displayed for browsing. Each participant receives handouts on the session topic for future reference. After the break, participants practice the skill(s) on each other or a mannequin.

Time is available at each step for group interaction and questions. The nurse-facilitator adapts the unit topic to respond to the

Figure 5–2
Benefits of Participation in Caregiver Training Program

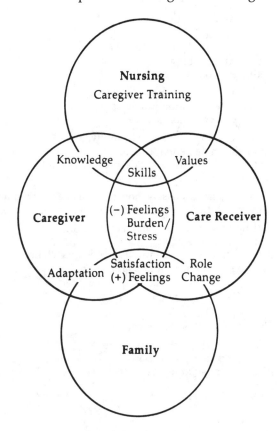

particular problems, issues, and questions raised by the participants.

In this type of group, it is critical to have a knowledgeable clinician who can relate skillfully, in a nonthreatening manner, with caregivers. We found that a gerontological nurse specialist is ideal for this position. Master's prepared nurses have substantive preparation in both the clinical and psychosocial aspects of their specialty field. Although many health education groups enlist various experts to discuss issues and present information, we purposely designed this curriculum to avoid this practice. Mahoney (1984) found that medical experts frequently have difficulty

Exhibit 5–1
Sample Agenda and Timetable 1

Sept. 15   Introduction
            Agenda Setting
            How do you find good medical care
            Why vital signs are vital
            Taking a blood pressure

Sept. 22   Taking a blood pressure (continued)
            Managing elimination problems
            Tips to prevent incontinence

Sept. 29   Confusion: What is dementia and what is not
            Coping with dementia/delirium
            Adding to the confusion: hearing and vision loss
            Tips, aids, and resources

Oct. 6   Using medications wisely: how to remember and sequence them
            Critical questions to ask before administering medication

Oct. 13   Getting around: Lifting and moving skills
            Protecting the caregiver's back
            Use and care of canes, crutches, and wheelchairs
            How to prevent and handle falls

Oct. 20   Beating the bed bath blues
            Special skin care for older adults
            How to give a backrub
            Changing a bed with someone in it

Oct. 27   Eating concerns, nutritional issues
            Feeding tips and suggestions
            What you must know about dentures.

            Program wrap up

relating to elderly consumers, especially in a group situation where participants raise many issues outside of the physician's specialty area. She encourages the use of a "continuity model" for consumer-oriented health education programs. In this model, a stable educator becomes very aware of the attendees' needs. Within the caregiver groups, this awareness helps the nurse to individualize the teaching given to participants, ensure their mastery of the tasks, and promote their positive self-esteem. This is not meant to imply that occasional use of an "expert" in some area cannot be used if this would best meet the needs of the group and facilitate the knowledge and competence sought.

Exhibit 5–2
Sample Agenda and Timetable 2

March 1   Introduction
           Agenda setting
           How do you find good medical care
           Why vital signs are vital
           Taking a blood pressure

March 8   Confusion: What is dementia and what is not
           Coping with dementia/delirium
           Adding to the confusion: hearing and vision loss
           Tips, aids, and resources

March 15   Using medications wisely: how to remember and sequence them
           Critical questions to ask before administering medications

March 22   Managing elimination problems
           Tips to prevent incontinence

March 29   Getting around: lifting and moving skills
           Protecting the caregiver's back
           Use and care of canes, crutches, and wheelchairs
           How to prevent and handle falls

April 5   Eating concerns, nutritional issues
           Feeding tips and suggestions
           What you must know about dentures

April 12   Beating the bed bath blues
           Skin care needs of older adults
           How to give a backrub
           Changing a bed with someone in it

           Program wrap up.

Implementing the Curriculum

A pilot project was implemented to test the curriculum and evaluate the impact of participation on caregivers' feelings of competence, stress, and burden. Three groups of family caregivers in southeastern New Hampshire and southwestern Maine participated. The pilot project fostered participant and community agency involvement from its inception. Meetings were held with leaders of the local professional nursing and social service agencies to inform them about the project and to solicit their help in recruiting participants. Brochures with registration forms enclosed were made available in physician offices, community health care agencies, churches, visiting nurse associations, senior citizen centers, and service programs for older adults. Posters were hung in drug stores, grocery stores, restaurants, laundries, and post offices. Announcements were placed in local daily and weekly newspapers, church newsletters, and the newsletter sent out by the area senior citizens council. Meeting times for the program were established through the registration form. The registration form queried potential participants for the most convenient time and location in which to schedule the group. Potential participants were then called to inform them of the dates, times, and locations of the meetings. This was a cumbersome process, but it was necessary because we had no sure way of assessing how caregiving responsibilities might affect time availability.

We found that one session per week, lasting two hours, provided the optimum opportunity for learning without significant disruption to the caregivers' routines. Interestingly, caregivers of mild to moderately impaired elders who could leave them alone while attending the class favored afternoon sessions (1–3 PM), while those who required someone to stay with their impaired family member preferred the evening (6–8 PM). Of the three groups that were held, one occurred in the spring and two in the fall. Caregivers were not interested in a summer program and we did not offer a winter session because of the risk of snow and potential driving hazards.

Two locations in which to hold the classes were carefully chosen. Both sites were long-term care facilities that offered accessible public transportation, parking, and a central location. The two nursing homes had excellent reputations in the community, welcomed the opportunity to host the program, provided equipment for the teaching demonstrations, and had sufficient space for the group meeting and skill practice. Equipment was borrowed from the University of New Hampshire Department of Nursing as well as from the long-term care facilities.

Participants

Eighteen people, ranging in age from the mid-30s to the mid-80s, with a mean age of 58, enrolled in the program. The typical caregiver was white, female, and married. Half of the caregivers worked, and of those employed, most worked more than 35 hours per week. All the participants were primary caregivers. Approximately 50 percent of caregivers shared their household with the older adult care recipient. All caregivers described their health as good. The majority of participants were related to the care recipient, primarily as spouses, daughters, or nieces.

Although the caregiver group was marketed to informal caregivers, there were some unexpected variations. Two of the women were licensed practical nurses (LPNs). One LPN was caring for her impaired husband while the other helped a 92-year-old confused woman. Both were over 70 themselves and noted that they predated the field of gerontological nursing. Now that they faced caregiving problems they wanted to learn about it.

Three participants were "anticipatory caregivers," a term used by Bowers (1987) to describe family members mentally preparing themselves to assume care responsibility for an aged parent. These three women expected to be the primary caregivers of their respective mothers within two years. Strikingly, these women all had prior experiences with the health care system that were negative. For example, one of the women had cared for her husband at home for one year during his terminal illness. She expressed much anger and frustration over her attempts to communicate caregiving problems to, and receive useful advice from, her husband's physician. Her goal in taking this course was to become better prepared for her mother's potential need for care by learning about available local resources and methods to interact more effectively with health care professionals. The other two women also had performed spousal caregiving in the past. The remaining participants were involved in current caregiving situations.

The Care Recipients

Care recipients were predominately female, with a median age of 86 years (range 50 to 92). Of the recipients, 75 percent were described by their care providers as having poor or fair health. Care recipients averaged four chronic health problems. The most common problems reported were stroke and musculoskeletal disorders. Major problems with IADLs in order of frequency were shopping, housework, meal preparation, and medication management. The most common problems with ADLs were bathing and toileting, with 75 percent needing help with bathing and over one-third experiencing bladder incontinence.

Caregiving Activities

The number of years spent in caregiving ranged from seven months to over ten years. Seventy five percent had been providing care for less than one year. Caregiving tasks ranged from complete physical care to anticipated caregiving with no actual care currently being given. Time spent in caregiving took from one to ten hours per day. Three quarters of the caregivers provided care seven days per week. The following case examples portray the physical demands and diversity of problems faced by some of these caregivers:

Selected Case Examples

Lucia, age 86, had been caring for her husband since his massive stroke ten years ago. She was solely responsible for his complete physical care and lacked any assistance from the home care system because his needs were considered routine "unskilled" care. Her husband depended on her to wash and lift him out of bed every morning, dress, feed, and give him his pills. He also had a problem with urinary incontinence. When asked about caregiver burden, Lucia disliked the concept; she viewed marriage as a responsibility to each other regardless of physical problems. Lucia did admit that they both had deteriorated during the last ten years. She came to the program specifically to learn how to become more efficient in her caregiving skills so that she would not become so exhausted. "It takes me all day to give him a bed bath and change the linen; I get winded and have to take some breaks. I remember seeing how fast the nurses changed the bed when he was in the hospital and wondered if I could learn how they did it," she said. Lucia did learn how to minimize her physical exertion not only for her husband's hygiene needs, but also to reduce her risk of a back injury.

Harry was in his mid-70s and cared for his dependent wife, a victim of parkinsonism for 12 years, a stroke two years ago, and now dementia. Similar to Lucia, he performed all of the household chores as well as attending to the personal care needs of his wife. As her mobility deteriorated, she fell on the average of once per week. Two months prior to the program, one of the falls resulted in a fractured arm. Harry was interested in learning about safe lifting and moving techniques as well as how to take his wife's blood pressure. Her medication regimen was complex and often caused the blood pressure to rapidly drop. In the past, she would tell him if she felt faint but now she was not reliable because of her confusion. Harry become quite proficient in his use of a transfer gait belt and sphygmomanometer.

Ellen, every day before work, traveled eight miles to administer insulin to her 85-year-old diabetic aunt. If she could not coordinate lunchtime coverage, Ellen spent her lunch hour with the aunt. She reported that her aunt had numerous insulin reactions and Ellen was worried that she might not be able to reach her in time during a snowstorm. Furthermore, Ellen's niece, a registered nurse in another state, had raised doubts about the appropriateness of the insulin injections. The aunt had methodically followed a diabetic diet for the last 15 years without any problems. During her hospitalization for a fall three months ago, she was started on insulin injections and discharged home on this therapy. Ellen specifically wanted to know if the insulin therapy should be questioned. The nurse validated the need to discuss her aunt's therapy. Ellen was initially rebuked by the physician for doubting his treatment. Ellen, however, received strong group support to continue to question the therapy. The nurse provided a journal article by a geriatrician on the subject matter to share with the physician as well as the name of a consultant for the physician and/or family to use for a second opinion. In addition, the session about finding good medical care and consumer rights reinforced the appropriateness of her action. Shortly thereafter, the physician changed the aunt's diabetic treatment back to diet control, thus eliminating the insulin reactions and Ellen's travel concerns and also restoring the aunt's confidence in her ability to live alone.

EVALUATION

The program was evaluated using several approaches in order to determine the appropriateness of the curriculum as well as the effects of the program on the participants. The curriculum content was evaluated during the program with a formative evaluation, and a summative evaluation was conducted upon completion of the program. Participants anonymously evaluated the course to ensure confidentiality and to promote honest criticisms. In addition, telephone interviews were conducted with all of the participants before they attended the first training meeting, and then again three and six months after completing the program. The telephone interviews were conducted by a research assistant who was purposely kept unfamiliar with the program in order to prevent any bias. Participants were informed that their interviews were confidential and would not be shared with the nurse-facilitator.

Curriculum Evaluation

During the first training program, the participants evaluated each session immediately after it was held. Since the program was being implemented for the first time, it was important to quickly detect any program weakness in order to have time for remediation. Participants, however, identified that the only problem was the evaluation process. They felt that the evaluation disrupted the social interaction and camaraderie that occurred at the end of the session. Consequently, the second and third groups evaluated the program only at the midpoint and after the last session.

The following are two examples of the comments received on the course evaluations:

> *Not only did I learn what I was hoping to but also I learned about aging in general; what to do to take care of myself to age better.*
>
> *So organized, every minute seemed valuable yet without pressure. I was comfortable asking all my questions and confident they would be answered.*

The nurse-facilitator kept a log of the program sessions including the type of problems identified, common questions asked, and reactions to suggestions. Several participants used the personal health record that was introduced in the first session. They shared their experiences with the group. Each had completed the care recipient's health history, including over-the-counter medications and insurance information as instructed. Two accompanied their older relatives on a medical visit and the other to the dentist. They each showed the record to the health providers and received help in updating the information. The dentist reinforced the nurse's message that many older people are not aware of the importance of informing their dentists about their medical problems and medications. When asked about their medical conditions by their dentists, many cannot recall their medications or diagnoses. Thus, the value of having a written information sheet was reinforced not only to those who were using it but to the rest of the group as well. Two other group members obtained durable medical equipment that was suggested. One member purchased a blood pressure set and brought it in to have the nurse ensure that he was using it appropriately. Participants also responded to referral recommendations and acted upon information received in the program. Two older care recipients were enrolled in an adult day care program part-time. Another group member obtained the services of a podiatrist who confirmed the nurse's assessment that her mother's foot problem was treatable. One of the anticipatory caregivers, who had to miss two sessions, not only requested the handouts but asked when the topics she missed would be covered in the next group (six months later); she made the sessions up the next time around.

Another participant brought in a complimentary letter to the editor from one of the local town papers that was written (unknown to us) by one of our former participants. The letter attested to the value of the program and encouraged anyone caring for an older relative to attend.

Eight months after the program was over, one of the participants, Lucia, called the nurse at home. She explained she was having difficulty finding one of the items demonstrated in the course: a sponge toothette for cleaning the mouth. When her husband started having bleeding gums, she had used the samples distributed by the nurse and found them to be effective. She was unable to find more at the local pharmacy, however. The nurse helped her locate a pharmacy where she could get more. This was an excellent example of how knowledge learned during the program came to be useful at a much later point in time. This anecdote raises the question of the timing of the evaluations. It is not unusual for short-term benefits to be attenuated over time (Montgomery & Borgatta, 1989). In the situation of Lucia, however, benefits of the program occurred long after the evaluation process was completed.

Caregiver Evaluation

The original evaluation design included a quantitative analysis of pre- and post-course scores using several standardized measures of self-esteem, caregiver stress, and burden. Given the rural location of the program, it was difficult to market and attract a participant pool large enough for a control group and inferential statistical analysis. Thus, a descriptive evaluation was conducted. Data obtained through questionnaires and telephone interviews were subjected to descriptive analysis.

All participants responded positively to the program. They strongly agreed to the statement asking if they would recommend this program to others in caregiving situations. Respondents ranked all topic areas as very useful with the subjects of how to take blood pressure, choose a physician, take medications safely, and provide good skin care listed as most useful. Only one suggestion was received for an additional topic area and that was to consider including an option for CPR classes. That recommendation may reflect the difficulty in some rural areas to gain access to CPR courses rather than the particular need to include it in a caregiving course. Several participants recommended that more time be spent on actual hands-on experiences. Others suggested that the length of the program be expanded.

The two major reasons participants attended the group were to learn nursing skills they could use and to learn about the health needs of a relative. When asked to what extent the group met these goals, all respondents indicated that their needs were very much met by the program. Given several options, the majority felt that it was very important that a nurse facilitated the group. All rated the opportunity to discuss issues with a nurse as a very important dimension of the group. Specifically not rated as important was the opportunity to talk with others about their experience, meet people in the same situation, or spend time with others. Participants clearly perceived this as a practical task-oriented group. Several were already attending support groups. When asked why they came to the caregiver training program, they indicated it was because they thought they would receive a different kind of information.

Reflections on the Program

A major barrier to doing an effective evaluation of the caregiving group was the small number of participants. Although many more caregivers expressed interest than the 18 who attended, they encountered difficulties we could not overcome. Transportation and accessibility are common themes in the rural health care literature and they influenced this program too. Older caregivers could not drive at night; others did not drive at all. Public transportation was limited and slow. Another barrier was the lack of someone to stay with the impaired care recipient while the caregiver attended sessions. This was the most frustrating barrier for caregivers. They wanted to attend the group but couldn't because they could not leave their older relative. How could they learn how to be a better caregiver when they couldn't get away? When offering this type of program in nonmetropolitan areas, it may be necessary to find ways to provide transportation and relief sitters before caregivers can take advantage of group interventions.

One of the most difficult tasks in providing services to rural older adults and their families is getting information to them about services available and in case finding, that is, identifying those who might best benefit from services (Young, Goughler, & Larson, 1986). Volunteer organizations may be effective mechanisms for informing older adults and their families about the availability of different types of programs. Although we contacted several home care and social service organizations, we did not contact volunteer programs. An organization that may be very effective in helping to promote health care programs in rural areas is the Cooperative Extension Agency. According to Van Hook (1987),

> *Ignorance of available services is viewed as the major barrier to service utilization in all areas, but the physical isolation and the historic unavailability of services may make lack of knowledge more of a detriment to program utilization in rural communities [p. 4].*

Health providers offering programs in rural areas must be innovative in developing marketing strategies that will reach and inform family caregivers.

Health care colleagues may need to be informed about the program and its assumptions so that they can be supportive. For example, a colleague reacted strongly when she heard that participants were taught how to take a blood pressure. She questioned why we would place so much emphasis on taking a blood pressure. Didn't we know that taking a blood pressure reveals little about the health of the individual? We had to explain that the goal of teaching blood pressure monitoring was to demonstrate to participants our commitment to sharing information. The willingness of the nurse to share the "mystery" of the blood pressure created a feeling of collaboration that might not have been achieved as effectively in any other way. We can only make the analogy to sexuality education with adolescents: the nurse was willing to "tell it like it is" and to "really share with them what they wanted to know." It demystified the meaning associated with the words "blood pressure" as well as providing an opportunity to clarify common misconceptions. It was the first time most of our participants had ever used a stethoscope or heard a pulse. They were genuinely excited about learning this skill and were very proud of their ability to do so.

Practice Implications for Rural Nursing

An interesting finding was that the majority of participants had been providing care for less than one year. Montgomery and

Borgatta (1989) noted that most caregivers seek help late in their caregiving responsibilities only after the strains and demands of caregiving become onerous. It may be that caregivers do not attend support groups until they experience the need for social-emotional support (Montgomery & Borgatta, 1989; Gallagher et al., 1989; Haley, 1989). The opportunity to attend a task-oriented program that "trains" them may have more appeal or legitimacy early in the caregiving process. If so, this kind of group may actually be able to postpone caregiver strain and lessen feelings of stress. Thus, caregiver training groups could be used as a mechanism of prevention as well as intervention.

Lack of access to health and social services in rural areas has been well documented. Moreover, case management for the frail elderly and their families has been recognized as a key method for negotiating the complexity of our health care system and ensuring appropriate coordinated service delivery. It is more difficult, however, to recruit and retain case management staff in rural areas than it is in urban ones. As Parker et al. (1990) state:

> *Case management in rural areas is difficult due to highly independent clients, limited services, and inadequate staffing. Yet paradoxically, these very difficulties make case management even more essential in rural areas [p. 108].*

Family members are intimately aware of the care recipients' preferences and provide a source of continuity amid professional staff shortages and turnover. Empowering family caregivers with information and the skills to negotiate the health care system establishes a strong foundation for managing care over a long period of time. Many caregivers have to retain primary responsibility for making decisions about chronic health management.

With the emphasis on family caregiving in the popular press, many families are concerned about future demands that may be placed on them to provide care for older family members. Men and women have delayed occupational advancement and relocation because of anticipated caregiving demands or current ones. The Family Caregiving Training Program may be an effective mechanism for preparing anticipatory caregivers. It has the potential for preparing adult children to move into the caregiving role. The program may help to raise issues that need to be considered in planning for a future role of caregiver.

Elder neglect has been linked with excessive demands on the caregiver, social isolation, and lack of knowledge of caregiving responsibilities. Preparing spouses and other family members for this role through anticipatory or current caregiver training may be an effective mechanism for preventing what Fulmer and O'Malley (1987) call "inadequate care of the elderly."

Hospitals and home health care agencies are appropriate organizations to sponsor family caregiver training programs. Offering a training program can provide links with the community, enhance the discharge planning process, facilitate transition to community-based care, and even serve as an income-producing program for the agency.

Research Implications

Only recently has the important role of informal caregivers been recognized. Providing adequate support groups for these caregivers is still an emerging development (Worcester, 1990). The training and support group described in this chapter was perceived by participants as very useful in helping them carry out their caregiving role. The number of participants and the rural setting, however, limit the program's generalizability. As mentioned in the caregiving literature, researchers on self-help groups have encountered methodological problems because of limited representativeness, lack of analysis of the care recipient's perspective, and omission of the total support network (Barer & Johnson, 1990). Future research focusing on these issues is needed.

This program, however, has avoided some of the weaknesses Clark (1983) identified as being commonly associated with support programs by specifying the philosophy and educational objectives of the program, documenting the process used in the group, establishing and testing a reproducible curriculum, and systematically collecting evaluation data. Moreover, we would like to foster replication and further analysis of this program by offering our manual and advice to others interested in caregiver training.[1] Only through continued development and evaluation of training courses for caregivers will we develop programs that will be effective in helping families meet the challenges associated with the care of their frail older members.

REFERENCES

AACN (American Association of Colleges of Nursing) (1989, September). *Issue bulletin: Nursing rural America to health.*

Archbold, P. (1980). Impact of parent caring on middle aged offspring. *Journal of Gerontological Nursing, 6*(2), 78–85.

Auerbach, A. (1976). The elderly in rural areas: Differences in urban areas and implications for practice. In L. Ginsberg (Ed.), *Social work in rural communities* (pp. 98–107). New York: Council on Social Work Education.

Baines, E. (1984). Caregiver stress in the older adult. *Journal of Community Health Nursing, 1,* 257–263.

Barer, B., & Johnson, C. (1990). A critique of the caregiving literature. *The Gerontologist, 20,* 26–29.

Barusch, A. S. (1988). Problems and copying strategies of elderly spouse caregivers. *Gerontologist, 28,* 677–685.

Bohland, J. R., & Rowles, G. D. (1988). The significance of elderly migration to changes in elderly population concentration in the United States: 1960–1980. *Journal of Gerontology, 43,* 145–152.

Bowers, B. (1987). Intergenerational caregiving: Adult caregivers and their aging parents. *Advances in Nursing Science, 9*(2), 20–31.

Bremer, A. (1989). A description of community health nursing practice with the community-based elderly. *Journal of Community Health Nursing, 6*(3), 173–184.

---

[1]For information on the Family Caregiving Training Program or to order the *Training Family Caregivers: A Manual for Group Leaders,* contact Raelene Shippee-Ricc at the University of New Hampshire Department of Nursing, Durham, New Hampshire 03825.

Brody, E. M. (1979). Aging parents and aging children. In P. K. Ragan (Ed.), *Aging parents* (267–287). Los Angeles, CA: University of Southern California Press.

Brody, E. M. (1985). Parent care as a normative family stress. The Donald P. Kent Memorial Lecture. *The Gerontologist, 25,* 19–29.

Brody, E. M. (1990). *Women in the middle: Their parent-care years.* New York: Springer Publishing Company.

Brody, S. J., Poulshock, S. W., & Masciocchi, C. F. (1978). Family caring unit: A major consideration in long-term care. *The Gerontologist, 18,* 556–562.

Brown, S. E., & Kelly, P. A. (1987). Responding to a community need: Preparation for parenthood for prospective adoptive couples. *Family and Community Health, 9*(4), 77–81.

Cantor, M. (1980). Caring for the frail elderly: Impact on family, friends and neighbors. Presented at 33rd Annual Meeting of the Gerontological Society of America, San Diego, CA.

Cantor, M. (1983). Strain among caregivers: A study of experience in the United States. *The Gerontologist, 23,* 597–604.

Clark, N., & Rakowski, W. (1983). Family caregivers of older adults: Improving helping skills. *The Gerontologist, 23,* 637–642.

Cutler, S. J., & Coward, R. T. (1988). Residence differences in the health status of elders. *Journal of Rural Health, 4*(3), 11–26.

Dennis, M. E. (1990). The older dyadic family unit and chronic illness. *Home Health Care Nurse, 8*(2), 42–48.

Drinka, T. J., Smith, J., & Drinka, P. J. (1987). Correlates of burden and depression for informal caregivers of patients in a geriatric referral clinic. *Journal of the American Geriatrics Society, 35,* 522–525.

Ermann, D. A. (1990). Rural health care: The hospital. *Medical Care Review, 47,* 33–73.

Fengler, A. P., & Goodrich, N. (1979). Wives of elderly disabled men: The hidden patients. *The Gerontologist, 19,* 175–183.

Fenton, M. V., Rounds, L., & Iha, S. (1988). Nursing center in a rural community: The promotion of family and community health. *Family and Community Health, 11*(2), 14–24.

Fickenscher, K. (1990, March). Research on primary care and rural health: Opportunities and challenges. *AHCPR Conference Pro-*

ceedings Primary Care Research: An agenda for the 90s. U.S. Department of Health and Human Services.

Fischer, L., & Eustis, N. (1988). DRGs and family care for the elderly: A case study. *The Gerontologist, 28,* 383–389.

Frankfather, D., Smith, M. J., & Caro, F. G. (1981). *Family care of the elderly. Public initiatives and private obligations.* Lexington, MA: Lexington Books.

Fulmer, T., & O'Malley, T. (1987). *Inadequate care of the elderly.* New York: Springer Publishing Company.

Gallagher, D. et al. (1989). Prevalence of depression in family caregivers. *The Gerontologist, 29,* 449–456.

George, L. K. (1990). Caregiver stress studies—There really is more to learn. *The Gerontologist, 30,* 580–581.

George, L. K., & Gwyther, L. (1986). Caregiver well being: A multidimensional examination of family caregivers of demented adults. *The Gerontologist, 26,* 253–259.

Giele, J. (1982). Family and social networks. In R. H. Binstock, Wing-Sun Chow, & J. H. Schulz (Eds.), *International perspectives on aging: Population and policy challenges.* New York: United Nations Fund for Population Activities.

Gombeski, W. R., & Smolensky, M. H. (1980). *Non-emergency health transportation needs of the rural Texas elderly. The Gerontologist, 20,* 452–456.

Greene, V., & Monahan, D. (1989). The effect of a support and education program on stress and burden among family caregivers to frail elderly persons. *The Gerontologist, 29,* 472–477.

Gubrium, J. F. (1988). Family responsibility and caregiving in the qualitative analysis of the Alzheimer's disease experience. *Journal of Marriage and the Family, 50,* 197–207.

Haley, W. (1989). Group intervention for dementia family caregivers: A longitudinal perspective. *The Gerontologist, 29,* 478–480.

Hasselkus, B. R. (1988). Meaning in family caregiving: Perspectives on caregiver/professional relationships. *Gerontologist, 28,* 686–691.

Hassinger, E. (1982). *Rural health organization.* Ames, IA: Iowa State University Press.

Hays, A. (1988). Family care: The critical variable in community based long term care. *Home Health Care Nurse, 6*(1), 26–31.

Hayslip, B., Ritter, M. L., Oltman, R., & McDonnell, C. (1980). Home care services and the rural elderly. *The Gerontologist, 20,* 192–199.

Hawranik, P. (1985). Caring for aged parents: Divided allegiances. *Journal of Gerontological Nursing, 11*(10), 19–22.

Hersh, A. S., & Van Hook, R. T. (1989). Summary: A research agenda. *HSR: Health Services Research, 23,* 1053–1065.

Hess, B. B., & Soldo, B. J. (1985). Husband and wife networks. In W. J. Sauer & R. T. Coward (Eds.), *Social support networks and the care of the elderly* (pp. 67–92). New York: Springer Publishing Company.

Hirschfeld, M. (1983). Home care versus institutionalization: Family caregiving and senile brain disease. *International Journal of Nursing Studies, 20*(1), 23–32.

Hogan, S. (1990). Care for the caregiver: Social policies to ease this burden. *Journal of Gerontological Nursing, 16*(5), 12–17.

Horowitz, A. (1985). Sons and daughters as caregivers to older parents. Differences in role performance and consequences. *The Gerontologist, 25,* 612–617.

Johnson, C. L., & Catalano, D. J. (1983). A longitudinal study of family supports to impaired elderly. *The Gerontologist, 23,* 612–618.

Jones, D. A., & Vetter, N. J. (1984). Survey of those who care for the elderly at home: Their problems and their needs. *Social Science and Medicine, 19,* 511–514.

Katz, S., Ford, A., Moskowitz, R., Jackson, B., & Jaffe, M. (1963). The index of ADL: A standardized measure of biological and psychosocial function. *Journal of the American Medical Association, 185,* 94–99.

Klaybor, M. (1988). A son's viewpoint. In J. Norris (Ed.), *Daughters of the elderly.* Indianapolis: Indiana University Press.

Krout, J. A. (1983). Transportation opportunity and the rural elderly: A comparison of objective and subjective indicators. *The Gerontologist, 23,* 505–511.

Lancaster, W. (1988). Marketing home health care to the rural elderly: From strategy to action. *Family and Community Health, 11*(2), 72–80.

Lassiter, P. G. (1985). Rural practice: How do we prepare providers? *Journal of Rural Health, 1*(1), 23–28.

Lawton, M. P., & Brody, E. (1969). Assessment of older people: Self maintaining and instrumental activities of daily living. *The Gerontologist, 9,* 179–186.

Mahoney, D. (1984). The development of an innovative health educational program for the well elderly. *Resources Educator,* ERIC ED 243010.

Mahoney, D., Shippee-Rice, R., & Pillemer, K. (1988). Training family caregivers: A manual for group leaders. Durham, NH: University of New Hampshire.

Marks, R. (1987). Stress in families providing care to frail elderly relatives and the effects of receiving in-home respite services. *Home Healthcare Services Quarterly, 8,* 103–130.

Maynard, J. (1990). Love, loss and the crossroads kitchen. *Metropolitan Home, 22*(10), 102, 104, 170.

Miller, B., McFall, S., & Montgomery, A. (1991). The impact of elder health, caregiver involvement, and global stress on two dimensions of caregiver burden. *Journal of Gerontology, 46,* 9–19.

Montgomery, J. E., Stubbs, A. C., & Day, S. S. (1980). The housing environment of the rural elderly. *The Gerontologist, 20,* 444–451.

Montgomery, R. J. V., & Borgatta, E. F. (1989). The effects of alternative support strategies on family caregiving. *The Gerontologist, 29,* 457–464.

Mossefin, C. (1987, Summer). *The challenge of rural nursing: Focus on rural health* (p. 4). Center for Rural Health Services, Policy and Resources, University of North Dakota.

Mutschler, P. (1985). *Working paper #26: Supporting families in care for the elderly. Volume I: What we know.* Waltham, MA: Brandeis University, The Policy Center on Aging.

Nelson, G. (1980). Social services to the urban and rural aged: The experience of area agencies on aging. *The Gerontologist, 20,* 200–207.

Norris, V. K., Stephens, M. A., & Kinney, J. M. (1990). The impact of family interactions on recovery from stroke: Help or hindrance? *The Gerontologist, 30,* 535–542.

Oleski, D. M., Otte, D. M., & Heize, S. (1987). Development and evaluation of a system for monitoring the quality of oncology nursing care in the home setting. *Cancer nursing, 104*(4), 190–198.

Parker, M., Quinn, J., Viehl, M., McKinley, A., Polich, C., Ditzner, D. F., Hartwell, S., & Korn, K. (1990). Case management in rural areas:

Definition, clients, financing, staffing and service delivery issues. *Nursing Economics 8*(2), 103–109.

Patton, L. (1989). Setting the rural health services research agenda: The Congressional perspective. *HSR: Health Services Research, 23,* 1005–1050.

Pearlin, L. I., Mullan, J. T., Semple, S. J., & Skaff, M. M. (1990). Caregiving and the stress process: An overview of concepts and their measures. *The Gerontologist, 30,* 583–594.

Phillips, L. R. (1989). Elder—family caregiver relationships. *Nursing Clinics North America, 24*(3), 795–807.

Phillips, L. R., & Rempusheski, V. F. (1986). Caring for the frail elderly at home: Toward a theoretical explanation of the dynamics of poor quality family caregiving. *Advances in Nursing Science, 8*(4), 62–84.

Poulshock, S., & Deimling, D. (1984). Families caring for elders in residence: Issues in the measurement of burden. *The Journal of Gerontology, 39,* 230–239.

Rabins, P., Mace, N., & Lucas, M. (1982). The impact of dementia on the family. *Journal of the American Medical Association, 248,* 333–335.

Rew, L., Fields, S., LeVee, L. C., Russell, M. C., & Leake, P. Y. (1987). AFFIRM: A nursing model to promote role mastery in family caregivers. *Family and Community Health, 9*(4), 52–64.

Rivlin, A. M., & Wiener, J. M. (1988). *Caring for the disabled elderly: Who will pay?,* Washington, D.C.: The Brookings Institution.

Schirm, V. (1989). Functionally impaired elderly: Their need for home nursing care. *Journal of Community Health Nursing, 6*(4), 199–207.

Scott, J. P., & Roberto, K. A. (1985). Use of informal and formal support networks by rural elderly poor. *The Gerontologist, 25,* 624–630.

Secretary's Commission on Nursing. (1988). Final report, 1. Washington, D.C.: Department of Health and Human Services.

Shanas, E. (1979). Social myth as hypothesis: The case of the family relations of old people. *The Gerontologist, 19,* 3–9.

Shanas, E., Townsend, P., Wedderbarn, D., Henning, F., Milhoj, P., & Stehouwer, J. (1968). *Old people in three industrial societies.* New York: Atherton Press.

Shaughnessy, P. W., & Kramer, A. M. (1990). The increased needs of patients in nursing homes and patients receiving home health care. *New England Journal of Medicine, 322,* 21–27.

Stafford, P. (1988). Caregiving and men's issues. In J. Norris (Ed.), *Daughters of the elderly* (pp. 179–184). Indianapolis: Indiana University Press.

Stoller, E. P. (1990). Males as helpers: The role of sons, relatives, and friends. *The Gerontologist, 30,* 228–235.

Stoller, E. P., & Earl, L. L. (1983). Help with activities of everyday life: Sources of support for the noninstitutionalized elderly. *The Gerontologist, 23,* 64–70.

Stone, R., Cafferata, G. L., & Sangl, J. (1987). Caregivers of the frail elderly: A natural profile. *The Gerontologist, 27,* 616–626.

Stone, R. I., & Kemper, P. (1989). Spouses and children of disabled elders: How large a constituency for long-term care reform? *The Milbank Quarterly, 67,* 485–506.

Stone, R., & Murtaugh, C. M. (1990). The elderly population with chronic functional disability: Implications for home care eligibility. *Gerontologist, 30,* 491–496.

Talbot, D. (1985). Assessing needs of the rural elderly. *Journal of Gerontological Nursing, 11,* (3), 39–43.

Thobaden, M., & Weingard, M. (1983). Rural nursing. *Home Health-care Nurse, 4,* 9–13.

Toseland, R. W., & Rossiter, C. M. (1989). Group interventions to support family caregivers: A review and analysis. *The Gerontologist, 29,* 438–448.

Troll, L. E. (1988). New thoughts on old families. *The Gerontologist, 28,* 586–591.

Van Hook, R. (1987, June 4). The crisis in rural health for the elderly. Statement before the U.S. House of Representatives Select Committee on Aging from the National Rural Health Associaton.

Weeks, J. R., & Cuellar, J. B. (1981). The role of family members in the helping networks of older people. *The Gerontologist, 21,* 388–394.

Worcester, M. I. (1990). Family coping: Caring for the elderly in home care. *Home Health Care Services Quarterly, 11,* 121–168.

Worcester, M. I., & Quayhagen, M P. (1983). Correlates of caregiver satisfaction: Prerequisites to elder home care. *Research in Nursing and Health, 6,* 61–67.

Young, C. L., Goughler, D. H., & Larson, P. J. (1986). Organizational volunteers for the rural frail elderly: Outreach, case finding, and service delivery. *The Gerontologist, 26,* 342–344.

Zarit, S. H., Reever, K. E., & Bach-Peterson, J. (1980). Relatives of the impaired aged: Correlates of feelings of burden. *The Gerontologist, 20,* 649–655.

Zola, I. (1990). Aging, disability and the home care revolution. *Archives of Physical Medicine and Rehabilitation, 71,* 93–96.

Agenda Setting Tool

Instructions:
1. In the left hand column please rank order the ten items you feel the most need for, or interest in. Place a 10 next to the subject of most interest, followed by a 9 for the next area of interest, 8 for the next and so on to a 1 for the item of least interest.
2. Place a check under the facts section which best describes your knowledge or information in each of the ten topics you ranked.
3. Place a check under the feelings section which best describes your feelings about each of the ten topics you ranked.

Rank	Facts			Feeling				
Interest Topic or Need	Have enough knowledge	Need more information	Would have no difficulty	Embarrassment	Fear	Would like to do but insecure	No intentions to do	Other (explain on back)
Taking a blood pressure and pulse								
Establishing a health diary								
Determining normal aging from illness								
Asking health professionals for information or asking questions								
Health care aids and appliances								
Lifting and moving dependent elders								
Resource information and referrals								
Disease management and information								
Modifying diets								
Feeding problems								
Pain management								
Confusion								
Bowel problems								
Sleeplessness								
Urinary incontinence								
Organizing caregiving								
Reducing caregiver strain								
Bed baths								
Changing an occupied bed								
Administering medications								
Catheter care								
Enemas								
Toileting								

6

Family Theory for Rural Research and Practice

Patricia Winstead-Fry

It is time for nurse scholars of family theory to provide some direction in the evolution of family theory. Kleinman (1986) documents the differences between biomedicine and social science that leave each unenriched by the other, even though the two disciplines overlap in important areas. He also makes the point that schools of nursing have been the most successful in integrating social science into health-oriented curricula. Most professional nurses have been exposed to McCubbin in undergraduate or graduate sociology classes and to Bowen in a family or psychiatric nursing course. Nursing is one of the few disciplines that provides the background to explore similarities and differences between ideas developed in the fields of biomedicine and social science.

The purpose of this chapter is to introduce the reader to a theory of family functioning that is appropriate for research and practice with rural families. The theory is a synthesis of Bowen's Family Systems Theory and McCubbin and colleagues' T-Double ABC-X Model of Family Functioning. A brief overview of both theories and an argument for synthesizing the theories for rural family research and practice will be presented in this chapter. The process used to synthesize the theories will also be presented, followed by a discussion of the synthesized theory. Finally, ideas about practice and research with the synthesized theory will be discussed.

OVERVIEW OF THEORIES

Figure 6–1 presents the genogram of the Lay family (Miller & Winstead-Fry, 1982, p. 107). According to Bowen's theory, one constructs a genogram to trace the multigenerational transmission of a dysfunctional process. Families evolve over time with a level of differentiation of self that is part of their biological makeup. The level of differentiation of self may be high or low. People with higher levels are goal directed, can manage life's stresses, can balance the emotional system and the intellectual system, and generally have fewer physical or emotional illnesses (Bowen, 1978; Kerr & Bowen, 1988).

When a family with a lower level of differentiation of self becomes anxious, there is an activation of behavior. If the anxiety persists, dysfunction in emotional life or social life occurs. For example in the Lay family, Dan is a problem child who currently keeps his parents up all night because he will not sleep.

A therapist following Bowen's ideas would use the genogram to trace the pattern of family conflicts that has led to the development of this symptom in the child. A triangle between the parents and the child would be the operating hypothesis. (A triangle is an automatic emotional reaction in which the parents ignore a conflict in their relationship by focusing on a problem in their child.) If one were to follow the emotional processes through the generations to the current nuclear family emotional process, one would find that the Lays were chronically anxious at the time of Dan's birth. Intervention would focus on decreasing the triangling between Dan and his parents by decreasing the triangles that exist within each of the parents' families of origin. By discussing family history and working with the parents to mend the emotional cutoff from their parents, the disruptive behavior caused by the triangle within the present generation (Dan and his parents) would decrease.

Figure 6-1
Family Genogram

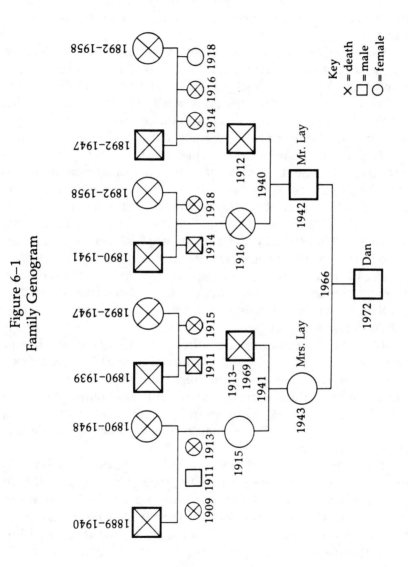

Key
x = death
□ = male
○ = female

Within Bowen's framework, the fact that both parents are only children (Figure 6–1) would be important because sibling position is expected to affect behavior. In this theory, family history and present symptoms are assumed to be related. The goals of therapy are not only symptom reduction, but also improved intergenerational relationships.

Since the introduction of the ABCX model in 1949 by Reuben Hill, it has undergone many modifications. For this paper the T-Double ABC-X version will be used (McCubbin & McCubbin, 1989). According to this theory, a family is coping and moving through a life-cycle stage, when a stressor occurs (A). The family is vulnerable to the event to the extent that it taxes their resources (B). The stressor may be any event that the family perceives as disruptive (C). The interaction of A, B, and C determine if there is a crisis (X). In the T-Double ABC-X model, other variables are introduced that make the adjustment to the stressor more or less problematic. If there is a pile-up of stressors (aA), the family may have more difficulty with the current stressor. The coping strategies that the family has learned and the social and psychological resources it can muster to manage the crisis are considered (bB). The meaning the family gives the stressor is also important (cC) in how they react to it. There is more latitude for outcomes other than dysfunction in this theory.

If the family resources are sufficient, the family will handle the stressor and move on. Such resources as intelligence, money, and social support are thought to buffer the impact of the stressor or to aid in resolving the stressor. In the appraisal phase, the family uses all of its skills and resources to figure out how to manage the stressor. The family will take some action. That action may lead to resolution of the event.

If the family appraisal of the situation is wrong, or the family is weak when the stressor occurs (because of pile-up), or the demand for change is beyond the imagination of the family members, adaptation to the event will occur. The family's basic resiliency, schema, problem-solving skills, coping skills, and the availability of social support will interact to produce an adaptation in the family which will allow it to go on functioning.

RATIONALE FOR THEORY SYNTHESIS

The rationale for synthesizing theories that developed in two different areas of scholarship will now be discussed. Bowen's theory is a psychiatric, medical model approach to family dysfunction. The basis of McCubbin's theory is the T-Double ABC-X Model which was introduced to sociology by Reuben Hill as the ABCX Model (1949). It has been researched and modified by numerous scholars of family life.

The Theory Construction and Research Methodology Workshop of the National Council on Family Relations is working to produce the *Sourcebook of Family Theories and Methods: A Contextual Approach* which will allow comparisons across models of family theory. One of the outcomes of this endeavor is a sense that family life scholars need to develop grander theories. As the work progresses, it is becoming increasingly clear that there are many overlapping concepts in the research literature. Some of these concepts are better defined and more measurable than others. It seems worthwhile to focus on building and testing the theories with the strongest concepts.

Bowen's ideas about differentiation of self and multigenerational transmission process are extremely difficult to measure quantitatively. McCubbin's model has numerous scales to measure aspects of the family life. To the extent that there is overlap between the two theories, some of Bowen's more difficult concepts may be measurable with scales developed within the T-Double ABC-X model. Such a synthesis would lead to a grander theory that is measurable.

Aside from arguments that grander theories are needed for family research and that nurses have a unique knowledge base from which to view family theory, there is a rationale based upon the characteristics of rural people that suggests a synthesis of Bowen and McCubbin may be profitable. One of the most compelling clinical situations this author has experienced was developing a genogram of a rural, farm family. As we began constructing the genogram, four generations of the family were in the room, contributing to the process. This was a totally different experience from practice in New York City. In the urban environment, clients are often unsure of their grandparents' names, number of siblings in that generation, and so forth. Typically, the client has to call a parent to get generational information that may be sketchy at best if there have been divorces or high mobility. Usually, there is a family "historian" who can provide the information needed to complete a three to four generational genogram of the family.

Developing the rural family's genogram was totally different. Transgenerational issues were immediately apparent as great-grandmother and grandmother shared perspectives about closeness and distance in the family. Generally, all generations had a good understanding of who family members are and which are close or distant to each other. Triangles and multigenerational processes could be seen during the development of the genogram.

Rosenblatt and Anderson (1981) and the U.S. Congress, Office of Technology Assessment (1990) cite data which show that rural couples are more likely to stay married than their urban counterparts. For purposes of this paper, a question needs to be raised about why these couples stay together. Is it a manifestation of fusion and lack of differentiation suggested by Bowen? Is it a reflection of the fact that farm life requires mutual dependence? Has the farm crisis of the 1980s caused families to come together for mutual support in order to survive financially, regardless of their emotional situations? The answers to these questions can best be pursued by a theoretical model that values stress and differentiation equally.

The final reason for suggesting the need for synthesis of the Bowen and McCubbin theories has to do with the characteristics of rural people. Before discussing these characteristics, it is necessary to clarify some definitions. A rural community is generally defined as one which has fewer than 2,500 residents. Rural does not mean farm. Of the total population of the United States, 5 percent live in rural communities, but only 2 percent live on farms (U.S. Congress, Office of Technology Assessment, 1990). Generally, rural communities are poorer, have more aged persons, and have fewer health and other services than their metropolitan counterparts. The trend of the 1970s for people to migrate to rural areas was reversed during the 1980s (Luloff, 1990).

While rural people are as diverse as any other group, over the years certain characteristics have been identified that are unique to them and to persons who move into rural areas. Ploch (1981) identified three groups of urban-to-rural immigrants. They are the "back-to-the-land social isolates," the "rural pragmatists," and the "middle aged and other urbanites turned rural romanticists" (p. 41). Regardless of which group the new rural person fits into, all accept rural values, at least as they perceive or romanticize them. So the characteristics of rural persons apply, with variability, to all of the people living in rural communities.

Rural persons are described as being more self-reliant and not easily accepting of help from others, especially from professionals of a higher status. These characteristics create an interesting dilemma for nurses. Often the first person called upon in an illness is the local nurse. Because there is a rural tradition of woman as healer, however, the nurse is not perceived as a valuable professional, but as a woman with special knowledge. The nurse is, therefore, expected to respond quickly and not to charge a fee for her services.

Long and Weinert (1987) and Shannon (1989) demonstrated that the definition of health for rural persons is very pragmatic. While their data was collected in Montana and Oklahoma, the conclusion that rural persons define health as being able to work and to get done what needs to be done rings true more universally. Commenting upon this definition, Bushy (1990) suggests that such a pragmatic orientation may influence patterns of health care utilization in that symptoms that do not decrease activity are ignored until serious illness requires care. She also points out that generally questions about mental health are ignored when rural persons are asked about health needs and services. Whether rural persons experience more mental illness is debated in the literature (Wagenfield, 1990).

One of the outcomes of living in a community of fewer than 2,500 persons is that everyone knows everyone else. This can be a source of strength. When knowing everyone combines with self-reliance and reluctance to accept help, however, the result can be underservice. It is likely that the health care providers' view that there is a large amount of depression, alcoholism, violence, and other ills that go untreated in rural society is related to the reluctance of rural persons to have someone they know help them.

The reluctance to seek help and the value on self-reliance are critical to the argument for synthesizing the theories of Bowen and McCubbin and McCubbin. Rural persons want to get a job done in a self-reliant manner. They are not likely to be interested in long-term therapy or in dependence on a therapist. Also, rural residents are frequently underinsured or uninsured; so they cannot afford much psychotherapy. The McCubbins' model offers an easily understood stress perspective on life's problems that is compatible with rural life. It is sensitive to economic issues which are at the heart of some of the stress rural persons experience. The McCubbins' model, however, was not developed for purposes of intervention. It is a research tool. Bowen's model, on the other hand is a therapeutic tool, which has the distinct advantage of using the therapist as a "coach" while the family does the work. Together, the two models provide the opportunity for presenting family problems in a stress framework, without placing the client in a dependent role. This approach should meet the needs of rural clients. Urban clients may also benefit from therapists who use the synthesized model. Because of the values that drive rural residents, however, the proposed model is thought to be especially significant for rural families.

PROCESS OF SYNTHESIZING THE THEORIES

The process of theory synthesis used is that described by Newman (1979) and Walker and Avant (1988). The basic process involves reviewing the main concepts of each theory and then diagramming the relationships among them. In order to think through the theories, several versions of the T-Double ABC-X Model were reviewed. While there was concern with some of the sample sizes, data collection procedures, and scales reported in the literature that supports the 1989 version, the theory was accepted as basically valid. A diagram of the T-Double ABC-X Model was first plotted out on a large piece of poster paper, leaving enough room to write around the concepts. Five case examples from family practice were reviewed. The five case examples were selected because there were genograms of the families, the families were good illustrations of Bowen's ideas, and a crisis brought the families into therapy. Using this clinical data, the core concepts of Bowen's theory were blended with the McCubbin and McCubbin model.

In order to generate the synthesized theory, the similarities and differences in the two theories needed to be outlined and studied. Briefly, the important similarities between the theories that emerged from the analysis include the following generalities. Both theories deal with family functioning, one more from the point of view of dysfunction (Bowen) and the other from the view of managing stress (McCubbin & McCubbin). Likewise both are visual theories, Bowen through the genogram and McCubbin and McCubbin through the diagram they present of the T-Double ABC-X Model.

Bowen posits that the intellectional and emotional systems are both important to functioning. Being interested in emotional dysfunction, he is less complete in his discussion of the intellectual system. McCubbin's model specifies the intellectual resources a family has in responding to crises (e.g. family typology and family schema as major factors in stress resolution). McCubbin and McCubbin, on the other hand, are less specific on the role of the emotions in resolving stress within the family, although concepts such as "pile-up" reflect the importance they give to the possibility of feelings becoming overwhelmed. The two theories complement one another in their subjectivity. Bowen's data are gathered while working with families who are experiencing some emotional upset. The McCubbins' and their colleagues' research is by-and-large paper and pencil testing resulting in subjective self-reports.

There are important differences between the theories. The McCubbins do not dwell on sibling position, a key concept for Bowen. However, one cannot help but wonder (given Bowen's data) what role sibling position might play in the McCubbin and McCubbin concepts of family schema and personal resources. The role of anxiety, key for Bowen, is less stressed by McCubbin and McCubbin, although they do refer to "physical and emotional health" as personal resources that affect the ability to respond to stressors (McCubbin & McCubbin, 1987, p. 17).

Another important difference in the two theories is causality. Bowen, reflecting his biomedical background, is deterministic and linear in his causality. In Bowen's perspective, lack of differentiation, in the presence of anxiety, will invariably cause dysfunction in some arena of life. McCubbin and McCubbin, on the other hand, use statistical probability to develop their model. Reliance on statistics creates a less deterministic theory. McCubbin and McCubbin also predict that even overwhelming events do not have to lead to dysfunction if the family has strengths.

Finally, the T-Double ABC-X theory is not a practice model. It is a carefully constructed research-based theory of "normal" family functioning. Bowen's, on the other hand, is totally practice-oriented. It evolved from practice and clinical research with schizophrenic families, and the best "proof" of the theory lies in its utility in practice. Empirical testing of Bowen's ideas is hampered by the lack of measurement tools and by the difficulties of sampling three generations.

In developing the synthesis, the only concepts that were problematical were "triangles" and "strains." Logically, a triangle is part of the current demand status of the family. However, because triangles can be quiescent until stress triggers anxiety, triangling was placed in the family appraisal of the situation portion of the model. The rationale being that quiescent triangles exist in the current status of the family. However, the impact of triangling on how the family appraises the situation is cogent to future family actions designed to deal with the stress.

Strains are defined as ongoing family tensions. After serious consideration, strains were thought to be manifestations of a triangling process, at least some of the time. For purposes of parsimony, the concept is included under the heading of triangles. It may be that there are ongoing family tensions, such as those related to chronic unemployment that are not part of a triangling process. These tensions, however, would be picked up in the tangible resource portion of the model.

Figure 6–2 presents a cleaned up version of the process used to synthesize the ideas. In actuality the large piece of paper used

Figure 6–2

Example of Process Used to Develop Synthesized Theory

CONCEPT: PILE-UP

"Everything happened at once."
"We were overwhelmed."
"Man, we had it!"
"I didn't think I had the strength to get through this."
"Last year's problems were practice for this tragedy."
"Just one thing after another . . . ."

CONCEPT: TRIANGLE

"My great-grandfather ran the show."
"My family has always worried about the youngest son."
"Whenever my mother-in-law cries, the whole family is upset."
"I don't understand why I can't get along with her—we really try."
"It is uncanny how the baby gets sick everytime I go for job interview."
"Our family agrees on everything."
"We aren't a very emotionally close family."

to outline the concepts had numerous erasures. Needless to say, families do not talk in theoretical language. However, they do say things such as, "Everything happened at once—too much," which can be labeled pile-up.

Figure 6–3 depicts the process of family adjustment to a crisis.

In the adjustment phase, the current status of the family consists of the interaction of vulnerability and multigenerational emotional process. These interactions are geometric, not additive. Vulnerability is defined as the interaction among pile-up, life-cycle stage, and ethnicity. Ethnicity is included in this model, even though it is not part of the McCubbin and McCubbin or Bowen theories because the characteristics of black and Asiatic families need to be acknowledged. The multigenerational emotional process includes family type and sibling position. It is the current status of the family that is jarred by a stressor event. The stressor may be anything. Death and divorce are obvious stressors. Lesser events such as holidays or the death of a pet, however, may serve as stressors for some families.

Once the stressor occurs, family appraisal of the situation begins. The appraisal is not an abstract intellectual act, but

Figure 6–3
Family Adjustment Phase of Stress

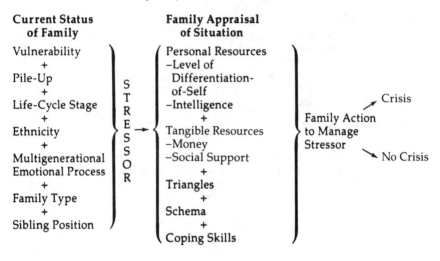

includes responding to the stressor while appraising it. The family appraisal of the situation consists of the interaction of personal resources which are the level of differentiation-of-self and intelligence, tangible resources which are social support and economic support, activation of triangles, family schema, and the coping and/or problem-solving skills that the family possesses. These appraisal parameters will interact to produce some action to manage the stressor.

The family may act by denying the stressor, by attacking the stressor, or by neutralizing the stressor. The only limit to the possible actions is the creativity and experience of the family. The family will do something at this point, whether well conceived or poorly conceived. Sometimes stressors just go away. For example, a lost child calls after several hours to say he is at a relative's house.

A family with sufficient resources, few triangles, a schema of themselves as effective, and a pattern of successful coping may handle a stressor in such a way that it is neutralized. In this event, no crisis occurs and the family returns to a new current demand status. If a family does experience a crisis, it may be resolved or unresolved. If the crisis is resolved, the family also returns to a new current demand status. As a result of dealing with the stressor or resolving the crisis, the family may function better, the same, or worse. Whatever the outcome, the family will go back to the business of living. The results of dealing with the stressor will not be seen until another stressor activates the family.

If the crisis is unresolved and continues, the family will increasingly experience a demand for change. This state of affairs initiates the adaptation phase. Figure 6–4 illustrates this phase. While crises are generally thought of as obstacles that families have to traverse before they move on, crises should not be viewed pejoratively. Some crises are inevitable, such as adolescence and aging. Other crises are actively sought by the family, such as moving to a new home or relocating for a better job. The nature of the crisis event is not as important as the amount of change the crisis requires of the family. During the adaptation phase, all of the components of the current status of the family and of the family appraisal of the situation continue to operate, but the demand for change pushes the family to realize that old ways are not working. The push from the demand for change creates a situation of narrowed focus, wherein the family's energies are mostly engrossed in dealing with the needed change. Within this intense field, the resiliency of the family, any triangles that are operative, the family schema, the coping skills and problem-solving abilities, and any social support interact to ultimately lead to an adaptation in the family. That adaptation will be the new current status of the family. The adaptation may be to the family's betterment. It may also, as Bowen highlights, lead to social, emotional, or physical dysfunction.

RESEARCH RESULTS AND IMPLICATIONS

Haber (1990) developed a scale to measure one aspect of differentiation of self, emotional maturity. Using that scale with some of McCubbin's and his colleagues' tools may demonstrate the interaction between the two theories discussed in this chapter. The Family Adaptation and Coping Evaluation Scales (FACES), now in its third revision, was developed using ideas of family therapists, including Bowen. FACES may be very useful in validating the

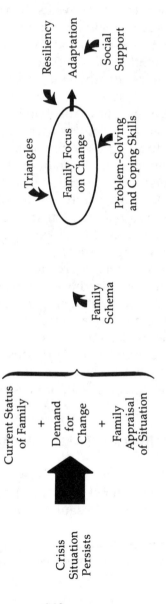

Figure 6–4
Adaptation Phase of Family Crisis

synthesized theory put forth in this book (Olson, Russell, & Sprenkle, 1983; Olson, Sprenkle, & Russell, 1979).

A suggested research study would involve testing the hypothesis that vulnerable families would have the lowest scores on Haber's Level of Differentiation of Self Scale (LDSS), secure and durable families would have middle scores, and regenerative families would have the highest scores. This hypothesis is based upon the observation that vulnerable families who are characterized as less in control, less active on their own behalf, and more self-blaming sound less differentiated to use Bowen's terms. Secure and durable families read as more middle level in differentiation of self. Regenerative families appear to be the most differentiated. They are characterized as planners, who have a sense of control about the good and bad life offers and who also have a sense of purpose.

Richards (1989) did a study of urban couples that has some of the features suggested above. She administered the LDSS, the Locke-Wallace Marital Adjustment Test (MAT), and the FACES III to 60 volunteer, married couples. This study used a canonical correlation method. For purposes of this discussion, the findings relative to the MAT will be ignored. Richards did not find a strong relationship between subscale scores on the LDSS and the FACES III. The relationships were in the predicted directions, except for adaptability which showed a negative relationship to the other subscales, that is, as adaptability scores increased, other subscale scores decreased. It should also be noted that Richards dealt with only cohesion and adaptability. She did not use these subscores to create the vulnerable, secure, durable, and regenerative family types. Given the theory she was testing, there was no need for her to address family type; so this is not a criticism of her work.

In order to explore if the synthesized theory presented in this chapter has heuristic value, rural persons need to be identified. It is important that the research participants identify themselves as rural. This identification is important because much rural research is conducted in the urban areas of rural states. For example, Burlington is the largest city in the rural state of Vermont. Whether residents of Burlington are truly rural persons can be questioned because IBM Corporation and the state university are located there.

From the perspective of testing a theory which purports to be advantageous for rural persons, it seemed imperative that not only census tract data identify participants as rural, but that the persons define themselves as such.

It would seem advantageous to explore concepts such as family support, community support, adjustment, and adaptation at first because they are basic to both theories. Also, there are instruments available to measure these concepts from McCubbin's and others' work. The Relative and Friend Support Index (McCubbin, Larsen, & Olson, 1982) measures family support. Scores from this scale might be compared to Haber's LDSS scale or to genogram data to test the theory presented in this chapter. Community support can be measured by The Social Support Index (McCubbin, Patterson, & Glynn, 1987). Adjustment can be measured by The Family Member Well-Being Index (FWBI) and adaptation by The Family Adaptation Checklist (McCubbin & Patterson, 1987). All of these scales are brief, generally consisting of eight to ten items. They can be compared with genogram material and other interview data.

The T-Double ABC-X model has been used in rural states, but the rural data has not been compared with the urban data. It is likely that the scales would need some re-working of norms and reliabilities to be useful in assessing rural families. To test that hunch, a small pilot study was carried out in Vermont. The participants were 25 men and women (19 women and 6 men) who lived in a rural area and who identified themselves as rural persons. For the pilot study, the Family Adaptation and Cohesion Evaluation Scale III (FACES III) was selected. The author selected this scale because of familiarity with it from previous studies. The sample ranged in age from 26 to 58 years. Protection guidelines for human subjects were followed.

Scores in the pilot study for cohesion ranged from 23 to 46, with a mean of 36.84, and a standard deviation of 6.4. For adaptation, scores ranged from 12 to 34, with a mean of 24.60, and a standard deviation of 6.5.

Olson, Portner, and Lavee (1985) report that the mean on cohesion for a comparable sample ($n = 2453$) was 39.8 with a standard deviation of 5.4. The mean of adaptation for the same sample was 24.1 with a standard deviation of 4.7. While the sample size of the pilot study is very small, the three-point difference in the cohesion scores and the wider standard deviation for both scores suggest that some adjustment of the scales may be necessary for use with rural persons.

IMPLICATIONS FOR PRACTICE

The distinction between adjustment and adaptation that this model offers is important for nursing practice. Nurses who work in emergency departments, intensive care units, and other crisis-oriented places see families who are in the throws of the adjustment phase. The current status of the family has been upset; the family appraisal of the situation phase is in process. Families at this time can look dysfunctional. They can be loud, assertive, and demanding—behaviors which are disruptive to a clinical unit and hard to deal with on the part of a staff. At this point, families need information. The family cannot form an appraisal of the situation without facts. Without an accurate appraisal, the family cannot use actions that are going to help the situation improve.

The state of affairs at the point when a family in crisis meets the health care system is very delicate. On the one hand, the professionals do not want to scare the family with dire predictions that may not come true. On the other hand, to play down potential difficulties denies the family the opportunity to appraise and to plan actions. The nurse must find a balance among his or her experience, the possible seriousness of the illness, and the family's need for information.

Generally, if a family can be guided to appoint a liaison person and the staff can provide one professional, a good line of communication may be established. The only rule in this phase of the communication is that the family must be allowed to select its own liaison person. This rule can be very trying for the staff if the family picks a fairly hysterical person, for example. In this situation, the staff needs to realize that families have tremendous reserves of strengths, no matter how disorganized they appear at the moment. The staff also needs to understand that if the hysterical mother is the liaison person, the family is used to getting information from her. They know how to "read" her and to interpret her. (Obviously, there are some situations so skewed that the staff will have to ask for another liaison person because the staff cannot communicate comfortably with the person the family selected.)

Olson et al. (1989) point out that most families solve crises and problems without resorting to community services or mental health professionals. Their findings offer an important caution when working with stressed families, as nurses and other health care workers do. American health care is aggressive. We want to do something for clients. It may be that supporting and encouraging the family and assuring them that they can get through the crisis may be enough intervention for some families. This conjecture needs to be refined in clinical practice.

It is during the adaptation phase that families are most likely to seek therapy. For the rural family, the need for therapy may be a further stressor, as their schema of themselves as self-reliant is challenged. The theory presented in this chapter allows the therapist to use many approaches; this is one of the benefits of this theory, and the therapist should consider a few options for intervention.

The therapist may test the family with FACES III to assess levels of cohesion and adaptability. The genogram will show patterns of closeness over generations. If there is a close agreement between the FACES III scores and the genogram, the therapist can be more sure of the "picture" of the family that is forming in his or her mind. By using this information and by focusing on the current stressors in the family, tasks can be assigned to various members that will work to mitigate the stressors while underlying emotional issues can be explored.

Genograms can also serve to outline successful family patterns. Constructing a genogram with a rural family that has four or five generations in the room can bring out family strengths that have been on the back burner. Most people tend to think that the crisis they are dealing with now is the worst crisis ever. However, such a response is a function of the narrowed focus that goes with the demand for change in the adaptation phase. In rural families, previous generations may have kept the family farm or business going through the Great Depression and the Second World War—

no small accomplishments! If several generations are working on the genogram, past successes can be used to bolster a family schema of competence.

This is a two-edged sword. If the family has been coping marginally for a couple of generations, a therapist can have a very depressed family group facing him or her as the genogram depicts a series of less than successful adaptations. The therapist, however, can use the family type to explore potential strengths that may be overlooked by the genogram.

A therapist could use the four family types, vulnerable, secure, durable, and regenerative, to plan interventions. Each type has strengths and weaknesses. The strengths can be the basis of generating family hope and activities. For example, if one were working with a family that had not coped well for a while and that family were of a secure type, one would use the sense of control and activity that typifies these families to move on.

The synthesized theory also suggests a crisis intervention approach. In crisis intervention, one of the most important and least discussed parameters for intervention is the sibling positions of the persons involved. Generally, oldest children are active problem solvers. If one of the parents in a family is an oldest, giving that person information and encouragement can be very helpful in resolving stressors. (Beware if both parents are oldests. There may be a covert power struggle going on that is making the stressor more upsetting than it might be otherwise.)

Similarly, youngest children are more used to having other people take care of them. In a family crisis, parents who are youngests may need more encouragement to do for themselves and may be overwhelmed if given too much information too quickly. Generally, going from simpler tasks to more involved ones brings these parents along. If there is a time-framed stressor (e.g., the bank will foreclose on the mortgage in 30 days) other persons may have to be invited *by the family* to help. In this case, the therapist's role is to support the family in identifying and seeking outside help.

Of special note in the model is the role of social support resources. These resources may take the form of a self-help group, such as Alcoholics Anonymous, or an aunt or uncle. For the urban trained therapist, the idea of having a relative take a child during a crisis may be unsettling. This is probably because extended family members of urban families often live far away and are barely known to the child. In rural areas, however, the extended family may live down the road, attend the same church and school. It is a simple, nondisruptive solution for some situations. For example, if a mother has to go to the city for surgery, the father may be left to run the family business alone. The need for the father to also take care of the six-month-old infant may so contribute to pile-up that asking another member of the family to take care of the baby is a functional thing to do. These arrangements are not demoralizing because the ethic of helping one's neighbors is often very strong in rural communities.

Professionals may want to participate in developing a support group for a special rural problem or they may want to facilitate bringing a national support group to the local area. There are so many support groups that many states have clearing houses to advise persons how to connect with an appropriate group. The use of support groups for rural persons is especially appropriate because of the value attributed to helping one's neighbors that typifies these people.

In summary, by synthesizing the Bowen Family Systems Theory and the McCubbin T-Double ABC-X Theory, a more measurable theory is offered for research. Also, the synthesis allows the practitioner a broader array of interventions because the strengths of the family are part of the assessment, as well as areas of dysfunction. The synthesis presented in this chapter needs to be further explored from both research and practice to ascertain its value.

REFERENCES

Bowen, M. (1978). *Family therapy in clinical practice.* New York: Jason Aronson.

Bushy, A. (1990). Rural determinants in family health: Considerations for community nurses. *Family and Community Health, 12*(4), 29–38.

Haber, J. (1990). The Haber differentiation of self scale. In C. Waltz & O. Strickland (Eds.), *The measurement of clinical and educational outcomes.* New York: Springer Publishing.

Hill, R. (1949). *Families under stress*. New York: Harper.

Kerr, M., & Bowen, M. (1988). *Family evaluation*. New York: W. W. Norton.

Kleinman, A. (1986). Some uses and misuses of the social sciences in medicine. In D. W. Fiske & R. A. Schweder (Eds.), *Metatheory in social science* (pp. 222–245). Chicago: University of Chicago Press.

Long, K., & Weinert, C. (1987). Understanding the health care needs of rural families. *Family Relations, 36*(1), 450–455.

Luloff, A. E. (1990). Small town demographics: Current patterns of community change. In A. E. Luloff & L. E. Swanson (Eds.), *American rural communities* (pp. 7–18). Boulder, CO: Westview Press.

McCubbin, H. I., Larsen, A., & Olson, D. H. (1982). F-COPES: Family crisis oriented personal scales. In H. I. McCubbin & A. Thompson (Eds.), *Family assessment inventories for research and practice*. Madison, WI: University of Wisconsin.

McCubbin, H. I., & Patterson, J. M. (1987). Family adaptation checklist. In H. I. McCubbin & A. Thompson (Eds.), *Family assessment inventories for research and practice*. Madison, WI: University of Wisconsin.

McCubbin, H. I., Patterson, J. M., & Glynn, T. (1987). Social support index (SSI). In H. I. McCubbin & A. Thompson (Eds.), *Family assessment inventories for research and practice*. Madison, WI: University of Wisconsin.

McCubbin, M. A., & McCubbin, H. I. (1987). Family stress theory and assessment. In H. I. McCubbin & A. I. Thompson (Eds.), *Family assessment inventories for research and practice* (pp. 2–32). Madison, WI: University of Wisconsin—Madison.

McCubbin, M. A., & McCubbin, H. I. (1989). Theoretical orientations to family stress and coping. In C. R. Figley (Ed.), *Treating stress in families* (pp. 3–43). New York: Brunner/Mazel.

Miller, S., & Winstead-Fry, P. E. (1982). *Family systems theory in nursing practice*. Reston, VA: Reston.

Newman, M. (1979). *Theory development in nursing*. Philadelphia: F. A. Davis.

Olson, D. H., McCubbin, H. I., Barnes, H. L., Larsen, A. S., Muxen, M. J., & Wilson, M. A. (1989). *Families: What makes them work*. Newbury Park, CA: Sage.

Olson, D. H., Portner, J., & Lavee, Y. (1985). *FACES III.* St. Paul, MN: University of Minnesota.

Olson, D. H., Russell, L. S., & Sprenkle, D. H. (1983). Circumplex model VI: Theoretical update. *Family Process, 22,* 69–83.

Olson, D. H., Sprenkle, D., & Russell, C. (1979). Circumplex model of marital and family systems I: Cohesion and adaptability dimensions, family types and clinical application. *Family Process, 18,* 3–28.

Ploch, L. A. (1981). Family aspects of the new wave of immigrants to rural communities. In R. T. Coward & W. M. Smith (Eds.), *The family in rural society* (pp. 39–53). Boulder, CO: Westview Press.

Richards, E. (1989). Self-reports of differentiation of self and marital compatibility as related to family functioning in the third and fourth stages of the family life cycle. *Scholarly Inquiry for Nursing Practice: An International Journal, 3*(3), 163–175.

Rosenblatt, P. C., & Anderson, R. M. (1981). Interaction in farm families: Tension and stress. In R. T. Coward & W. M. Smith (Eds.), *The family in rural society* (pp. 147–166). Boulder, CO: Westview Press.

Shannon, A. (1989). Educators innovate to match changing needs: Preparing nurses for rural health care. *American Nurse, 21*(2), 10.

U.S. Congress, Office of Technology Assessment. (1990). *Health care in rural America.* OTA-H-434. Washington, D.C.: U. S. Government Printing Office.

Wagenfield, M. O. (1990). Mental health and rural America: A decade review. *The Journal of Rural Health, 6*(4), 507–522.

Walker, L. O., & Avant, K. C. (1988). *Strategies for theory construction in nursing.* Norwalk, CT: Appleton-Lange.

Part II

Consumers and Providers

7

Telephone Reassurance:
A Social Support Intervention

Holly A. Cozzi-Burr

Telephone reassurance can increase options for social support of the elderly. Social support becomes increasingly important as a person's level of impairment or isolation increases. The literature supports the view that some elders need additional social support.

Issues of aging, independence, and support are what compelled a holistic study of the population of those over the age of 65 on Maine's Mount Desert Island (MDI) and a pilot telephone reassurance project. This community of elders was chosen because of this writer's familiarity with this aggregate in her work as a community health nurse for the Community Health Agency on the island.

For some older, healthy adults, a sense of well-being is promoted through activities such as club meetings and exercise groups. For those who cannot leave home or are dependent upon others for care, however, being old and feeling trapped are synonymous. In either case, assessing factors that affect the health status of the elderly population can provide a profile of needs and resources which might otherwise get lost in the existent health care framework (Ruffing-Rahal, 1987).

COMMUNITY ASSESSMENT

Maine coincides with the rest of the nation in showing a trend toward the aging of the population as a whole. At present, one of every eight people (12.5 percent of Maine's population) is age 65 or older. Maine ranks eleventh nationally for the size of its population of elders. According to Mezey, Rauckhorst, and Stokes (1980), about 95 percent of the population age 65 and over are never institutionalized. In Maine, only 7 percent of the elderly are in nursing or boarding homes. The majority of the aged are assisted by friends and family in their own community without need for support services (Bureau of Maine's Elderly, 1987). The independent living status of Maine's aging population is being threatened by several social factors. Some of these negative influences on independence are increasing chronic illness, reduction in social security and health care benefits, rising cost of insurance, upward spiraling cost of living, increased number of dual income households, and the mobility of the society in which we live. The need for a clear understanding of what forms of support the elderly perceive as helpful to them in maintaining their independence made this an appropriate area for study.

In order to gain an impression of what the elder community identified as priorities, a questionnaire was formulated and distributed at two senior citizen clubs, one Meals for Maine service site, and one adult fitness class. Personal assessments were then conducted in the homes of people living in three different elderly housing sites. People to be interviewed were selected from volunteers answering the survey.

Leaders, or key informants of the aggregate, were identified and interviewed by this writer to shed light on how the needs of that population could be met. This group of leaders consisted of the presidents of two senior groups, the Meals for Maine site coordinator, a representative of the Maine Housing Authority, and the outreach worker and the care manager for the Eastern Area on Aging.

A profile of the needs and resources of elders on the island was catalogued according to Dorothy Orem's self-care nursing model. Orem's model was chosen as an appropriate framework for the project because it does not assume illness, is aimed at maintaining wellness and client independence, and is focused on the priorities and goals of the client (Cozzi, 1988). The following were some of the key issues for elders that surfaced in data from the questionnaire: lack of transportation and domestic services, inadequate snow and ice removal from commonly used walkways, lack of routine social contact, and inadequate linkages between natural and formal support systems to ensure adequate care of isolated elders (Cozzi, 1988). The following diagnoses, found from the questionnaire and personal assessments, form a partial list of the problems shared by the elderly people on the island:

1. self-care deficit related to mobility into community groups
2. self-care deficit related to access to professional and service people
3. self-care deficit related to coping with environmental hazards
4. self-care deficit related to adequate housing (Cozzi, 1988).

This writer conducted focus groups during the summer with three major senior groups on the island. The groups addressed were the Bar Harbor and Southwest Harbor senior groups and the Tuesday Meals for Maine group which combines seniors from all over the island. The intent of the focus groups was to achieve consensus about the meanings of priority issues identified by survey respondents. Open-ended discussions were held on 14 areas of need identified in the questionnaire. The idea of a telephone reassurance program crystallized through discussion of the other key issues as a logical way to meet some of the needs identified. A secondary gain of convening focus groups was that the elder community became a co-participant in program planning. By involving the elders in the planning, a program could be developed that would speak to the priorities identified by the community.

The target population of the telephone reassurance pilot program resides in Maine. People age 65 and over in Bar Harbor comprise 20.6 percent of the population or 820 people (1985 Census of the Population). By 1995, it is anticipated that there will be a 110-person increase in the age 65 and over group (Office of Data, Research, and Vital Statistics, 1987). It is unknown how many people in this age group in Bar Harbor are homebound, live alone, or are chronically ill. This writer found, however, that 75 percent ($n = 99$) of the survey respondents live alone. Additionally, she found that approximately 8 percent of the elderly receive services from the Community Health Nurse Agency and 100 percent of these people are chronically ill or housebound.

Prior to the telephone reassurance pilot project, the only type of support offered in the Bar Harbor area for people considered to have a need due to isolation or illness was the Senior Companion Program. In the companion program, senior volunteers visit with clients at their homes in order to develop relationships, bridge problems of social isolation, and assist with needed services such as shopping. Unfortunately the program has a deficit of volunteers on MDI and a waiting list of recipients who have a need for socialization or help with activities such as reading, writing, transportation, or cleaning. This lack of volunteers may be due to the required commitment of 20 hours per week and the low financial reimbursement available for the senior companion activities.

Other factors which contribute to the need for more social support were found from this writer's surveys and interviews. The chief theme emanating from the needs assessment was isolation, particularly of homebound elders who are unable to participate in senior clubs, and of newcomers to senior housing who are not privy to informal networks. Breakdown of informal networks, the strain of relinquishing a social role, risks of living alone while awaiting alternate living situations, diminished resources, and depression are all factors in the elder population that demand creation of more support networks (Cozzi, 1988).

PILOT PROGRAM

The pilot program was based on the following goals and objectives:

1. To develop a social support network for homebound elders who live alone.
2. To identify a referral service for elders in need of support services.
3. To identify those in need of telephone reassurance.

These goals and objectives were to be met by soliciting volunteers and providing training, supervision, and coordination of schedules and activities and by piloting the telephone reassurance program for one month. The Community Health Agency (CHA) was to function as an intermediary referral service for program participants.

PROGRAM MODEL

Telephone reassurance is a recognized intervention used to bridge a void that many frail, disabled, or isolated people experience. Telephone reassurance is a program whereby a recipient is called once a day at a specific time by a volunteer. In this writer's variation of the concept, Care-Call, the volunteer inquires briefly as to the homebound participant's well-being and needs and passes along any requests for services from the participants (i.e., snow shoveling, meal delivery, or nursing care). If the phone is not answered, a designated contact person is notified, who makes a personal visit. Participants must inform volunteers when they will not be home in order to ensure that calls are not made to empty households. The length of program use can vary according to need.

The notion of telephone reassurance was conceived by Grace McClure during the 1960s. McClure's experience of finding a friend, who had been unresponsive to telephone calls for days, succumbed to mishap, precipitated the social contact service (Gelfand, 1984). Telephone reassurance programs have been replicated across the country and may be found in other agencies where services are provided to the elderly. Telephone reassurance is identified in the 1981 amendments to the *Older Americans Act* as part of the in-home assistance that local Areas on Aging must provide (Huttman, 1985).

Telephone reassurance programs have a high rate of volunteerism as they make few demands on volunteers. The Eastern Maine Medical Center (EMMC) in Bangor has a telephone reassurance program. Its Telecare program has been in existence for ten years, operating with two volunteers per day, seven days per week, 360 days per year. Responsibility flows in both directions in the

EMMC model; participants are required to call in to the Telecare volunteer station.

Variations of the telephone reassurance concept such as "Dial-A-Listener" and "Telephone Club" of New York exist as social support programs utilizing volunteers (Huttman, 1985). The System to Assure Elderly Services (STAES) developed in St. Louis, MO, has been a successful solution to self-care problems of seniors there. The STAES senior volunteers may provide direct service, reassurance, or act as an "information network" (Morrow-Howell & Ozawa, 1987, pp. 17–20). "Care-Ring," another outreach social support network for the lonely also gives positive attention to the volunteers through training sessions and planning (Paull, 1972). The major differences between telephone reassurance and other social support programs using volunteers are (1) telephone reassurance demands relatively few resources, and (2) volunteers are not funded.

PLANNING

The planning phase was the most time-consuming facet of operationalizing the program on MDI. An effective reporting system had to be implemented to ensure accountability of the volunteers to the agency and to the community at large. Volunteers were given a card with the participant's name, telephone number, address, days and times to be called, two contacts, and any information pertinent to the participant's situation. A form was provided for the caller to record dates of completed calls, dates calls were pre-arranged not to be made, or dates a contact had to be notified. The volunteer was to mail this form to the program coordinator monthly.

A protocol for volunteers was developed as a specific guide for calling participants. The protocol instructs the caller to allow the phone to ring at least ten times, lists possible reasons for no answers, gives a format for notifying a contact person or the police department, and states what action to take in case of personal unavailability.

Office protocol for the CHA entails the secretary logging incoming referrals, both for Care-Call and for other services, and involvement of the professional staff for follow-up with program clients or volunteers when the project coordinator is unavailable.

Other documents used by Care-Call include an informational brochure, an admission form, a note to the contact person, and a letter that confirms a participant's discontinuation of Care-Call.

Another facet of planning was solicitation of volunteers and program participants. A local newspaper was contacted and an interview concerning the program appeared in the paper. During the start-up phase, telephone contact was made with individuals in the community known to be active in a wide range of volunteer activities.

RECRUITING AND TRAINING VOLUNTEERS

A speaking engagement was arranged with the Bar Harbor Senior Citizens group to solicit volunteers and to promote Care-Call. Since the group was part of the aggregate from which the need for telephone reassurance surfaced, the group was well informed. Eight people were added to the volunteer list as a result of the presentation, the newspaper article drew five volunteers, one community member volunteered her spouse, and one person volunteered as a result of personal solicitation.

Fourteen volunteers attended the Care-Call training session. Good training and clear guidelines for volunteers were essential to the success of Care-Call. The program coordinator used a blend of lecture, discussion, and simulation to train the volunteers. To foster a cooperative effort and enhance motivation and individual confidence while diminishing isolation (de Tornyay and Thompson, 1987), group training at the senior housing sites was presented for volunteers who were mobile. One homebound volunteer received instruction at his residence by the program coordinator.

Biographical information about the volunteers contributed during the initial training revealed that all but one of the 16 individuals had previous volunteer experience. The members included a retired licensed practical nurse, a retired fireman, a retired teacher, a disabled certified nursing assistant, a retired nurse, and several homemakers. Of the 14 female volunteers, one member is in her 30s, the others are beyond retirement age. Two of the volunteers are male. At the end of one month, 14 members were active in calling participants and two volunteers held substitute status.

RECRUITING PARTICIPANTS

Participants were solicited through letters written to local head nurses, social workers, discharge planners, two local nursing homes, the Eastern Area on Aging outreach worker, the local hospice director, the Bar Harbor Housing Authority, and the Physician Group Practice.

All referrals to the pilot program were made through the CHA and screened by the coordinator. Participants were contacted and a home visit was made by the program coordinator to complete the intake process. The only criterion for participation is that the recipient live alone.

IMPLEMENTATION

On November 1, 1988, four participants began to receive calls from Care-Call volunteers. When a new assignment was made, the coordinator would contact the volunteer by phone with participant data and instructions as to the day and time to begin calls. Participant data cards were then mailed to the volunteer and duplicates retained in both the office Care-Call Kardex and the coordinator's at-home Kardex. During the implementation phase, blank Care-Call applications and information sheets were distributed to the local discharge planners to facilitate the referral process. Posters advertising Care-Call were placed in two Bar Harbor grocery stores, two senior housing sites, and the Bar Harbor Town Office building.

The pilot program targeted a small number of people, representative of the aged population of MDI, for whom there was some gap in services and for whom a friendly check-in call would be welcome (Table 7–1).

Table 7–1
One-Month Overview of Pilot Program

Participants:
Total number of participants: 6
Discharged from Care-Call: 1
Total calls received: 103
Age: 65+
Sex: 99% female

Primary reasons for accepting service:
40% isolation
40% chronic illness
20% homebound

Frequency of service:
80% seven days per week
20% one or two days of the weekend

Other agencies/services involved:
5 cases

MANAGEMENT

Weekly telephone contacts were initially made to the volunteers to gather calling statistics and flush out any concerns or questions. The effort to provide a positive working relationship and enhance job satisfaction has proven to be fruitful, as the volunteer retention rate has been 100 percent.

Promotional opportunities have included speaking engagements at civic organizations, a series of newspaper articles, and interviews with both cable and local television stations. Promotion was woven into both the planning and implementation phases to generate referrals and public support. Promotion and recruiting of participants was restricted to Bar Harbor for the pilot program. Fund-raising efforts were conducted by the coordinator and included both letter writing and speaking engagements at civic meetings. Operating expenses for the program have been limited to the cost of postage for volunteer mailings and printing informational material. Funds are managed by the financial officer of the CHA.

EVALUATION

An ongoing monitoring process speaks to why the project has progressed toward identified goals. All program activities are logged in the coordinator's notebook. Information concerning sources of referrals, participant concerns, reasons for discontinuance, costs in terms of time and money, as well as statistics are routinely reviewed.

The initial evaluation examined the program's impact on individuals. Questions focused on participant experiences and satisfaction with the program as well as volunteer satisfaction with their role and accountability. Because the population was small, data from call recipients were collected by telephone interviews with all participants. Program volunteers were requested to anonymously complete a questionnaire and return it to the program coordinator.

Although there were no potential participants who declined, a consideration during the evaluation process was that, because of the beliefs and values of some people, the role of being a Care-Call participant might not be acceptable. Some individuals might identify being on the program roster with the stigma of being feeble and choose not to participate.

Evaluations showed that Care-Call has acted as a social support mechanism. One sign of the program's success is that volunteers perceive that participants are "happy to receive a call" and report feeling endeared to the participants. In the nine questionnaires returned to the coordinator, each volunteer responded with such common assessments as: "people need to be thought about and to know someone cares when they are alone . . . ," "participants have a daily contact with the outside world," "this work can be done by anyone who can dial a phone," "the feeling of caring," "it's good to be needed," "it's good to get involved," "to hear another's voice must give a sense of security to those who live alone." Additional questionnaire data suggest the adequacy of the orientation and program structure.

Another sign that Care-Call is appreciated is that the participants during telephone interviews state that they "look forward to the next call," "fear" a mishap, and like the security of knowing that someone "checks-in." A recurrent theme verbalized was reciprocity. In cases when a volunteer forgot to call his or her participants, the participants called the coordinator with concerns about the well-being of the caller. Other dominant themes of the participants' interviews were guilt for "troubling someone to call," and dependence on the volunteer versus self-reliance.

The CHA has received few requests for referrals for additional services. It is reasonable, therefore, to assume the agency will not have to take on an expanded role as a screening and referral service.

One strength of the program is the type of volunteer to whom the program appeals. Volunteers are empathetic, motivated to help, and very reliable. The high level of retention is due also largely to the fact that this is independent work that can be done out of the volunteer's own home. The notion of the volunteers as individuals with needs for connection to others was also highlighted as a reason for their call to service.

In summary, the evaluation process points to Care-Call as an effective intervention which was engineered to address factors influencing social support. In an effort to invigorate the art of "neighbor helping neighbor" (Morrow-Howell, Ozawa, 1987, p. 20), Care-Call preserves important social values and aids in overcoming problems caused by environmental and situational deficits.

As a direct result of community support and participant/ volunteer satisfaction, Care-Call expanded to include all towns on MDI in January 1989. Since that time, a new volunteer coordinator has been trained to assume responsibility for orienting and managing the volunteers, making assignments, and keeping records. Promotional efforts are continuing with support from community groups. There has been a 75 percent increase in volunteers and a 200 percent increase in participants. A total of 3,468 calls has been made to participants, and several calls to contact people have resulted in appropriate referrals for hospitalization or other needed services.

SUMMARY

A need for island people to maintain personal ties in the face of a changing population is a fitting standpoint from which to explain the success of the telephone reassurance effort on Mount Desert Island. By working together with the aggregate to facilitate change older individuals recognize as necessary, an appropriate solution has been implemented to a care dilemma facing elders, their aging children, their neighbors, and community services which sometimes struggle to provide support with minimal funding. Telephone reassurance is a low cost program that appeals to people who have time to volunteer and to organizations that can contribute funds for community projects, and which represents a need valued by the population for whom the program is targeted.

Telephone reassurance, as a social support program, has utilized an opportunity to establish goodwill in the community, and it forms a basis for bridging a gap between island residents, agencies, and organizations and augments existing support networks. By forming linkages in the island community, the interface of the older person, health, and environment may be documented. One possible consequence of involvement with participants in the program might be to hypothesize about the health consequences of social isolation and types of support (Seeman, Berkman, 1988). The need for a clear understanding of the population, who because of the changes of aging will need various forms of support, will aid in fostering the self-care the community is capable of mobilizing.

REFERENCES

Bureau of Maine's Elderly (1987). *State Plan: 1987–1989* (DHS Publication No. 1327.1001). Augusta, ME: State House.

Cozzi, H. (1988). *Community Assessment of the Elderly.* Unpublished paper.

de Tornyay, R., & Thompson, M. A. (1987). *Strategies for teaching nursing.* New York: Wiley.

Gelfand, D. E. (1984). *The aging network: Programs and services* (2nd ed.). New York: Springer.

Huttman, E. D. (1985). *Social services for the elderly.* New York: Free Press.

Melosh, B. (1982). *The physicians hand.* Philadelphia: Temple University Press.

Mezey, M. D., Rauckhorst, L. M., & Stokes, S. A. (1980). Community and home assessment. In B. W. Spradley (Ed.), *Readings in community health nursing* (pp. 154–156). Boston: Little, Brown.

Miller, J. B. (1976). *Toward a new psychology of women.* Boston: Beacon Press.

Morrow-Howell, N., & Ozawa, M. N. (1987). Helping network: Seniors to seniors. *The Gerontologist, 27*(1), 17–20.

Office of data, research and vital statistics. (1987, October). *Population estimates for minor civil divisions by county.* (No. 1305-1065).

Paull, H. H. (1972). Treatment for loneliness: A plan for establishing a social network of individualized caring through care-ring. *Crisis intervention,* 63-83.

Ruffing-Rahal, M. A. (1987). Resident/provider contrasts in community health priorities. *Public Health Nursing, 4*(4), 242–246.

Seeman, T. E., & Berkman, L. F. (1988). Structural characteristics of social networks and their relationship with social support in the elderly: Who provides support. *Social Science Medicine, 26*(7), 737–749.

8

Crisis Intervention and Suicide Prevention from a Rural Perspective

Deborah A. Clark

Wagenfield, in his presentation to the Conference on Rural Community Mental Health, characterized rural culture as follows:

> *On the broadest possible level, rural values tend to emphasize several themes: man's subjugation to nature, fatalism, a present-time orientation, an orientation to concrete places and things, a view of human nature as basically evil, human activity as being, not doing, and human relationships having their basis in personal and kinship ties. [Falcone & Rosenthal, 1982, p. 4]*

In contrast, urban areas are stereotypically seen as liberal, future-oriented, impersonal, tolerant, and progressive. Rural communities have been characterized as laid back, non-competitive and low stress. They appeal to individuals wanting to quit the "rat race." There are, however, many misunderstandings about rural communities and life-styles. Rural living does not necessarily mean stress-free living. A *Harvard Medical School Mental Health Letter* states that the suicide rate is lower in rural areas than in cities (Grinspoon, 1986). Yet the Center for Disease Control's *Suicide Surveillance 1970–1980* in 1985 listed the Western region of the

United States as having an overall suicide rate of 14.8 per 100,000, while the national rate was 11.9 per 100,000. Each of the rural states out West has a suicide rate higher than the national rate. In the Northeast, the rural states of Maine and Vermont also have a higher suicide rate than the nation as a whole. The idea of a lower suicide rate in rural areas is a myth and the prevalence of suicide in rural areas is certainly a subject warranting further investigation.

SUICIDE IN RURAL MAINE

When exploring predominate feelings and factors contributing to suicidal behavior, depression, isolation, despair, lack of resources, and loneliness are terms that are frequently mentioned. These same feelings are also mentioned when describing some characteristics of rural populations. Interestingly, these characteristics can also be applied to the elderly who are, in actuality, a group at higher risk (with a national suicide rate of 19.2) than the young as reviewed by Voirst (1986).

In a 1968–1975 study of suicides in Maine, more than half of the 16 counties had a suicide rate well above the state and national average. These eight counties are the least populated ones, with the majority of the people living in isolated, remote areas. In addition, four of these counties have unemployment rates above the state average and incomes below the state poverty level (Tukey, 1981).

In Maine, 57 percent of all suicides are by firearms. There has been an increase over the past ten years nationally in the use of firearms for suicides. The use of firearms poses a major problem in the area of intervention, as this method is more lethal, and offers fewer chances for intervention or rescue. Firearms are common household items in rural communities. Suicide rates by gender in Maine (1985) match the national figures, with males accounting for 77 percent and females accounting for 23 percent. More females in Maine, however, are using firearms rather than poisoning, the most common method used by females nationwide.

Although the suicide rate during the first six months of the year in Maine is similar to the national trend with a peak occurrence in April, the last six months vary by having another peak in November.

In looking at the high suicide rate in rural counties in Maine, Tukey (1981) asked, "what factors, external to isolation and being rural, exist in these counties with high rates that persist?" (p. 14). Ten years later suicide prevention professionals are still asking the same questions. If we continue to believe the myth that rural settings have lower rates of suicide, we will continue to have difficulty answering Tukey's question as we will not be seeing an accurate picture of the situation.

A RURAL SUICIDE PREVENTION PROGRAM

Dispelling myths is an ongoing educational process. When confronting the issue of suicide prevention, programs need to be developed for rural areas. Some of the rationale and steps that went into establishing the Somerset County Crisis Stabilization Unit in Maine will be discussed next.

It is important to examine how programs are introduced into a rural area. Successful introductions of mental health programs into a rural community appear to depend primarily on mental health personnel being informed and sensitive. Well-developed knowledge of the community's social and power network is vital. The community is more likely to support a program which it perceives a need for and which it feels it has helped design.

During the initial start-up period of the crisis stabilization unit, many meetings were scheduled with groups already established in the area. Nothing much seemed to be accomplished during these meetings, with individuals being very polite, but reserved. As the meetings broke up, people would stay to talk with the speaker on a one-to-one basis. It was usually during that time period that much more was accomplished. Rumors were dispelled, and questions were asked that would not have been asked within the larger group. It was also important to seek advice from local individuals on practical matters not related to program design such as, "Where do you order your supplies?", "Where's the best place locally to get . . . ?", "Who do you think I should talk to about . . . ?" The director of the chamber of commerce was a wealth of information on such practical matters and paved the way for introductions to individuals we may not have otherwise met. He was also able to provide a historical background that we would not have found in any survey or needs assessment. This networking was extremely helpful in attempting to avoid pitfalls and identify power networks. In a rural community it is essential to tie in with existing agencies and to explore what we in the mental health field may view as nontraditional resources when developing new programs. Mental health, social service, and education programs are viewed as more traditional resources, but these services are often understaffed and underfunded in rural areas. The chamber of commerce, police departments, and some of the social and civic organizations may be viewed as more nontraditional resources, but they are often more directly connected with the social and power networks in rural communities. These organizations often have great potential for fund-raising and generating community support that are vital in keeping a program operating. Start-up time is generally more extensive in rural than in urban settings as it is more than the program itself being evaluated. The individuals running the program are examined carefully in terms of their commitment to the community as well as to the program. It may take an outsider longer to be accepted in a rural area, but once that acceptance does occur it is usually prolonged and intimate. When the program coordinator was seeking letters of support for additional funding, a former client wrote to the state mental health department that the coordinator was warm and down to earth and not the least bit professional. This letter was actually quite a compliment as professionalism had a negative connotation for this client. Had the funding source not understood this connotation, that letter would hardly have been taken as one of support.

Somerset County in north central Maine is geographically remote and about as large as the state of Connecticut with a population of only 45,000. More than half the population resides in six major communities. The remaining 20,000 people reside in small communities, rural plantations, and townships. In 1984 the unemployment figures were 13 percent with most of the employed population working in forestry, papermaking, and shoe manufacturing.

In an attempt to address the needs of the population, the state of Maine funded a mobile crisis unit in 1981. The initial grant was for $79,000. The expectations were for the unit to be staffed 24 hours a day and dispatched through the sheriff's office as that was where people were likely to call for assistance with any type of crisis. Crisis workers would respond to calls in individual homes, churches, police stations, or wherever the crisis was occurring. Law enforcement staff would accompany workers to any potentially violent situation. The unit was originally staffed by two full-time and two part-time crisis workers. Shift hours were 8:00 AM to 4:00 PM, 2:00 PM to 10:00 PM, and 10:00 PM to 8:00 AM. Workers would rotate weekend duty, thereby covering the unit 24 hours a day, seven days a week. When originally staffing the unit, major consideration was given to candidates with some experience in handling psychiatric emergencies. Since, at that time there were no other programs in the state of Maine doing on-site crisis intervention, it was difficult to find individuals with crisis intervention experience. Of the four original crisis workers, three had master's degrees (one nurse, two counselors) and one had a bachelor's degree. All but one had direct experience in psychiatric emergencies. The one who did not have this experience left the unit within the first six months. The unique nature of this program required much inservice training. The lack of similar programs in the area resulted in many things being learned by trial and error. During the second year of operation, the unit joined the American Association of Suicidology (AAS). This association proved to be an extremely valuable resource. Annual conferences were attended by the coordinator and crisis centers in other states were visited. With consultation from AAS, a training program was developed which met AAS standards for crisis center training programs (Wilson, Hoff, Tapp, & Wells, 1981). Part of that training program included a test used as a screening tool in interviewing potential crisis workers. The test is designed to test knowledge, attitude, and skills in the area of crisis intervention. This test has been an effective tool in hiring staff and assessing training needs of crisis workers.

Funding began in July 1981 but the unit was not fully operational until April 1982. It was determined that it would take the first year to become established within the community, so cost-effectiveness that first year was not a factor for continued funding. Although the community had been involved in the original planning of the unit, there was still a great deal of skepticism regarding our overall operation. The coordinator was "from away" and many expressed concerns that they had seen these programs come and go and were hesitant to invest too much until they felt the unit would (1) meet their needs and (2) be around for a while. An advisory board was established composed of individuals within the community to assist during this initial time period.

It was important that the law enforcement officials saw the crisis unit as a help rather than a hindrance. Many officers felt initially that the crisis unit workers might "get in the way" of them doing their jobs. The first few incidences in which a crisis worker was present to "talk down" an irate spouse or a suicidal individual went a long way toward establishing credibility for the unit. Word-of-mouth traveled as fast for those occurrences as it did for not so successful incidents.

It was important in establishing creditability to be forthright with the community regarding what the unit could do and what it could not do. There were initially some unrealistic expectations by other local agencies regarding the services that we could provide. Educating the community as to the goals of the unit and the constraints of the unit was an ongoing process and often accomplished with subtleness. Traditional educational workshops were often met with resistance. Presentations the unit felt would be useful and those the community wanted were not often the same. Whereas the unit was looking toward more theoretically based workshops, the requests were geared more toward a practical "how to" approach to problems. It was essential to meet the community's requests first.

Following the first few years of the unit's existence, with the connections made to AAS, the staff began to realize that many of the concepts used in the foundation of the unit were based upon studies with urban populations, and the rural setting seemed markedly different. For example, it was originally speculated that most of the calls would come after hours. In actuality most of the calls came between 9 AM and 11 AM. Perhaps in a setting with few traditional resources, people do not necessarily have a nine-to-five mentality.

The crisis unit has continued to grow throughout the last ten years. In 1987 it was certified by the AAS, becoming the only certified crisis center in Maine. Maine, like many other states has been undergoing financial difficulties which have had many ramifications for mental health programs. There has been a thrust toward scaling down state mental hospitals and looking toward the community to support and provide for the needs of individuals in psychiatric crisis. In 1990, the crisis unit applied for and received a grant for an emergency residential component. This two-bed program offers crisis stabilization for those needing 24-hour supervision. The length of stay ranges from two to seven days.

A brief treatment program was also started in response to an increasing need for more services in the area. The treatment program generates some income; it is the only component of the crisis unit charging a fee.

The current operating budget of the crisis unit is $340,000. Monies are received from the county commissioners, United Way, fees for workshops, hospitals, individual grants from Probation and Parole, Bureau of Mental Retardation, fund-raisers, and donations.

The current staff, including the brief treatment and residential components, consists of three full-time and ten part-time workers. Students from a local social work program do internships on the unit. The crisis unit continues to operate 24 hours a day.

SUMMARY

Working in a rural setting can be a challenging and exciting venture. Innovative approaches are called for when working with a population facing isolation, limited traditional resources, and poor transportation services. An understanding and respect for the rural culture is needed when planning and implementing programs in rural areas. Further study is needed to identify the unique risk factors experienced by rural populations and to develop specific interventions to be used in rural environments.

REFERENCES

Falcone, A. M., & Rosenthal, T. L. (1982). *Delivery of rural mental health services.* New York: Synapse.

Grinspoon, L. (1986). *The Harvard Medical School Mental Health Letter, 2* (8).

Suicide Surveillance, 1970–1980. (1985, April). Centers for Disease Control.

Tukey, G. M. (1981). *Suicide in the state of Maine: A statistical study 1968–1975.*

Voirst, J. (1986). *Necessary losses.* New York: Ballentine Books.

Wagenfield, M. O. (1977, May). *Cultural barriers to the delivery of mental health services in rural areas: A conceptual overview.* Presented to the Conference on Rural Community Mental Health, National Institute of Mental Health, Rockville, MD.

Wilson, K., Hoff, L. A., Tapp, J. T., & Wells, J. O. (1981). *Organization certification standards manual for crisis intervention programs.* Colorado: American Association of Suicidology.

9

Innovative Approaches to Emotional Support and Mental Health Needs in a Rural Setting: Initiation, Implementation, and Expansion

Beverly J. Chasse
Diane York
Mary Bayer
Ruth Davis

PROLOGUE: MELANIE'S STORY

Professional and volunteer support team members and their clients exemplify Martha Rogers's theory of unitary human beings in which people are seen as open energy systems. This energy is ever flowing, omnidirectionally between people and between individuals and their environments. At various times Patient Support Team members have, themselves, been recipients of support, and after receiving, have passed the energy along by reaching out to others. The story of Melanie exemplifies this interchange.

When she became a recipient of the Patient Support Team's efforts, Melanie was in her late 30s. She was a 1960s "flower child," living by herself one summer in a tent. Her oldest child, conceived in the Rockies, was named Coyote. Later, she and her

173

husband joined a very conservative church. Members wore plain clothes, lived together in a trailer park, worked communally giving their income to the church, and kept only enough to provide for their basic needs. Church women dressed alike, in long, grey skirts with plain blouses, and kept their heads covered. Although she later expressed disillusionment at the subservient role women were expected to play, Melanie acquiesced to church teachings for several years. During this time, Melanie was estranged from her mother and siblings. Eventually, she and her husband, Tim, left the church, and slowly rebuilt ties to their families.

Two years out of the church, Melanie felt that life was opening up, beginning anew. Only fatigue and some nagging discomfort in her abdomen marred her joy. She was treated for hypothyroidism, but the symptoms continued. Finally, in May, an acute episode of nausea, vomiting, and abdominal pain brought her to the hospital. Emergency surgery to relieve a bowel obstruction also revealed a malignant tumor in her right colon with metastasis to her liver.

Initially shocked and devastated by the diagnosis, Melanie soon chose to adopt an "I'm going to fight and win" attitude. Interaction with the nurse counselors, Beverly Chasse and Jo Brinkman, and the Patient Support Team, strengthened a resolve which she chose to maintain throughout the rest of her life.

Along with standard medical treatment, including chemotherapy, she used visualization techniques taught by the nurse counselor, attended the hospital's cancer support group, read inspirational literature, spent a week at an Indian healing center in Boston, and, along with her husband, attended a Bernie Siegel workshop.

She developed a strong bond with the Patient Support Team volunteers, and chose to spend some of her limited energy as a team member. Often it takes time to become part of a group, but Melanie and the team both felt, from the beginning, that she was where she belonged. Over the next few months, she was able to attend several team meetings, and occasionally to volunteer her services to the hospital. When her limited energies did not allow her to stay for the whole morning, the hour or two she could spend visiting others as part of the team were very meaningful to her.

In the late winter/early spring of 1990, Melanie had her last hospital visit. She was dehydrated from vomiting and diarrhea, probably a toxic reaction to chemotherapy. Several days after admission, she suffered a series of seizures, and then for several days was barely responsive. There was a general feeling among medical staff and her family that the end was at hand. An unoccupied room across the hall from hers was made available to her husband and daughters, then 13 and 11. The nurse counselors and Patient Support Team volunteers provided snacks and often spent time with the girls while their father sat at their mother's bedside. Slowly, Melanie began to rally. Tim was still unwilling to leave Melanie alone, but badly needed some respite and time to focus on the needs of his daughters. Support team members spelled him at Melanie's side, and her mother arrived to be with her and to help at home.

The next two months were Melanie's last hurrah. Her room filled with cards, posters, pictures, seed catalogues, and other personal items. Friends arrived and took her for rides around the hospital in a large rolling recliner. Always a lover of flowers, she monitored the growth and blossoming of the geranium seedlings on the window sill at the end of the hall. Once, with IV pole and Tim in tow, she attended an hour of a cancer support group meeting. Efforts of the Patient Support Team and some staff members concentrated on affirming Melanie, wife, mother, glowing individual, not Melanie, the cancer patient.

As the weeks passed, Melanie increasingly talked of going home. Although chemotherapy had been discontinued as futile, she talked of experimental regimes and liver transplants. In this period, the nurse counselor, Bev Chasse pushed her to look at the possibility of death, preparations she might wish to make "just in case," and the meaning for her family if she were to die at home. Prior to this time, Melanie had not been able to discuss her greatest fears with Tim, feeling that she must keep up her fighting spirit, even with him. Now, with Bev initially acting as go-between, they were able to talk about their greatest fears, and a few days before she died, she was also able to discuss her death with her children.

Initially "going home" was a short visit for lunch with Tim, her daughters, her mother, and the nurse counselor. Slowly walking from room to room with the aid of her walker, reconnecting with this much loved place, brought tears to her eyes. Two other visits over the next few weeks preceded her actual discharge from the hospital in late April.

Two weeks later, Bev got a call from Tim saying that Melanie was "different," moaning, but not alert. After a call to her physician, she was given additional pain medication. Later, both her physician and her primary nurse from the hospital stopped by to see if Melanie or Tim needed anything. Later when Melanie's breathing became shallow, Tim called Wendy, the primary nurse, and she was there when Melanie died. At Wendy's suggestion, Jo Brinkman, the nurse counselor, was called. Jo stayed with Tim while he woke his daughters, told them the news, and, with Melanie's mother, they said their last goodbyes.

Melanie's story illustrates a personalized form of care developed at Franklin Memorial Hospital. The supportive caring that Melanie and her family experienced is the result of a program begun by a nurse, Mary Bayer. Mary, like many nurses, was concerned that health care is increasingly technological and depersonalized, with providers of health care specializing in specific diseases, body systems, or phases of the life cycle. Traditional support systems within families and communities have been fractured for many, or no longer exist for others. Even the promise of an increased life span and improved functioning, the gift of technology, brings a set of problems. Nurses are increasingly challenged to find new approaches to help patients deal with chronic disease, and hopeful, but painful treatment regimes. Even terminal illness presents complex decisions about where and how one will die.

In rural America, personal stories are often played out against a background of struggle within the health care system. The literature abounds with reports of economic woes, difficulties in attracting and retaining qualified professionals, and maintaining their skills in the face of low patient volume. This, combined with growing rural poverty, presents a bleak picture for the future of small hospitals.

In spite of these difficulties, personal problems, as well as personal possibilities stand out in an area where long-term relationships and community ties are the norm. Although the care provided is less complex than at many urban hospitals, it can be of high quality, and the family atmosphere close to home and loved ones offers its own therapeutic benefits. Smallness is an advantage when it results in a sense of family among hospital staff and allows the institution to provide unique services in response to community needs.

The hospital-community link is a vital one in rural areas. Often the hospital is one of the community's largest employers. James Alberns, a rural hospital administrator, points out that "the loss of a hospital just further weakens the fabric of the rural area" (Moore, 1988). In the same article, William Schoen, chief executive officer of Health Management Associates in Naples, Florida, states that a rural community that loses its hospital "must rethink whether it should even be a community." Richard Margolis, a journalist specializing in rural life, speaks eloquently to this in a February 16, 1990, article in the Bangor (Maine) Daily News. He states that small hospitals provide "a certain kind of curing and caring" that cannot be found in big city hospitals, and further states that small hospitals must be viewed in human, as well as financial terms, not left solely to "the mercy of the marketplace."

It is this "special kind of curing and caring" that can make rural hospital nursing deeply rewarding. A relatively stable client and co-worker population allows for the building of strong bonds and supportive, continuing relationships. From this base, problems and projects that require long-term effort can be launched and carried to completion. A thin bureaucratic layer allows nurses at the bedside not only to participate in, but also to provide leadership in areas in which they have interest or concern. Middle managers who are also involved in direct client care and know the day-to-day problems encountered by staff, can find their management inspired by the courage and triumphs of clients and families.

The close and continuing relationships experienced when a few people must work closely together over time inevitably create some friction. In a stable rural community, waiting for a co-worker to move on or to retire may be a long wait. Problems skirted today will inevitably pop up in a similar situation next week or next month. Rural institutions with an eye toward service and customer satisfaction have a vested interest in cooperative employee relationships. The nursing shortage has strengthened nursing's voice within the institution. Increasingly, problem solving at the lowest levels is actively encouraged and supported. This presents both a challenge and an opportunity for those of us in rural hospitals. Problem solving can be difficult and uncomfortable. It also holds out promise for creating a nurturing atmosphere for clients and staff, an atmosphere that is optimal for healing.

The thin layer of bureaucracy, along with the possibility of being personally known and trusted by administration and co-workers in a small institution, can provide many opportunities for creativity. Areas that need attention, or where care can be improved, usually outweigh the available people to work on them. Limited resources in a rural area make it unlikely that health prevention or promotion activities are being duplicated nearby. A nurse with special interests, skills, and knowledge can become a local expert, in demand to share that expertise within the hospital and often the greater community. These opportunities for professional growth are often supported, actively or tacitly, by small hospitals unable to attract known experts and eager to expand or improve existing services.

THE NEED

Hospitalized patients frequently find themselves in crisis situations, often in a crisis which cannot be resolved adequately through the intervention of either the attending physician or the general duty staff nurses alone. In large hospitals, such patients and their families are usually able to obtain crisis intervention services through the medical center's department of psychiatry.

However, in small rural hospitals, where there is neither a department of psychiatry nor an on-site crisis intervention team, patients who experience the emotional trauma which frequently accompanies physical illness or injury are usually without the service which might help them to resolve the crisis more easily.

In the late 1970s, Franklin Memorial Hospital, a 70-bed acute care hospital in Farmington, Maine, experimented with the development of a unique role for a psychiatric nurse, in a position designated as "nurse counselor." The nurse was an American Nurses' Association certified psychiatric/mental health nurse who reported directly to the director of nursing.

Her job description excluded any direct care-giving such as delivering medications or doing treatments, but, rather was intended as a liaison nursing position between nursing staff, physicians, patients, families, and other departments within the hospital. The intent was that the nurse counselor would be able to do some interpretation of diagnosis and prognosis as well as patient/family teaching and counseling. Another role of the nurse was to provide inservice education to the nursing staff regarding interpersonal relationship skills and crisis intervention techniques.

THE ASSESSMENT PHASE

During the initial assessment phase, the nurse counselor met with staff of the various departments within the hospital, investigating how those departments dealt with a variety of crisis situations within the hospital and posed the question, "What is missing?"

The nursing department articulated a need for emotional support for the nursing staff during periods when there were stillborn babies, or when large families were gathered to be supportive to patients in the intensive care units, or when young patients were dying. Other departments echoed similar needs.

The volunteers indicated an interest in learning how to be more supportive to families when there was impending death in the hospital. Most of the volunteers were feeling highly inadequate with families, who often were persons they knew from other settings in the community.

However, this information and cooperation was not gained easily during the first few months. Even though members of various departments were willing to share some of their concerns, the comments were often directed toward the needs they perceived in *other* departments. The nurse counselor was aware of being watched and observed at every turn. Tales of how "certain board members had been against the appointment" began to surface. One prominent physician met her in the hall, looked her over and stated, "So you're the new hot shot, eh? Well, you'll have to prove yourself to me!" and walked away.

As situations came to her attention, the nurse counselor discreetly intervened with patients and families. During the first month, an elderly man was dying and his wife and only daughter were desperately wanting him to live. The nurse spent some time alone with the man, finding out that he felt guilty in dying since his family kept saying they couldn't get along without him. The nurse was able to help him to find the courage to share his feelings with the family. The intervention was successful and patient and family expressed gratitude not only to the nurse, but to the physician as well. The physician, who was skeptical at first, began to refer difficult patient and family situations to the nurse counselor, who was able to handle them effectively.

Another important key to the initial success of the program was the nurse's willingness to be called in during nights and weekends when particularly traumatic events would occur. Her office, which was located near the emergency room, soon became a gathering place for families to wait apart from the general waiting room in the emergency unit.

Because she had a telephone there, families were able to make private calls without subjecting themselves to the eyes and ears of onlookers. Her participation with families also took the pressure from the emergency room personnel, freeing them to busy themselves with attempting to save the life of the patient, yet knowing that families were in capable hands. If the attempt was unsuccessful, the nurse counselor was present while the attending physician spoke with the family. She would then stay on, talking with families until they were ready to leave the hospital. She also spent time in being emotionally supportive to staff after unsuccessful resuscitations or traumatic deaths.

In order to share her knowledge quickly with others in the hospital, during the first few months the nurse counselor began a series of inservice meetings with nursing, social service, and ancillary staff on the topic of coping with death, dying, and crisis. These sessions were held weekly in the afternoon at change of shift for an hour to an hour and a half, and were attended by staff members from many departments. A social worker and a few nurses became very interested in the work and the nurse counselor made a point of supporting them and, when possible, working through them rather than intervening directly with patients herself. Helping other staff to feel effective during difficult situations began to remove the mystique from the intervention theories and, before long, many staff were interacting positively in situations they had shied away from in earlier times. The nurse counselor was always available as a consultant and role model, but attempted to discourage the idea that she was the only person who was able to do this work effectively. She was also quick to share experiences that she found difficult or unsuccessful so that others could readily see that she did not always have all of the answers.

At the same time, the local university invited the nurse counselor to begin teaching a course on the topic of death and dying. Initially about 35 students signed up for this course and within a year and a half the class had become very popular, often drawing as many as 200 students each semester. The students were general college students, as well as members of the community including teachers, emergency technicians, nurses, social workers, and graduate students in need of an elective course.

Within a few months of the initiation of this position, the nurse counselor was frequently invited to speak to a variety of civic groups in the community. She eventually gave presentations at family practice physician conferences, home health agencies, funeral service groups, and the Chaplaincy Program of the hospital.

VOLUNTEER TRAINING

The workshops and lectures soon attracted a group of persons who wanted to volunteer their time in a meaningful way. At the same time, the nurse counselor became aware that there were many occasions in which she would be able to use additional persons for crisis intervention. One person was unable to handle the situation effectively when there were multiple injuries in the emergency room, or when patients who did not necessarily need a professional person could benefit from emotional support from an empathic person. It was decided to attempt an experiment: using specially trained volunteers in a supportive role to patients, with the nurse counselor serving as a supervisor and role model.

Ten volunteers were selected. These volunteers were persons who were already "natural helpers," persons upon whom others frequently called for emotional support and assistance in times of crisis in their lives. The nurse counselor held a series of 3-hour workshops weekly for six weeks with these ten volunteers. The workshops were devoted to teaching crisis intervention techniques, listening/communication skills, and some basic theories about death and dying. The composition of the group in terms of personal life experience was to play an important role in the development of a variety of self-help/support groups for patients and families in the future.

THE SUPPORT TEAM BEGINS

After completing the six-week training sessions, the ten volunteers were coupled into pairs of two and each pair was assigned a full day of volunteering at the hospital, Monday through Friday. The volunteers wore colored lab coats over street clothes when they reported for duty. This identified them as a unique group apart from others already involved in the hospital.

Each day one pair of volunteers would report to the nurse counselor for a briefing during which time the nurse counselor would outline the names and present short histories about the patients who were to be visited by the volunteers on that day. In addition to the planned visits, other priorities were identified throughout the day, which the volunteers would respond to immediately. At those times, the volunteers were instructed to come immediately to the emergency area and receive directions from the nurse counselor who usually wanted them to be supportive of anxious families.

At frequent intervals during the day, the nurse counselor would make contact with the volunteers to advise and support their work with patients and families. At the end of each day the pair of volunteers would meet again with the nurse counselor for a debriefing session and at that time priorities for the following day were identified.

Group meetings were held at monthly intervals. All ten volunteers would meet with the nurse counselor and with members of the Social Service Department for general conversation and discussion regarding the effectiveness of their work. Viewing inservice education videotapes and talks from outside speakers would often be a part of these meetings also.

The group named itself the "Patient Support Team" and within two to three months, they had attained a distinguished reputation within the hospital and the community at large. Prospective members for the team began approaching the nurse counselor asking how they too might become Patient Support Team volunteers.

At one of the group meetings the criterion for new membership was established by the team. This included taking the nurse counselor's "Death and Dying" course taught at the local university. After successful completion of the course, the candidate would then be assigned to an experienced Patient Support Team member. For a six-month period the trainee would be expected to report on a weekly basis for duty, always working with the experienced team member, under the supervision of the nurse counselor. At the end of that six-month period, the candidate would appear before the entire Support Team and satisfactorily answer a series of questions posed by the team. After completing this process, the candidate would then be awarded a certificate as a Patient Support Team member and be allowed to work under the supervision of the nurse counselor.

In the first year of the nurse counselor/support team concept, three of the local clergy also joined the support team. These clergy members were also a part of the Chaplaincy Program at the hospital, a volunteer group from the community which provided a chaplain to the hospital each week.

Frequently these chaplains would invite the nurse counselor to speak at a regular hospital chaplain meeting to share insights and knowledge with the group. In a situation where there was an impending death or serious crisis with a patient who did not have a regular church affiliation and who wished to speak with a clergy person, the support team clergy were able to fill this role. At times when there was no church affiliation and the family was expressing the need for a clergy person to conduct the funeral, one of the support team clergy members was invited to become involved with the patient and family prior to the death. This gave the clergy person an opportunity to gain insight into the patient's personality and past life, thereby enabling him or her to deliver a personal eulogy and funeral service as well as provide emotional support to the family at the time of the death.

SUPPORT GROUPS

As the nurse counselor's reputation grew within the community, she received many requests to do out-patient counseling for a variety of patients who were at home in the community. Among these were stroke patients and their families, cancer patients and their families, and parents whose children had been killed. After discussion with the Patient Support Team and the administration of the hospital, the nurse counselor decided to begin some support groups which would meet on a regular basis at the hospital and would be open to patients and families who were hospitalized as well as to persons living in the community.

Two women on the support team who had previously suffered strokes, along with the nurse counselor and the director of social service, began a monthly support group for stroke patients and their families. At the same time, two cancer patients and another support team member, who had at an earlier time undergone successful surgery for removal of cancer, began a support group for cancer patients and their families.

This group met twice a month in the hospital conference room and frequently included patients who were actively receiving treatment in the acute care setting. Not only did the support team volunteers involve themselves in the group, they also accompanied cancer patients to nearby medical centers when they went for radiation therapy and/or chemotherapy. A team member who was undergoing chemotherapy for Hodgkins Disease spearheaded a program offering to fit wigs to any newly diagnosed cancer patient who was scheduled for chemotherapy and was facing a hair loss. This woman would meet with the cancer patient and bring a supply of wigs in the hopes of matching the patient's hair color, texture, and style prior to the initiation of chemotherapy.

At the end of the first year the nurse counselor was also seeing several families who had recently lost children. She met with these parents on an out-patient basis as individual couples. In the interim, a couple who had lost a teenage daughter in a boating accident several years earlier joined the team. Again, after several discussions within the support team itself, the volunteers plus a couple who had lost a baby agreed to form the nucleus of a Bereaved Parent Group, which began meeting on a monthly basis at the hospital.

The local public health nurse, who was caring for many seriously ill children in the community, as well as supporting parents of babies lost to sudden infant death syndrome, agreed to serve as a co-facilitator of the group along with the nurse counselor. The group drew a number of parents from the community who had lost children of a variety of ages and in many different situations.

As word of the support team and the support groups formulated by this team grew, the nurse counselor and support team members began receiving invitations to speak at rural hospitals in many different parts of the state. They found that other small hospitals were struggling with similar problems and were looking to the group for advice and suggestions as to how they too could begin being more supportive of their patients and families. Several hospitals within the state of Maine have since adopted programs that are similar to the program established at Franklin Memorial Hospital.

BEREAVED PARENTS AS TEACHERS

The Bereaved Parent Group soon became an important factor in the community. After several months of meetings just to share feelings around the death of a child, the group realized that couples in the community continued to have children die. The group felt that their experiences in coping with the loss of a child might be able to help other groups within the community.

In addition to making themselves available to be called into the emergency room at the time of a sudden death of a child, the Bereaved Parent Group also extended itself in an educational mode to various persons within the community such as physicians, clergy members, funeral service providers, and ambulance personnel. They held a series of meetings with these groups, outlining the interventions that they had received which they felt were helpful. Then the parents discussed those interventions which they felt were not helpful at the time of the death of their children.

With the funeral service group, the point was made that parents of dead children have a great need not only to see their children, but to hold their children in their arms following the death. Parents shared their wish to dress their little ones for the last time prior to placement in the casket. Several family members wished that they had been more involved in the preparation of the child's funeral in instances where well-meaning grandparents or friends had taken over, leaving the parents feeling impotent and empty. This behavior had greatly prolonged the parents' grief work.

Because of the conversations with the funeral directors, a number of important changes have been made in our community. Funeral directors have become comfortable with allowing parents to spend long times next to the caskets of their children, and are increasingly involved with surviving siblings and friends, encouraging them to put school pictures and notes and drawings and other meaningful items in the casket prior to its final closing. On many occasions, the entire parent group has attended the funeral and the burial of children, encouraging the newly bereaved parents to do or say whatever they feel is right for them.

The Bereaved Parent Group is frequently invited to speak at various groups throughout the state and has been an important factor in raising the consciousness of health care providers by helping them to cope more effectively with the death of a child. The group came each semester to the nurse counselor's Death and Dying class at the university and spent entire sessions sharing their stories with the students. Feedback from students has been that this class was one of the most moving and effective ones that they experienced in the class and has led to important behavior changes among the students each semester.

As the interest in the support team grew, many new persons were able to complete the rigorous requirements for membership. With a larger group, support team members are able to take turns being on call for emergencies over the weekend, and can be called in at off hours, frequently even in the middle of the night, in order to help patients, families, and hospital staff. After a traumatic death experience in the emergency room, for example, the nurse counselor and/or support team volunteers are able to spend time not only with the family of the deceased person, but also with emergency room and ambulance personnel in order to do a "debriefing" allowing the caregivers an opportunity to vent their feelings of frustration and failure, and to receive support from the group.

In a few short years the hospital was able to close the gap between the services that were provided and the services that were needed in crisis situations. It then could claim a smoothly running intervention program which also serves as an important public relations mechanism between the hospital and the community. The nurse counselor position became a pivotal point in the coordination of problem solving interventions, ongoing inservice education, and as a referral source enabling a skilled volunteer group to continue providing many hundreds of hours each month to a rural community hospital.

THE CHANGING OF THE GUARD

During the fifth year of the support team concept, the original nurse counselor decided to resign in order to pursue new goals. She was able to leave knowing that an important project was underway and that her successor would be building on a firm foundation. This was eight years ago. The successor to this position was privileged with team members who possessed a great deal of skill, experience, and hunger for new knowledge. Status quo is not an option with such motivated individuals.

The new nurse counselor took initiatives designed to enhance the program including biannual retreats to share experiences with each other. Such retreats afford the volunteers an opportunity to focus on themselves, to receive. A cookout contributes to a festive atmosphere during these times of spirit replenishing. The team also takes advantage of educational offerings throughout the state and attends as a group. These opportunities are financed through donations made directly to the support team, generally at the request of a family whose loved one the team has "worked" with. Camaraderie and team spirit are heightened, as well as knowledge gained on these outings.

The professional staff of the hospital, having had their consciousness raised, began to identify still more support needs. Nurses, particularly, were gaining confidence in their capabilities in this support role and managing many instances themselves. Often the team was being activated only for the major support needs such as the death of a child or trauma involving multiple victims (and multiple families). A referral was also initiated during those times when staff or patient acuity dictated that nursing staff's efforts focus on assessment and the tasks involved in meeting the patient's physical needs, while delegating support needs to the team.

Referrals from the professional staff have gone from quickly summoning a support team member during critical situations, to recognizing more subtle indications of needs. They refer patients who are faced with difficult decisions, such as the realization that nursing home placement is their only alternative. They notice that a young woman is admitted with an asthma attack around the anniversary of her husband's death, and team members are called upon to facilitate the woman's grief. When a young couple must spend their anniversary in the hospital because the wife is on intravenous medications because of an exacerbation of Crohn's disease, the team brings a card table adorned with a lace tablecloth and candles. An uninterrupted anniversary celebration is begun.

Staff of departments other than nursing also have become attuned to the nature of the support team work. Laboratory personnel drawing blood from a young patient whose treatment for leukemia is coordinated through a larger city medical center, note the child's mother weeping silently. The mother sobs: "I haven't allowed myself to cry all through this, because I was afraid that my faith wasn't strong enough." The nurse counselor facilitates her grief surrounding her child's diagnosis and treatment. She also assists with arranging a meeting with her clergy.

The x-ray technologist refers the 42-year-old woman who had a positive breast biopsy, and is now in for a bone scan, when she bursts into tears. A support team member stayed with her throughout the procedure and discovered that she had refused support at the time of her positive biopsy because of her own denial of the diagnosis. The bone scan broke through her defense. The patient goes on to attend the Cancer Support Group regularly throughout mastectomy and chemotherapy. Two years later, she is a Reach to Recovery volunteer for the American Cancer Society.

The two previous examples are typical of outpatient referrals from ancillary departments. The emergency room physicians and nursing staff refer directly to the nurse counselor or activate the Patient Support Team. Referrals come from many sources. Inpatient referral need only be cleared through the primary nurse, who decides if the patient's physician need also have input.

DEVELOPMENT OF THE NURSE COUNSELOR'S PROFESSIONAL SKILLS

As the program expanded, the need for the nurse counselor to enhance her skills and knowledge became an issue. She pursued further training through the Elizabeth Kubler-Ross Center in Headwaters, Virginia. This began with participation in a Life, Death, and Transition workshop, a five-day residential, experiential, intensive workshop. These are held throughout the United States and Europe as well, with a goal of resolution of "unfinished business." These are generally attended by persons seeking some resolution of an overwhelming emotional trauma or professionals seeking both self-growth and skill enhancement in working with this population. The nurse counselor found many ways in which the externalization process used in these workshops could be adapted to her work and to the work of the team, and so pursued further training in facilitating this process.

The hospital also supported the nurse counselor's attendance at the Advanced Training Program for the Professionals in Clinical Application of the Simonton Approach. This program is offered through the Health Training and Research Center in Little Rock, Arkansas. This intensive four-day seminar is designed to equip professionals with specific techniques for intervening in life-threatening illness in an effort to aid the recovery of the patient, focusing on emotional needs with the goal of increasing hope and improving the quality of life.

These two major programs, as well as numerous inservices on a more local, smaller scale, demonstrate the extent to which the hospital administration is supportive of this position. The programs ensure the nurse counselor's skills and knowledge are current, and, therefore, the training presented to volunteers and staff, continues to be effective and of high quality. Rural hospitals face a challenge in ensuring such standards are maintained. This is particularly true in this instance, where the nurse counselor is seen as a local expert on the areas of death and dying, and, with the support team, now looks out of state for offerings. The challenge is being met by the sharing of this expertise with other mental health professionals to avoid the one-local-expert syndrome and by attempting to join forces with area health care organizations to finance educational offerings on a local level.

The nurse counselor is now offering a Death and Dying course at the hospital for current and potential support team members. This course is opened to Behavioral Health Services and nursing staff as well. The plan is to continue to offer a Death and Dying course at the hospital on a regular basis, with continuing education and college credits available. This course examines developmental concepts of grief, factors that influence the outcome of grief, stages of dying, languages of dying patients, stages of grieving, commitments to dying persons, hopes and how they change, hospice vs. acute care, death of a patient, death of a child, and one's own death and attitudes.

The nurse counselor is now a member of a Critical Incident Stress Debriefing (CISD) team. These teams have been established to provide a form of crisis intervention specifically designed to assist emergency workers to reduce the number of psychological casualties among their ranks.

A critical incident has been defined by Dr. Jeffery T. Mitchell as, "Any situation faced by emergency service personnel that causes them to experience unusually strong emotional reactions which have the potential to interfere with their ability to function either at the scene or later . . . . All that is necessary is that the incident, regardless of the type, generates unusually strong feelings in the emergency workers." Through the CISD process, emergency personnel are provided a tool to potentially alleviate overwhelming emotional feelings and physical symptoms. The CISD also addresses very real issues that contribute to the loss of valuable employees, thereby salvaging not only careers, but resources, knowledge, expertise, and human caring.

The CISD team consists of a three-member response team. Debriefers are volunteers who are familiar with emergency services. They are carefully selected from the following career groups:

- mental health professionals
- psychologists, social workers
- emergency medical service personnel
- fire service personnel
- chaplains
- EMS instructors

Following application and selection, debriefers receive training in the area of stress and the CISD process. They are committed, not only to the recognition of critical stress in emergency workers, but to provide a means to improve the quality of life for its victims.

A formal debriefing session is optimally conducted 24 to 72 hours following an incident. It should generally not be postponed for longer than one week. On occasion, psychological intervention may be needed on a scene, but a formal debriefing is best held after a 24-hour normalizing period following the incident. The CISD process is available to any emergency service requesting the team services. All information discussed during the debriefing is strictly confidential.

Community providers are so aware of the invaluable service of this team that they themselves now recommend the team's involvement in major traumatic instances. The ambulance on its way in with a SIDS victim asks for assurance that the team has been contacted. A firefighter told of children trapped in a residence engulfed in flame, requests the team be notified. Funeral home directors and clergy members accept an invitation to the Bereaved Parents Group to hear what has and has not been helpful in these parents' experiences. Mental health providers request the nurse counselor's expertise with a client who has experienced multiple major losses. School guidance counselors request the nurse counselor's input in planning development of a crisis team. The reciprocity and, again, caring among residents, care providers, businesses, and institutions represents and is representative of the sense of community experienced in this rural setting.

EXPANSION OF SERVICES

Franklin Memorial Hospital developed other progressive programs in the attempt to keep pace with the community's needs. The nurse counselor role was one of the first positions initiated which focused on the emotional and/or mental health aspects of patient care. The success of the nurse counselor led to a larger case load than one professional could manage. The Patient Support Team's inception developed out of the increasing demand, as well as from a recognition that well-trained volunteers could often make contributions of a high quality. Volunteerism in itself generates enthusiasm in both the staff and volunteers and provides an opportunity for community involvement in its hospital.

The recognition that patients' support needs were being met so well with this position in place, led to exploration of other areas. The staff identified areas where they were not managing services as well as they would like. Emergency Mental Health Services emerged as another major area where improved care could be addressed. The development of this service is discussed next.

Emergency Mental Health Services

Funded through a Maine State Bureau of Mental Health and Mental Retardation Grant, the Emergency Mental Health Service called upon both hospital and community resources to work collaboratively to meet the emergency mental health needs of the community. The nurse counselor joined with the staff of Social Service, as well as many of the community mental health providers, in a training program to provide crisis intervention out of the hospital's emergency room. The local mental health clinic provides those services on a nine-to-five, Monday-through-Friday basis. Now they would be available 24 hours a day, seven days a week. The service was established six years ago. It has undergone changes to improve delivery, and it remains a viable service.

Philosophy. A community mental health perspective may describe mental health in terms of a balance of stressors and supports that exist between a client and the biopsychosocial environment. Mental illness may be viewed as a negative balance in this relationship, and may be more positively balanced by interventions in primary and secondary prevention activities. Primary prevention focuses on mental health promotion and illness prevention, while secondary prevention activities involve early assessment, diagnosis, and treatment of those clients with acute mental health difficulties or illnesses (Flaskerud & Servellen, 1985).

Process. A Certificate of Need was submitted to the state by the 70-bed community hospital. It was approved. A state-supported grant was awarded for the development of an emergency mental health service. Issues relating to program development, management, staff recruitment and training, and clinical functions were coordinated by hospital-employed clinicians and a medical director of the program. Some of these issues addressed the need for psychiatric supervision of clinicians; coordination of the program with other community mental health resources; and how to meet the expanding need for crisis intervention services as state hospitals for the mentally ill decreased their availability of hospital beds. A 24-hour service was developed, with an accessibility to any client who came to the hospital emergency room in a psychiatric/ mental health crisis. An on-call system used first response mental health professionals, which included psychiatric nurses. They provided direct client assessment at the emergency room. Additional on-call backup was provided by psychologists and a psychiatrist for any consultation requested by the first response clinicians. Such consultation is required in the involuntary committal process. Full- and part-time clinical staff were available in addition to on-call personnel.

The Nurses' Role. As first response providers, psychiatric nurses are in a unique position in a potential mental health crisis. Their educational preparation provides them with an ability to consider an individual client's physical, emotional, and spiritual needs, within the context of the needs of the community. The following paragraphs describe more specifically those psychiatric nursing interventions in primary and secondary prevention in the emergency mental health service described previously.

Primary prevention activities encompassed a variety of both client and community interventions. For example, information on the mission and accessibility of the service were described during an interview with a local radio show host, as part of a continuing weekly series on health-related topics. Another community presentation by the psychiatric nurse—on eating disorders—was done in collaboration with a hospital nutritionist.

Consultation was another activity used on the primary prevention level. The "client" presented in a variety of ways: for example, as a nursing staff member requesting assistance to set behavioral limits on the inappropriate behavior of an inpatient on the medical floor; or as a hospital department head seeking support in dealing with a particularly sensitive issue regarding a staff member. Community clients include the police or sheriff's department requesting assistance in forming a protocol for the supervision of suicidal inmates. Another example of a client was a school district crisis management team requesting information on how to access the service.

Crisis intervention services were a part of a primary prevention effort, with the goal of illness prevention, and included psychiatric liaison activities. Emergency room requests for emergency mental health evaluations were a particularly valuable entry point for crisis intervention. For example, a hospital employee overwhelmed by personal and/or family stress or a college student in crisis, referred by a college counselor, was seen immediately in the emergency room. Assessment and intervention activities were begun. Psychiatric nursing interventions were aimed at the most effective way to decrease the potential or present use of maladaptive coping behaviors by the person in crisis.

Other nursing interventions at the primary prevention level included assistance in the formation of coalitions, task forces, or support groups. Membership in a local substance abuse coalition fostered a sense of team partnership and collaboration between persons concerned with the impact of chemical use issues on both the individual and the community. The networking between coalition members facilitated a consistent and united approach to the prevention of substance abuse.

Psychiatric nursing interventions also included secondary prevention activities in rapid accessibility to treatment from a wide spectrum of therapeutic approaches and arranging for psychiatric hospitalization when needed. Clients could rapidly access the emergency service and be assessed within 30 minutes after the on-call first response provider was notified. This access facilitated an early case-finding approach, as clients were not deterred from seeking treatment by a lengthy wait.

Following patient assessment and evaluation, the client participated in a written treatment plan to meet his or her needs. A treatment plan could include referral to a local counseling center, private therapist, a therapy group, or support group. If indicated, the psychiatric nurse could intervene by recommending voluntary or involuntary hospitalization and discuss this further with supporting staff on second response emergency call.

Other Services Expand

Chemical dependency services became the next target area. Community needs were assessed to be that of inpatient medical detoxification, without traveling 80 to 100 miles and more to outpatient services. A Certificate of Need was approved by the state for two detoxification beds. The professional hired to serve the detoxification patients also received training for provision of emergency mental health services.

A Young Widows/Widowers Support Group was offered for a two-year period. There was a population of six to 12 persons identified with this immediate need. The group's attendance ranged from two to 15 with an average of five. It was discontinued as the population changed, but would be restarted should the need arise. The nurse counselor attended initial meetings of an ongoing Crohn's Syndrome Support Group, also in response to a population's voiced needs. This group began with the intent to be a self-help group with shared responsibilities for facilitation, and continues to meet regularly three years later. A Cardiac Support Group became incorporated into the hospital's Cardiac Rehabilitation Program. This is activated as the population dictates.

The support groups currently functioning are the Bereaved Parent Support Group and the Cancer Support Group. The Bereaved Parent Support Group is open to parents and grandparents who have lost a child of any age to any cause. Attendance ranges from ten to 30, with an average attendance of 15 persons. Cancer Support Group attendees include patients with cancer, those whose loved ones have cancer, those who have lost loved ones to cancer and caregivers seeking both support for themselves as well as improved care approaches for their patients with cancer.

Both groups are deeply committed to maintaining a confidential, nonjudgmental environment in which to share feelings, ideas, and experiences. The underlying philosophy of the Cancer Support Group is that individuals can and do indeed have an effect on their illness or their wellness and that "beating it" means living fully and consciously every moment one has. They have enjoyed many survival stories and have shared the sadness of loss as well. The Bereaved Parent Group shares a sense that this is the one place where someone really does have some idea of what they are going through. They share among themselves what has helped them to survive and to recover to whatever degree possible.

The need for more integration among the hospital's mental health services became apparent as their numbers continued to grow. A new department was created, Behavioral Health Services, which integrated Emergency Mental Health, Chemical Dependency, Patient Support, and Social Services. The intent is to cross-train staff in each of these areas, and for all to participate in covering emergency mental health services. This process is ongoing and includes the goal of each mental health professional being adequately trained to respond to off-hours support needs and coordinate support team involvement as necessary.

The routine for the Patient Support Team has not changed a great deal. This is not due to an "if it works, don't fix it" approach. The service continues to be critiqued at the monthly meetings and now at the Behavioral Health Services meetings as well, and minor adjustments have been made as needed. Documentation, as is so with other areas of health care, is increasingly scrutinized. Consideration is being given to use of a sticker to be placed in progress notes upon a patient's or family's referral to the Patient Support Team. This need is recognized mainly when volunteers, who do not have access to patient charts, are called in during off-hours. They then report to the patient's nurse, who charts their involvement. This requires perusal of all progress notes to see who on the team is involved. Documentation in these instances is often limited to "Patient Support Team with family," leaving much to the imagination about how the family/patient was perceived by the support team member involved. It is wonderful to be at a point where fine-tuning is now needed.

REWARDS:
MAINTAINING MOTIVATION OF VOLUNTEERS

The expansion of services was linked with the expansion of volunteer numbers and activities. Rewarding these people was a joyful responsibility. The Patient Support Team has given an average of 2,700 hours annually over the last three years. The team member's hours are maintained in a log which is completed for each hospital contact. These volunteers are included in the recognition extended to all other hospital volunteers. Currently, this includes an annual recognition dinner held at a local restaurant, complete with certificates of appreciation presented by the hospital president. This dinner is held during National Volunteer Appreciation Week.

Volunteers are invited to hospital activities such as the annual Christmas Party free of charge. Volunteers, in general, are viewed with a great deal of respect both within the institution and the community. Many of them are retired professionals and their participation expresses the deep sense of commitment of the helping profession. Others of them have had specific life experiences that have left them with a feeling that they want to give something back of what they received in a time of need. They reflect the attitude of Alcoholics Anonymous whose underlying philosophy that to keep it, you must give it away. Still others of these volunteers simply desire to extend themselves beyond tasks and become more deeply involved in persons' lives.

The support team volunteers are distinguishable throughout the hospital in their gold-colored jackets and are deeply appreciated by staff for the skill and caring they bring to patients. Nursing recognizes their contribution. This is particularly gratifying because nurses are generally capable and knowledgeable in areas of patient support. Most nurses realistically accept that they are not always in a position to be available to their patients' emotional needs. The nurse counselor and support team members closely coordinate their activities with the patient's primary nurse. The nurse is viewed as the pivotal caregiver who is in the best position to assess total patient needs. An attitude of mutual respect and appreciation with a shared goal of optimal patient care enhances this working relationship.

Currently the team's certified members include a retired nurse whose brother died of cancer and whose husband is a volunteer; a retired laboratory technician whose husband died suddenly, shortly before retirement, and who has several family members who have died of cancer. A young woman with an undiagnosed, painful, and occasionally restricting neuromuscular disorder who also had breast cancer treated with lumpectomy and radiation has been a member for several years. A retired schoolteacher and her retired postmaster husband joined the team. Their 20-year-old daughter died in a boating accident 14 years ago. They helped start the Bereaved Parent Group. Another couple on the team consists of a retired housekeeper and her retired auto mechanic/truck driver husband. She is a cancer survivor of 20 years, he a cardiac patient and recovering alcoholic. They had a stillborn child and a 24-year-old son who died in an auto accident. They also helped initiate the Bereaved Parents Group, as well as the Cancer Support Group. A young woman who had major surgery at this hospital with a likelihood of a cancer diagnosis and who remembered the team's support is a member. She is a unit secretary in the hospital.

SUMMARY

Franklin Memorial Hospital has been a forerunner in recognizing and reaching out to meet the emotional needs of patients and their families. Anxiety and suspicion on the part of some staff in the early years has given way to the cry of "where are the nurse counselors, where is the Patient Support Team?" when a crisis arises. Each volunteer who completes the arduous certification process and goes on to work semi-independently, demonstrates the extent and quality which volunteer service with careful professional direction and support can provide.

Franklin Memorial Hospital deals creatively with an aspect of patient care that is critical to and synonymous with community hospitals—caring. Consideration of the individual as such, with their families considered in their total care, and friends and community considered as their "extended family," contributes to the uniqueness of health care(ing) in a rural setting.

REFERENCES

Flaskerud, J., & Servellen, G. (1985). *Community mental health nursing: Theories and methods.* Connecticut: Appleton-Century-Crofts.

Moore, M. (1988). A round table discussion—Rural health care in America. *Federation of American Health Systems Review,* 39–43.

Reilly, W. E. (1990, February 16). Benefits of small, rural hospitals cited. *Bangor Daily News.*

Part III

Management

10

The Role of Rural Community Hospitals: Opportunities and Challenges for Rural Health Nurses and Nursing

Julia C. Tiffany
Margaret Hourigan

Several authors (Christianson, Moscovice, Wellever, & Wingert, 1990; Ermann, 1990; Moscovice, 1989; Joint Task Force of the National Association of Community Health Centers and The National Rural Health Association, 1989; Moscovice & Rosenblatt, 1986; Mullner & Whiteis, 1988) identify problems facing rural hospitals and health care providers today. Physicians, nurses, and other health care providers serving in rural areas suffer particular frustrations as a result of professional isolation, limited support services, insufficient continuing education opportunities, limited peer contact, and excessive work loads and time demands. Financial problems result from the need for rural hospitals to serve large populations of uninsured, underinsured, elderly whose care is reimbursed by an inequitable Medicare system. As a result of economic constraints, many rural institutions lack complete facilities or suffer from outdated physical plants and inadequate equipment. Many also experience limitations in their ability to provide support services because of difficulties in recruiting personnel. Rural hospitals face hardships when competing for nurses and other care providers because of rising salaries, shortages, and increased demands for care. These factors combine to foster a perception that rural hospitals and thus rural health care providers offer poor-quality care.

The literature depicts the small rural community hospital as an institution bordering on collapse evidenced through closed beds, cuts in services, and dwindling staffs. It describes these hospitals as bereft of medical staff and, as a result of economic conditions, unable to keep up with technology and resources needed to attract physicians.

Although little is mentioned in the literature regarding successful small rural community hospitals, it is the authors' experience that such organizations do exist. They not only provide health care to their communities, they also provide jobs for local residents and financial support to local businesses. Our experience shows that rural community hospitals can not only survive but thrive when the board of trustees, the administration, and the medical staff develop and enact a common philosophy, work cooperatively to settle problems, respect each others' unique roles and contributions, and actively anticipate future needs and changes in health care. This common spirit is demonstrated through the employment and retention of highly qualified personnel, purchase of state-of-the-art equipment, creation of an environment that exacts excellent patient outcomes, promotion of a professional nursing staff of expert generalists, and fostering of a lean, efficient management team.

A MODEL FOR SUCCESS IN A
RURAL COMMUNITY HOSPITAL

A 50-bed community hospital in Western Maine is one example of a successful rural community hospital. This hospital enjoyed an 84 percent occupancy rate during 1990. It has sustained continued growth and development over the course of many years. Understanding its history, developmental process, and characteristics may be helpful to other institutions and practitioners bent on providing rural health care.

The hospital, accredited by the JCAHCO (Joint Committee for Accreditation of Health Care Organizations) and licensed by the state, is part of a corporation that also owns a 109-bed nursing home, a nine-bed boarding home, and two medical office buildings. Its birth demonstrates the collegiality and spirit perhaps reflective of other rural communities. In 1947, a group of local businessmen, intent on drawing new industry into the area, determined that the community needed more physicians in order to be more attractive. They additionally determined that, in order to attract physicians, the community must have a hospital.

With Yankee independence and a desire for autonomy, they chose not to apply for federal funding through the Hill-Burton Act but rather raised necessary monies from community donations and private loans. The effort proved successful. The next ten years evidenced the opening of a 25-bed hospital and the recruitment of six physicians.

In 1968, the current chief executive officer (CEO) was hired. While management theory alludes to the benefits of high-level administrators moving on after eight to ten years, the longevity and influence of this CEO has been a powerful force in the hospital's development and continued success. On accepting the position, he negotiated that, for the first time, a physician would be a voting member of the board. He and the board then articulated a mission statement that has continued to guide and influence the hospital's growth even to this day. The hospital's mission is simply, tacitly, and philosophically to provide state-of-the-art equipment and highly qualified people for the delivery of health care to the community.

At the time of the CEO's appointment, the hospital was medically staffed by five general practitioners and an orthopedic surgeon. Early on, the CEO determined the need to upgrade the laboratory and radiology equipment in order to expand diagnostic capabilities. By 1972, a board certified radiologist, a pathologist, and a general surgeon had joined the medical staff.

Assuming that a physician office building adjacent to the hospital would attract even more physicians, the CEO convinced the board to make such a purchase. In 1973, two internists joined the medical staff.

During the 1970s, the hospital expanded by developing physical therapy and respiratory therapy departments. A library was built and other resources were developed to ensure continued staff development. Increasing staff and services precipitated the need for a new and larger physical plant. The year 1979 evidenced the completion of a 50-bed facility funded, again, solely through community donations and private loans. Continuing development and growth through the 1980s has resulted in a current medical staff that includes five internists, three general surgeons, three orthopedic surgeons, two anesthesiologists, four family practitioners, two radiologists, a urologist, two pathologists, four emergency physicians, and an occupational health physician.

This 50-bed hospital offers a breadth of facilities, programs, and services more typically seen in larger institutions. The physical plant houses a four-bed maternity unit which includes a recently redesigned family centered birthing room, a 42-bed medical-surgical unit, and a four-bed special care unit, as well as an emergency department, operating suite, and ambulatory surgical unit. Services provided by the hospital include emergency transport, an outpatient chemical dependency treatment program, and an occupational health program which includes inpatient and outpatient physical therapy, sports medicine, and health education. The radiology department includes equipment and personnel capable of x-ray, nuclear diagnostics, mammography, and ultrasound. The department contracts out for needed computerized tomography. The social service and discharge planning departments ensure continuity in patient care.

A combination of forces and factors have coalesced to influence and ensure this hospital's success. Strong and consistent leadership exhibited through the board and the CEO, a clear and viable mission, community support evidenced through contributions and through use of the hospital, a modern physical plant, and state-of-the-art equipment have joined to create an environment which draws quality personnel. Quality personnel attract patients. Patients generate income which can be used to further develop the facilities. Success breeds success.

Because of rising health care costs and weakening rural economies, many policymakers and rural health leaders today are suggesting that the country cannot afford to sustain rural services. They argue that rural communities and third-party payers cannot afford to sustain rural health care—particularly those services requiring hospitals. Goldsmith (1989) predicts that "except for major regional institutions, the acute-care hospital as we know it will probably not survive. . . . The hospital of the future will reach out into homes and residential communities" (p. 195). With an increasing emphasis on ambulatory care centers, outpatient services, and home care, one might ask whether or not, with the exception of large full-service institutions, hospitals of *any* kind and in *any* location are dinosaurs in their own time.

In order to comprehend the question surrounding the place of rural hospitals in our system, it is necessary to understand the history and context of American health care and the roles of physicians and hospitals in bringing us to both the heights and the depths evidenced in our health care system today.

THE ROLE OF HOSPITALS IN AMERICAN HEALTH CARE

Though a myriad of health-related disciplines evolved and developed throughout the 20th century, the physician remains, to this day, central to the delivery of health care in this country. Health care equates with medical care. The American people would have it no other way. As Goldsmith (1989) describes, "health services are a neighborhood business, beginning and ending with a doctor and a patient" (p. 105).

While physicians are central to health care, hospitals are central to physicians. Moscovice and Rosenblatt (1986) depict the doctor-hospital dyad as "a closely knit, symbiotic relationship. . . . Doctors need the hospital because of its income potential for their practice and also because of their desire to deliver comprehensive health care to their patients." (p. 26). Starr (1982) states that "we now think of hospitals as the most visible embodiment of medical care in its technically most sophisticated form" (p. 145).

Hospitals have undergone a radical metamorphosis within the last 100 years. In that time, their role and significance to health care in America has changed dramatically. Goldsmith (1989) suggests that hospitals evolved as "creatures of the Industrial Revolution. They were intended to be warehouses for unfortunates dying of tuberculosis, smallpox, pneumonia, and other infectious diseases" (p. 106).

Starr (1982) documents well the transformation of hospitals from "places of dreaded impurity and exiled human wreckage . . . (to) the most visible embodiment of medical care in its technically most sophisticated form" (p. 145). Following the Civil War and into the early 20th century, increasing industrialization drove large numbers of people into urban areas, preventing their traditional reliance on family and community for care when ill or injured. Crowded conditions in urban areas spawned new illnesses and health problems.

The advent of antiseptic surgery performed under anesthesia offered physicians and patients a plethora of new treatment options. Performing surgery in the home or office where patients and physicians had traditionally met proved unrealistic and inadequate. Increasingly, physicians looked to hospitals to serve as a central location for treating patients. Growth in the volume of surgeries served as the basis for hospital expansion and profit. With greater pressure for admission, hospitals shifted from terminal care for the poor to acute care for the populace.

During the same time, changes in nurses and in nursing played a significant role in the metamorphosis of hospitals and in the successful outcomes evidenced by the advances in medical care. Heeding the lessons and role-modeling of Florence Nightingale, American nurses established training schools and actively recruited "wholesome daughters of the middle class" (Starr, 1982, p. 155) into nursing. Nursing's attention to and concern with cleanliness, ventilation, nutrition, and psycho-social as well as physical concerns markedly improved patient survival, recuperation, and well-being.

Medicine itself remained in a very formative and, therefore, vulnerable stage during this period. Physician leaders concentrated on delineating, organizing, and standardizing medical care and medical education—thus "staking-out" medicine's central role in the delivery of health care. Changes in and the evolution of nursing, therefore, served as a threat to the development of medicine.

The societal context of the late 1800s and early 1900s prescribed clear differentiation regarding male and female roles and relationships. Men were literal and figurative "captains of the ship" in all aspects of life. As a result, and by way of following societal mores, female nurses acquiesced to the domination of male physicians both individually and collectively. As new health care disciplines evolved during the 20th century, they too accepted the central role of the physician. In hospitals, physicians controlled admissions and determined even the minutia of patient care. Thus, hospitals evolved as medical institutions. Admitting physicians became the hospital's chief source of income and, eventually, their entire reason for existing.

Unlike other bureaucracies in America, hospitals remained, for the most part, independent and parochially controlled. Until the early 1920s, physician staff appointments to hospitals were limited to a small, professional elite. General practitioners, particularly those in more rural areas, grew increasingly anxious as they practiced under the simultaneous pressures of overwork, lack of access to new technology, and loss of patients to hospitals and specialists in urban areas. The American Medical Association (AMA) responded to these physicians' anxieties by advocating for the development of local, autonomous hospitals. The association held that every doctor should have a hospital within his or her easy access. In the absence of an organized health care system, these hospitals, though small in size, reflected the needs and priorities of their respective communities as determined by local physicians and hospital administrators (Stevens, 1989).

Spreading hospitals over the country encouraged, or at least allowed, doctors to practice in rural areas. This move enhanced the distribution of health care to the broad population. Americans began to depend on easy access to physicians and to hospitals. Health care came to be seen as a basic right rather than a privilege.

Americans bestowed great confidence in the capacity of physicians to prevent and cure disease. Medical research generated new knowledge and precipitated the evolution of new fields and areas of specialization within medicine. Increasingly, medical diagnosis, monitoring, and treatment involved technological innovations and complex interventions on acutely ill patients who would have, in an earlier time, died from their diseases and injuries. Medical care previously provided in homes and private offices moved into hospitals. The number of hospitals escalated rapidly as did the importance of their role in the delivery of American health care. Starr (1982) states, "hospitals replaced private practitioners as the most powerful force in the . . . medical system" (p. 359).

In the 1920s, efforts mounted by the American College of Surgeons, sought to reform and standardize hospitals. Nationwide, hospitals adopted the prescribed standards in an effort to preempt more thorough government regulation. Over time, hospitals, as described by Starr (1982) "came to present the familiar American paradox of a system of very great uniformity and very little coordination" (p. 177). Emulating one another, hospitals offered the same services regardless of the overall needs of their communities.

Each war in our history has served as a bridge to better and more advanced health care. Following World War II and for the first time in our history, public monies, under the Hill-Burton Act of 1946, poured into hospital construction in response to diagnostic and treatment innovations spawned by the need to treat large numbers of critically injured and ill people. These monies also served to generate much needed new businesses and new jobs.

The decision to provide construction funds for community hospitals put the power and resources of public finance solidly behind the development and expansion of hospitals. In order to minimize the threat of politics at the bedside and thus the inviolate patient-doctor relationship, Hill-Burton, following precedent and pressure from the AMA, specifically barred any federal regulation of hospital policy. The interrelationship and interdependence among patient, physician, and hospital remained sacrosanct even during this initial time of public finance.

Through the 1950s, the public continued to demand increasingly greater access to medical services and thus to hospitals. Americans wanted the full benefits of modern medicine readily available and close to home. Costs soared with demand and with care innovations and capabilities. Three distinct sectors of medical care evolved, each having its own impact on the delivery and construct of health care. First, complex and expansive medical centers focused on generating research and providing training. Second, large numbers of practitioners followed patients to the suburbs where they established private, office-based practices. Finally, and by far the smallest in number and lowest in prestige, a few physicians sought to provide care in rural and inner-city settings (Starr, 1982).

Inequities evidenced during this time did not go unnoticed. Policymakers and the public began to recognize that abundance and scarcity existed side by side. Starr (1982) describes, "medicine had been a metaphor for progress, but to many it was not becoming a symbol of the continuing . . . irrationalities of American life" (p. 363). To equalize the distribution of health care, Congress, in 1964, adopted recommendations from the Debakey Commission which called for an infusion of federal funds to establish regional health centers—local diagnostic and treatment stations and medical complexes.

Recognizing the inequities inherent in the health care system, increasingly broad constituencies additionally demanded a compulsory health insurance system—a system that would meet the needs of the elderly and the poor. In 1965, the American health care system underwent a revolutionary change. President Johnson signed Medicare and Medicaid into law. Buoyed by popular approval, Medicare, with its uniform national standards for eligibility and benefits, provided hospital insurance programs and government-subsidized voluntary insurance to cover health care costs for those on Social Security. Medicaid, providing health care benefits for the needy, left to the states decisions regarding how extensive service to the poor would be. Both assuaged the American ideal of altruism by caring for the needs of the elderly and poor.

While expanding funding, the government sought to reassure physicians and hospitals that it would make no effort to control them. To appease concern and resistance, it adopted the practice of paying according to costs rather than according to a schedule of negotiated rates. This approach proved extremely favorable to physicians and hospitals alike. Both Medicare and Medicaid gave physicians and hospitals the license to spend (Stevens, 1989).

Medical costs rose uncontrollably. Through Medicare and Medicaid, the federal government had declared that, regardless of income, health care was the public's right (Stevens, 1989). The government then proceeded to allocate ever-increasing funds to ensure that right.

During the 1970s and into the 1980s, hospitals and physicians alike grew increasingly dependent on third-party reimbursement through Medicare, Medicaid, and insurance companies. By 1980, more than 92 percent of hospital expenditures flowed through third-party payment systems (Blaney & Hobson, 1988). Unlike other economic models driven by a balance of supply and demand, however, health care demand and use rose despite rising costs. Cost containment in health care became a national issue in public and private sectors. The health care financial environment, delineated by retrospective reimbursement and readily available capital for expansion and renovation, mandated attention and the need for change.

In 1982, Chrysler Corporation, frustrated by escalating health care costs, began to collect detailed information on their employees' use of the health care system. They developed audits, screened hospital admissions, and pressed for outpatient services whenever feasible in an effort to gain some semblance of control over health care costs. During its first year, Chrysler reported savings of $20 million over its original health care budget. Its second year evidenced a savings of $58 million (Stevens, 1989).

Government too responded. The Tax Equity and Fiscal Responsibility Act (TEFRA) of 1982, in response to a hospital sector inflationary rate three times higher than the overall rate of inflation and in response to fears that the Medicare program would be shortly bankrupt, called for the development of a prospective payment system for Medicare. In early 1983, the federal government, moving with unusual speed and unanimity, reversed key economic incentives which had previously driven the behavior of hospitals and physicians. Instead of reimbursing hospitals on a cost-incurred basis, Medicare now reimbursed hospital care through a set of predetermined fees which varied according to diagnosis. The system rewarded hospitals for early discharges and encouraged them to weigh the benefit of technically dependent and expensive interventions (Mullner, Rydman, & Whiteis, 1990). Prospective payment and cost containment have now become the focus of, and a driving force behind, health care for the 1990s (Kalisch & Kalisch, 1986).

DILEMMAS AND CHALLENGES IN RURAL HEALTH CARE

Rural hospitals, and thus, rural health care, are struggling to survive as we enter the 1990s. A confluence of regional and national developments creates the context and establishes the reasons for current problems in rural health. The deterioration of rural economies, demographic trends toward older, poorer, and underinsured rural populations, and reduced opportunities for public support through tax revenues and donations, fuels the struggle (Patton, 1989). Additionally, rural hospitals evidence difficulty in their ability to respond to pressures created by changes in the American health system. Recent shifts from inpatient to outpatient settings juxtaposed by rapid advances in and increasing dependence on medical technology have resulted in an increased need for capital, precipitating competition for patients (Moscovice, 1989). Increasingly, rural hospitals must compete for patients as rural residents prove willing to travel long distances for care in urban medical centers (Amundson & Hughes, 1989).

Norton and McManus (1989) found that in 1985, only 20 percent of the nation's physicians practiced in rural areas. Throughout the history of medicine's development, and increasingly today, physicians rely on hospitals in order to provide the sophisticated and technologically dependent form of health care expected of and aspired to by medical practitioners and their patients. Problems faced by rural community hospitals may thus play a significant role in precipitating difficulties experienced in recruiting and retaining physicians.

Rabinowitz (1988), reviewing the geographic origins of medical students, noted a decline in the number of medical school matriculants from small towns and rural areas. History evidences that students from rural areas are more likely to return to practice in rural areas. Rabinowitz suggests that this shrinking pool of applicants may reflect problems in teaching and counseling in rural secondary schools.

Prior to 1988, the National Health Service Corps placed physicians in rural areas as part of a pay-back system for the cost of their medical education. Today, however, the corps seems in the process of being dismantled as a result of recent budget cuts and the establishment of new priorities. In 1988, 1,700 physicians were placed in rural areas by the corps. This number decreased to 900 in 1989 and 500 in 1990 (Joint Task Force of the National Association of Community Health Centers & the National Rural Health Association, 1989).

Data on rural hospitals for the period spanning 1979 to 1985 evidences perplexing information. During this time, the physician-population ratio stood at 163:100,000 in urban areas but 53:100,000 in rural areas—an impressive difference especially given travel and distance imperatives. Though 25 percent of all Americans lived in rural communities, these areas received 42 percent fewer health dollars and 50 percent fewer social service dollars when compared with urban areas. During this time, 50 percent of the hospitals in America were defined as rural though they held 23 percent of the beds, admitted 20 percent of the inpatients, performed 17 percent of the surgeries, and delivered 19 percent of the babies. While occupancy rates decreased from 76 percent to 65 percent for hospitals across the country, occupancy of rural hospitals fell to 56 percent (Moscovice, 1989; Winter, 1990).

Using these data as rationale, Congress created a two-tier system of reimbursement when implementing the TEFRA-mandated prospective payment system for Medicare recipients. Under this system, Medicare paid from 35 percent to 40 percent less for a service in a rural hospital compared with the same service in an urban hospital. The impact on rural hospitals proved debilitating. One hospital, for example, found itself spending $.24 out of every dollar to cover the Medicare shortfall (Chase, 1989).

Between 1980 and 1989, 163 rural community hospitals closed. Six hundred more face closure in the next five years

(DeLeon, Wakefield, Schultz, Williams, & VandenBos, 1989). Medicare's prospective payment system and inequities in financial reimbursement are identified as critical factors precipitating these closures (Christianson, Moscovice, Wellever, & Wingert, 1990; Ermann, 1990; Moscovice, 1989; Patton, 1989). What is the impact of so many rural community hospitals closing?

In addition to generating financial difficulties, the two-tier system of Medicare payment generated a perception of rural community hospitals, practitioners, hospital administrators, and even rural residents as second-class. Patton (1989) describes the effect of this perception when he states, "Medicare's prospective payment system (PPS) proved to be an explosive political catalyst. . . . PPS quickly became a metaphor for the federal government's insensitivity to rural needs. In short order, rural hospitals launched . . . a seemingly uncoordinated but relentless lobbying campaign" (p. 1007).

Government responded. In 1986, the Senate created a Rural Health Caucus, followed in 1987 by the House of Representatives' establishment of a Rural Health Coalition. These bodies represent special interest groups composed of those concerned with the availability of quality health care in rural areas. By 1989, 50 percent of the Senate and 20 percent of the House held membership in one of these committees (Patton, 1989).

Legislative actions also attempted to improve the operating environments of rural hospitals. In 1986, the 99th Congress passed an act to assist rural hospitals with capital payments. Congress also instituted a special category for sole community providers. The 100th Congress reduced, though did not eliminate, the urban-rural differential in Medicare payments to rural hospitals (Moscovice, 1989).

In 1987, the Executive Branch of the government responded to the plight of rural hospitals, health care providers, and residents by creating the Office of Rural Health Policy housed within the Public Health Service. The Omnibus Budget Reconciliation Act of that year directed the office to evaluate the financial viability of small rural hospitals, determine their ability to attract and retain physicians and other health professionals, determine access to quality health care, establish and maintain a clearinghouse for collecting and disseminating information on rural health care issues, and advise the secretary of the department of Health and Human Services regarding the effects of policies and proposed statutory changes on rural health (DeLeon et al., 1989). Even with these changes and interventions, however, Moscovice (1989) opines that rural hospitals remain at risk.

What does it matter whether or not rural hospitals face enormous problems and potential closure? Is a hospital essential for the provision of health care in a community? What is the effect of a rural hospital's closure?

The literature and this country's approach to current problems in health care center on economic concerns and viability. There is little evidence that research and policy attend to patients' or communities' perceived needs or desires. In order to explore the implications and feasibility of downsizing and limiting access to hospitals, the authors examined a cross-section of hospitalized patients on one day in the above-mentioned 50-bed rural hospital. Time negated the ability to explore outpatient and emergency services and to describe those services offered residents of the nursing home or the boarding home.

A DAY IN THE LIFE OF A
RURAL COMMUNITY HOSPITAL

On this particular day in January 1991, the hospital served 48 inpatients. An assessment of the diagnoses, treatment modalities, care requirements, demographics, and social dynamics of these patients suggests seven major categories delineating the reasons for their hospitalization:

Treatment of Acute Illness or Injury

- A 21-year-old male recovers from surgery which repaired a liver laceration and accomplished a spleenectomy following blunt abdominal trauma from a skiing accident.
- A 40-year-old female receives IV antibiotics and oxygen therapy to treat her bilateral pneumonia.

Elective Surgery

- A 27-year-old male is admitted with degenerative disk disease for elective laminectomy surgery.

Treatment of Complications of Chronic Conditions

- A 95-year-old woman is admitted from a nursing home with an unspecified infection requiring antibiotic IV therapy. She suffers from congestive heart failure and renal failure and requires medication adjustment and stabilization.

The Need for Diagnosis and Referral

- An 83-year-old man is admitted from the boarding home after he attacked two residents and a staff person. His admission seeks to assess the reasons for his apparent dementia and aggressive behavior and to make plans for alternative placement in a facility that can handle his behavior.

- A 38-year-old female is admitted with diarrhea and weight loss. She requires fluid and electrolyte stabilization prior to undergoing diagnostic work-up to rule out Crohn's disease.

Social-Circumstance Preventing Discharge or Referral

- A 10-year-old boy is admitted for antibiotic therapy to treat osteomyelitis. Although responding well to the therapy, social circumstances prevent his discharge home. His exhausted HIV-positive mother must care for her husband, the boy's stepfather, who is dying from AIDS.

- A 75-year-old male is admitted from home to treat a chronically dislocated hip. He requires placement in a nursing home because his wife of many years has begun divorce proceedings. She refuses to provide appropriate information and institute procedures needed for placement. The Department of Human Services is called in and must begin the lengthy process of assuming guardianship in order to place him in a nursing home. The man has been held in the hospital for three months.

Inadequate Alternative Care Facilities

- A 25-year-old, ventilator-dependent patient with multiple sclerosis has been a patient in the hospital for four years. Few nursing homes in the state are staffed and equipped to care for ventilator-dependent patients and those that are have long waiting lists.

Obstetrical Services

- The obstetric unit holds three patients on this day. None have experienced a normal, uncomplicated birth. One is delivered by

Caesarian as a result of minimal variability on fetal monitoring during labor. A second, admitted for treatment of pregnancy-induced-hypertension, has a Caesarian because of signs of increasing toxicity. The third, diagnosed with epilepsy, weighs 300 pounds and is admitted for induction of labor.

Did these people need hospitalization? Did they need hospitalization in their own community? If they did require hospitalization, what would the implications have been for transporting them to a distant medical center? The literature suggests that it might be economically beneficial to deliver more home health care and/or to transport patients to centralized medical centers, which because of their large volume, could deliver higher quality care (Christianson et al., 1990; Ermann, 1990; Goldsmith, 1989; Moscovice, 1989).

In assessing the needs of patients and reasons for admission on one day in the life of a small rural hospital, it is clear that several required intravenous (IV) therapy. Increasingly, entrepreneurial businesses are developing which provide high-technology interventions such as IV, oxygen, and respiratory therapies in the home (McLaughlin, 1990). Community health nursing is also developing expertise and increasing capabilities in these areas. However, most patients requiring these treatments must still be admitted to hospitals, at least for a short time, for diagnosis, stabilization, and the initiation of therapies. For acute illness, sustained nursing observation is critical in order to assess and treat the physiological and psychological responses to the illness and to medical intervention. As we increase our home care capability, many of these patients will enjoy earlier discharge and treatment in the comfort of their own homes with follow-up by community health nurses and local physicians. The ramifications of high technology therapies delivered in the home appear, on first perusal, to be ideal. It will take time, however, to develop sufficient numbers of personnel and agencies who can provide home care for the patients who require highly technical treatment. Distance factors mandate numbers of personnel available and their ability to travel between patients. Patient acuity demands flexibility and, in many cases, round-the-clock coverage or availability to deal with treatment problems or change in condition. Community resources are not yet fully organized for, or economically capable of, meeting these needs. Current reimbursement protocols produce barriers. Additionally, there will continue to be numbers of patients who lack the necessary family or friend support systems and physical environments required for home treatment. As we develop in this area, we must continue to assess the economic ramifications, quality, and sequelae of home treatment. This is particularly true in rural areas where the caregiver-to-patient ratio may need to be high because of distance between patients.

A key force that drives health care toward increasing home care is the assumption that the cost of delivering care in the home will be cheaper than the cost of delivering the same care in a hospital. However, the charge to one patient from the cited rural Maine hospital who received IV antibiotic therapy at home over the course of 17 days was $4,800 or $284 per day. The charge for her five-day stay in the hospital for diagnosis and initial treatment of her infection was $860 or $172 per day. The assumption that health care delivered at home will be less expensive requires more research and analysis.

Could patients have been transported to a distant hospital? First of all, one must determine if the patient could have survived. In most of these cases, the answer is probably "yes" perhaps with the exception of the man who sustained a liver laceration and ruptured spleen as the result of blunt trauma. However, transportation particularly from rural areas requires long periods of absence from the community for ambulances and emergency personnel. This absence reduces the overall emergency coverage available to the community and may jeopardize others who require emergency care. Many rural emergency services are small and staffed primarily by volunteers who hold other full-time jobs. If these people are finding that they need to increase the time required to meet the demands of providing emergency services, they may resign leaving communities further bereft of emergency transport services.

Additionally, patients cared for in their own communities are afforded the support and comfort of family, friends, and an environment that is known and comfortable. Transportation to distant centers would prevent this psycho-social support so important to recovery and healing. Can we afford to attend to this "soft part of the healing process" or will American health care be driven only by the physical and economic dimensions of illness and injury? Is this another schism, another dilemma?

During our assessment of patient needs and reasons for hospitalization, it became evident that some remained hospitalized because of extenuating social situations or because of the unavailability of alternative care resources. A wide chasm in care capabilities exists between acute-care hospitals and long-term care facilities. Some patients require extensive discharge planning to mobilize and integrate the varied services they require in order to sustain them in the community. The contemporary use of hospitals goes beyond the simple diagnosis and treatment of physical illness and injury. The hospital serves patients who have nowhere else to go. It serves patients who have no one else to care for them.

OPPORTUNITIES FOR NURSING
IN RURAL HEALTH CARE

Most of the literature regarding rural health care exists in hospital and health economics journals. Nursing literature, and particularly research relating to rural health, remains in an early stage of development. It does hold promise for the future, but much yet remains to be done.

Parker, Polich, Olson, and Hay (1989) and Pickard (1989) speak of the need and strategies to recruit and retain nurses in rural areas. Motta (1989), publishing in a nursing journal but not speaking specifically of nursing, delineates the need for and impact of networking to save money and consolidate resources. She describes pooling specialized personnel such as nurse anesthetists, staff developers and educators, and those involved in quality assurance and peer review. These personnel are hired by and deliver services to members of the networking institutions.

Nurse service providers including Jezierski (1988), Lassiter (1985), and the *Journal of Emergency Nursing* (1988) and nurse educators including Reimer and Mills (1988) profile characteristics of rural health nursing and document the educational needs for rural health nurses. Rural clients, their health needs, and the demands on nursing are distinct. With limited facilities available; isolation; transportation hardships related to distance, geography, and weather; environmental and occupational risks; rural people, according to Jezierski (1988),

> *tend to be, out of necessity, singular, independent people who are conservative about seeking health care. . . . They have learned to make it on their own and tend to deal with crises themselves. They will delay seeking medical help hence their problems can be more serious when they do seek it [p. 327].*

Lassiter (1985) speaks of the kin and friendship networks in rural communities which provide strong sanctions regarding behaviors and strongly influence, both positively and negatively, peoples' health practices. These family-like relationships influence nurses, themselves relatives, neighbors, and significant others to people they serve as professionals. Confidentiality and trust become issues.

In describing the characteristics of rural health nursing, the cited authors note challenges related to both diversity and infrequency in dealing with many patient care needs. Weiss, for example, in the *Journal of Emergency Nursing* (1988) describes the challenge as needing to "function as master of all trades" (p. 21A). Bauman, in the same article notes, "working the emergency room gets kind of hard when you only put in one chest tube every two years. . . . You get a little rusty" (pp. 24A–25A). Ruiz, in the same journal article, appreciates the peace, serenity, and atmosphere of her community and hospital where people are on a first-name basis and where little turnover results in the feeling of family. She misses contact and networking with other nurses and notes a dearth in educational and formal growth opportunities. Salvatore, in the same article, states

> *you'll learn something every day . . . you must be willing to train all the time and review constantly . . . you have to*

*feel comfortable working alone . . . you feel more in con-
trol of patient care . . . you know your patients . . . you
have to be very flexible . . . and very organized . . . it's
real nursing [p. 30A].*

Reflecting on the preparation and educational needs of rural
health nurses, Lassiter (1985) cites the need for competencies in
assessment of both individuals and communities; expanded knowledge of family and group dynamics; abilities with culturally oriented interviewing and with interview data analysis; leadership
skills which include knowledge and ability with budgeting, fund-
raising, and staff management; and appreciation of the dynamics of
planned change.

In our opinion, rural health care holds incredible potential
for nursing. It affords an arena for experiencing and influencing
health care in an area where there exists a plethora of gaps and
needs. We must, however, recognize certain realities in our own
profession, in the health care system, and in our society at large.

Nurses are primarily salaried employees of large, hierarchi-
cally and economically oriented institutions. This reality and history has sheltered us from the need to pay primary and close
attention to the economics of health care in our daily work lives.
We have had and taken the opportunity to focus our attention and
practice on individual (including family) human needs in a rather
idealistic way. Nursing espouses values which focus on the delivery of total patient care and to the right of all people to equal
health care. We become frustrated in institutions and practice
settings that decrease or negate our ability to deliver the kind of
care we value and instinctively know influences patient outcomes.

Even with expanding numbers of nurses educated at the graduate level, as a profession, we remain woefully undereducated
regarding health care financing and health care policy. Because
most nurses are salaried by institutions, we have not had to experience and deal with the repercussions and realities of instituting
new systems and models for health care delivery. As hiring institutions increasingly demand that nurses be accountable for their
time and the nursing interventions that fill the day of patient care,

we continually struggle with setting priorities and separating what is "necessary" from what is "nice." Although we struggle with the frustration of not being able to deliver what we have come to define as holistic health care, we continue to hold on to a value system and a pattern of caring that goes beyond attending only to the "narrow now." Slowly, more of us become entrepreneurs and change-agents even as pre-prescribed roles, payment structures, and practice policies challenge us at every turn.

Literature attests to the need, particularly in rural areas, to assess individual and community needs and to create new models for health care delivery in order to meet these needs. Because nursing holds to a holistic value system and a practice model that goes beyond the "narrow now," it is common and natural for us to involve patients in identifying their needs and participating in their own care. It, therefore, seems natural for nursing to more consciously, publicly, and actively extend this individually focused skill and our research into the community. Assessment of community needs in rural areas will partner us with residents and foster the design and creation of new models of health care responsive to citizens rather than solely to the whims of practitioners, policymakers, and economists.

For nursing to be effective participants in creating new models for health care, the authors believe that we as nurses must come to grips with the realities of our status, patterns, and relationships as a developing profession. Historically, we have acquiesced and abided by a model of physician domination and control of health care (medical care). As we increasingly determine and work toward autonomy and independence, we are blocked by this model. Indeed, we find that we live in a society that strongly values and holds on to the centrality of the physician in health care. Even as we seek recognition and reimbursement for the care we provide, we are dependent on a physician's order for the determination of that care. At best we are interdependent with physicians. In many areas, we are indeed dependent.

As we deny, resist, and are frustrated by this notion of dependence, we fail to explore and appreciate its repercussions and even possibilities. For physicians to be successful in their medical care, they must depend on (especially in hospitals but also in the community, clinics, and other areas where their care is delivered) nurses for continued and skilled assessment, appropriate intervention, and timely feedback. Without nurses, some patients would die or at least not thrive. To ensure benefit from the plethora of highly technical and complex medical interventions increasingly common today, physicians would have to remain at the bedside. The polarity between our concept and ideal of being independent from physicians and the reality of our being dependent on them has generated an adversarial relationship between medicine and nursing. As adversaries, we do not and cannot work together to create new models for care.

Nursing faces challenge and opportunity in another arena. Nursing, medicine, and the plethora of new disciplines rising in the field of health care remain mired in what we have come to term *the acute care syndrome.* Though we acknowledge that our greatest contemporary challenges lie in treating and dealing with the repercussions of chronic illnesses, every exacerbation of a chronic illness is reacted to as a whole new phenomenon rather than as the continuing evolution of a life process. Our health care system and especially our systems for paying for health care remain geared to acute and crisis-oriented intervention. Goldsmith (1989) writes, "our contemporary care system, hospital and health insurance alike, tends to ignore the disease until it reaches that life threatening stage" (p. 107). While we pay lip service to the need for primary prevention through health promotion and teaching, nursing has gained proficiency and been recognized as expert in illness care and teaching. We have, as a society and as a profession, lost the thread spun by early community health nurses—teaching and meeting health care needs before they become acute problems. Can we create ways to regain this focus?

Our current situation in health care cries out for the development of alternative models and sites for care of people with chronic conditions. We need alternative institutions and modalities that can bridge the gaps currently in evidence between home care, hospital care, and long-term care. Nurses work with people in need of care wherever they are. We move easily into a variety of settings. Society, patients, and other practitioners acknowledge this capability though we have as yet failed to value and capitalize on it. Nurses are "naturals" for designing and implementing new models for care both institutionally and in the home or community. We must face and deal with the barriers that confront us, however, which include practice restrictions, payment structures, and a society that views anything other than physician-managed care as second rate.

Change in our health care system will come only through partnerships and the establishment of a health care agenda that not only values but demands change. Nurses in their daily practice naturally bring people together and coordinate care. Can we adapt these skills to meet the larger health care needs of society?

CONCLUSION

Rural health nursing and rural health nurses stand at the threshold of unique challenges and opportunities. Although many difficulties face us as a profession and as a society, rural health nurses are in a particularly ripe position. Though isolated and faced with many divergent needs, they hold recognition and respect in their communities. Gaps in care and the solidarity evidenced in many small communities lend themselves to the creation of new models for health care. It would not be surprising to find that this is already occurring in many areas. We need to find ways to share and to learn from one another. We must find ways also to share beyond the boundaries of nursing. It is only through bridging to and with other disciplines and consumers that we will move beyond the crises and complexities that face us today in health care.

This book serves to begin the journey of articulating the realities and opportunities facing rural health and rural health nurses. This chapter focuses on the role of small, rural, community hospitals. It asks whether or not rural residents and health care providers can survive without hospitals. It describes problems facing rural communities and rural health care providers, positing whether or not hospitals can survive. Exploring the answers to these questions opens areas that hold great promise and potential for nursing. Can we meet the challenge? Will we?

REFERENCES

Amundson, B., & Hughes, R. (1989). Are dollars really the issue for the survival of rural health services? *Rural Health Working Paper Series, 1*(3), 1–14.

Blaney, D., & Hobson, C. (1988). *Cost-effective nursing practice.* Philadelphia: Lippincott.

Chase, G. (1989, December 20). Hospital officials set to lobby for funding. *Sun-Journal, Lewiston, Maine, 3.*

Christianson, J., Moscovice, I., Wellever, A., & Wingert, T. (1990). Institutional alternatives to the rural hospital. *Health Care Financing Review, 11*(3), 87–97.

DeLeon, P., Wakefield, M., Schultz, A., Williams, J., & VandenBos G. (1989). Unique opportunities for health care delivery and health services research. *American Psychologist, 44*(10), 33–71.

Ermann, D. (1990). Rural health care: The future of the hospital. *Medical Care Review, 47*(1), 33–71.

Goldsmith, J. (1989). A radical prescription for hospitals. *Harvard Business Review,* May/June, 104–111.

Jezierski, M. (1988). Rural nursing: The challenge. *Journal of Emergency Nursing, 14*(5), 326–328.

Joint Task Force of the National Association of Community Health Centers and the National Rural Health Association. (1989). Health centers in rural America: The crisis unfolds. *Journal of Public Health Policy,* 99–116.

Journal of Emergency Nursing. (1988). An inside look at rural nursing. *14*(5), 21A–36A.

Kalisch, P., & Kalisch, B. (1986). *The advance of American nursing* (2nd ed.). Boston: Little, Brown.

Lassiter, P. (1985). Education for rural health professionals: Nurses. *The Journal of Rural Health, 1,* 24–28.

McLaughlin, M. (1990). Bringing it all back home. *New England Business,* 29–34.

Moscovice, I. (1989). Rural health: A literature synthesis and health services research agenda. *HSR: Health Services Research, 23*(6), 891–930.

Moscovice, I., & Rosenblatt, R. (1986). A prognosis for the rural hospital: Are rural hospitals economically viable? *The Journal of Rural Health, 1,* 11–33.

Motta, G. (1989). Networking saves money and enhances patient care by consolidating resources. *Journal of Enterostomal Therapy, 16*(3), 95–96.

Mullner, R., Rydman, R., & Whiteis, D. (1990). Rural hospital survival: An analysis of facilities and services correlated with risk of closure. *Hospital & Health Services Administration, 35*(1), 121–137.

Mullner, R., & Whiteis, D. (1988). Rural community hospital closure and health policy. *Health Policy, 10,* 123–136.

Norton, C., & McManus, M. (1989). Background tables on demographic characteristics, health status, and health services utilization. *HSR: Health Services Research, 23*(6), 725–756.

Parker, M., Polich, C., Olson, D., & Hay, M. (1989). A rural hospital responds to the nursing shortage. *Nursing Economics, 7*(4), 215–217.

Patton, L. (1989). Setting the rural health services research agenda: The congressional perspective. *HSR: Health Services Research, 23*(6), 1005–1051.

Pickard, M. (1989). Protecting the supply of rural nurses. *Health Texas, 7,* 14, 24.

Rabinowitz, H. (1988). Rural applicants. *The Journal of Medical Education, 63,* 732–733.

Reimer, M., & Mills, C. (1988). Rural hospital nursing as an elective. *The Journal of Rural Health, 4*(2), 5–12.

Starr, P. (1982). *The social transformation of American medicine.* New York: Basic Books.

Stevens, R. (1989). *In sickness and in wealth.* New York: Basic Books.

Winter, R. (1990). Rural hospitals. *The American Legion, 129*(4), 25–27, 64.

11

Swing Beds: Providing Extended Care in Rural Acute-Care Hospitals

Mary Val Palumbo

DESCRIPTION OF SWING BEDS

Swing bed programs were established in 1973 when the U.S. Department of Health began experimenting with the idea of providing long-term care in small, rural, acute-care hospitals. "The experimental programs were premised on the assumption that it is more cost effective to provide long-term care in acute-care hospital beds in low-occupancy hospitals in rural areas than to construct new nursing home beds" (Shaughnessy, 1985, p. 303). The Omnibus Reconciliation Act of 1980 authorized Medicare and Medicaid reimbursement for skilled and intermediate nursing services provided by rural hospitals with fewer than 50 beds that met criteria for establishing a swing bed program. The title "swing bed" refers to a change in the level of nursing care without the patient being moved from the facility or even the bed. As of 1989, 1,100 small rural hospitals had been certified by Medicare to

This chapter is based on a manuscript entitled "Providing extended care in the acute care setting," that appears in *Geriatric Nursing* May 1991. This version appears with the editor's permission.

provide swing bed services (Shaughnessy, Schlenker, & Kramer, 1990).

Swing beds have proven to be financially beneficial to small rural hospitals while improving the care provided to patients requiring extended hospitalizations. Prior to swing bed programs, many patients who no longer required acute-care nursing services were unable to be discharged because of the limited number of skilled nursing home beds. Consequently, the hospital lost money because there was no Medicare reimbursement for the patient awaiting placement. With the swing bed program, the hospital receives reimbursement and the patient receives services that are tailored to his or her needs. Patients also appreciate being able to stay close to home in their community hospital while receiving rehabilitation or terminal care services.

SWING BEDS VERSUS NURSING HOMES

Although it may appear that a swing bed program would be in competition with local nursing homes for clientele, this is not the case. "The two provider types have gravitated to reasonably complementary roles in most communities, with swing bed hospitals serving the subacute or near-acute patient market and community nursing homes serving the chronic care or more traditional long-term care market" (Shaughnessy et al., 1990, p. 67).

The quality of care in nursing homes versus swing beds has also been investigated by Shaughnessy and others. The sample in Shaughnessy's study reported in *Health Services Research* (April 1990) included approximately 2,000 patients from 44 swing bed hospitals and 49 nursing homes in 18 states. Results indicated that,

(1) Relative to nursing home care, swing bed care is more effective in enhancing functional outcomes and discharge to independent living and in reducing hospitalization for long-term care patients, and (2) nursing home care appears more desirable than swing-bed care for long-stay chronic care patients with no rehabilitation potential [Shaughnessy et al., 1990, p. 65].

DESCRIPTION OF A SWING BED HOSPITAL

Envisioning the setting of a small rural hospital may provide insight into the challenges and joys of a swing bed program. Copley Hospital is a 50-bed nonprofit institution located in Morrisville, Lamoille County, Vermont. The inpatient system provides primary and secondary care and the hospital is part of a referral system for tertiary care at a medical center that is one hour away. The outpatient system includes 24-hour emergency service with a physician-staffed emergency room. A Birthing Center and Special Care Unit make up approximately ten of the 50 beds, the rest are for medical/surgical care. The hospital serves the ten towns of Lamoille County plus three adjoining towns. Lamoille County is rural by almost any standard. While three of the county's towns have populations of over 2,500, no town has a central population density this large. These towns, therefore, are considered rural by the U.S. Census Bureau (Malone-Rising, 1987).

The occupants of Lamoille County earn their living mainly from light industry, including crafts, repair work, and the service professions. Seasonal and year-round farming (i.e., maple sugaring, garden produce, Christmas trees, and dairy) supplement many family incomes; however, the prevalence of these as primary occupations is declining. The fact that the area's many lakes and mountains have attracted increasing numbers of seasonal residents, tourists, and skiers must not be overlooked when considering the county's employment opportunities and the clientele of Copley Hospital. The appealing mountain scenery contributes to challenging travel during the winter and "mud season," and there are many unpaved roads in the county.

ONE EXPERIENCE OF NURSING RESPONSE
TO SWING BEDS

The idea of swing beds initially was met with skepticism by our nursing staff. Many of the nurses preferred working with the younger acutely ill patients. The swing bed patient was perceived as being elderly, "no code," needing more care, and being a poor rehabilitation candidate. Prior to the swing bed program, our nurses were caring for elderly patients requiring extended, rather than acute care, but in a way that left the staff frustrated and the patients' needs unmet. Fulmer et al. (1986) point out that 60 percent of hospitalized patients are elderly yet few nurses identify themselves as gerontological nurses. Much work needed to be done at Copley to present the swing bed patient in a positive way. One example of this was that right from the start our swing bed patients were referred to as residents and the program was named the Resident Care Program. This name was chosen after an interview with a swing bed patient in another hospital revealed the patient's dislike for the label "swinger."

In order to facilitate the transition to the swing bed program, the position of resident care coordinator was created. This position was to be filled by a registered nurse who would act as primary nurse for all the swing bed patients and coordinate their admissions, care, and discharges with the rest of the health care team. This position is one that should be filled by a nurse who not only enjoys working with the elderly but also has a strong knowledge base in the special needs of the geriatric patient. Experience in rehabilitation nursing is desirable and strong physical assessment skills are essential since these residents are seen less frequently by their physicians than are other patients. The ability to be a team member is important, but leadership and assertiveness skills are also critical requirements.

Our resident care coordinator's first job was to develop standards of care for the residents. Inservice education helped the staff to differentiate the needs of the extended care patients. A major area of concern was the functional assessment. Since patients come to an acute-care hospital with problems requiring immediate nursing actions, priority is given to assessments that relate to the patients' current or potential conditions. How far the patient walks each day or whether or not he or she can transfer into a tub is not a priority when lower lobe breath sounds cannot be auscultated. Consequently, in the course of an acute hospitalization, the assessment of functional level is often neglected.

Residents, however, needed a new admission form and Kardex that stressed assessment of their functional level. The nursing

Kardex had to summarize the resident's abilities so that a nurse who was unfamiliar with the resident (e.g., an agency nurse hired for the day) could easily understand the resident's routine. A long-term care Kardex was introduced to replace the acute care one that stressed schedules for preps and laboratory tests and pre- and post-operative changes in diet and activity. The new Kardex also had room for the care plans of the entire health care team. The new admission form followed a head-to-toe format similar to the acute-care nursing admission form currently used, in order to facilitate an easy transition for staff nurses. Assessments of mental status, dentition and oral cavity, skin condition, mobility, and continence were expanded.

Once functional level was assessed properly, a care plan was developed that would maximize the resident's functioning (Figure 11–1). Residents were encouraged to dress each day and eat their meals with others in a dining area. Principles of restorative feeding were incorporated into care plans for residents with a "self-feeding deficit" nursing diagnosis. The use of restraints was held to a minimum as the staff learned to trust their assessments of the resident's ability to ambulate. Acute-care problems, such as accidental disconnecting of IV's, falls, and confusion due to oversedation from postoperative narcotics, were less of a problem with the residents because of their more stable conditions. Residents wheeling themselves through the halls became a familiar sight. Assisting the residents to dress themselves in street clothes was a new skill for many of the acute-care nurses. It often required more time than was anticipated. Adjustments in the nurses' patient care loads were necessary.

Our nurses gradually learned to replace the time they usually spent on vital signs, assessments of unstable conditions, and charting with teaching and encouraging self-care as well as providing rehabilitative and preventive nursing care. A new respect for the different skills needed to provide long-term care emerged. As Smits (1987) summarized in her comparison of the quality of care in nursing homes and swing bed programs,

> *Perhaps the most important lesson to be learned . . . is that nursing home care, when objectively analyzed, cannot*

Figure 11-1
Total Plan of Patient Care

BLADDER
___ B.R.
___ Bedpan
___ Urinal
___ Commode
___ Catheter
___ Size
___ Date Change
___ Irrigation
___ c
___ ē
___ Incontinent
___ Self control
___ Total care
___ Assist

FRACTIONAL URINE
___ Self
___ Assist/supervise
___ Total care
___ Schedule

BLADDER TRAINING
___ Date Started
___ Date Completed

BOWEL
___ B.R.
___ Bedpan
___ Commode
___ Incontinent
___ Self control
___ Assist
___ Total care

BOWEL TRAINING
___ Date Started
___ Date Completed

FLUIDS
___ Restrict
___ Force
___ Intake
___ Output
___ Diabetic fluids

EATING HABITS
___ Feeds self
___ Prepare food
___ OOB in chair
___ Feeder
___ Tube feeding
___ Size
___ Date Change
___ Assist
___ D.R. ___ B ___ D ___ S
___ Supplement feeding
___ Salt substitute
___ Sugar substitute

EYE SIGHT
___ Right
___ Left
___ Both
___ Cataracts
___ Wears glasses
___ Blind
___ Right ___ Both
___ Left ___ Legally

HEARING
___ Partially deaf
___ Right ___ Left
___ Totally deaf
___ Uses hearing aid

LOCOMOTION
___ Walks
___ Crutches
___ Cane
___ Walker
___ Bed to chair
___ Lift to chair
___ Wheelchair
___ Stretcher
___ With 1 assist
___ With 2 assist
___ Fully ambulatory

DEXTERITY
___ Right hand ___ Left hand

PARALYSIS
___ Rt. Arm ___ Lt. Arm
___ Rt. Leg ___ Lt. Leg
___ Rt. side of face
___ Lt. side of face
___ Quadriplegia
___ Paraplegia

POSITION
___ Change by self
___ With 1 assist
___ With 2 assist
___ Q 2 hrs.

RESTRAINTS
___ Bed ___ Chair
___ Waist ___ Jacket
IMPORTANT: CHECK EVERY HOUR AND RELEASE EVERY TWO HOURS

SIDERAILS
___ Constantly
___ At night
___ Omit

SUPPORTIVE
___ Bed cradle
___ Foot board
___ Trapeze
___ Pillows
___ Bed board
___ Brace
___ Foam rubber
___ Special mattress
___ Water mattress
___ Water bed
___ Alter pressure pad

SPECIAL EQUIPMENT
___ Prosthesis
___ Self
___ Assist
___ Total care
___ Type

BRACES
___ Self
___ Assist
___ Total care

MENTAL ATTITUDE
___ Oriented
___ Well adjusted
___ Moody
___ Cheerful
___ Depressed
___ Confused
___ Alert
___ Agitated
___ Forgetful

ALLERGIES

SPEECH
___ Speaks well
___ Mumbles
___ Aphasic
___ Language spoken

BATH
___ Tub
___ Shower
___ Self care
___ Assist
___ Total care
___ Bed

MOUTH CARE
___ Dentures
___ Upper
___ Lower
___ No dentures
___ No teeth
___ At bedside
___ Self care
___ Assist
___ Supervise
___ Total care

SKIN
___ Routine
___ Special
___ Decubitus
___ Site:
___ Contractures
___ Site:

DRESS
___ Shoes
___ Stockings
___ Clothes
___ Self care
___ Assist
___ Supervise
___ Total care

GROOM
___ Comb/brush hair
___ Shave
___ Nails
___ Feet
___ Hairdresser
___ Self care
___ Assist
___ Supervise
___ Total care
___ Podiatrist

PRIVILEGES
___ Bed rest
___ To B.R.
___ Up ad lib
___ OOB schedule
___ Up with assist

ACTIVITIES
___ P.T. ___ Time
___ O.T. ___ Time
___ S.T. ___ Time
___ Escort needed
___ Self care
___ Church Services
___ LOA permission

234

Reprinted with permission of the Briggs Corporation, Des Moines, Iowa.

AGE	BIRTH DATE		S	M	W	D	RELIGION:	HOSPITAL AFFILIATION		DIET
ROOM	NAME						ANNOINTED DATE:	PHYSICIAN	PHONE #	LEVEL OF CARE

Discharge Planning:

Discharge Planning Up-Date:

Nursing

Goals

Short Term:

Long Term:

Problems and Needs

Plan of Approach

Nursing

235

Figure 11-1 (Continued)

Dietary _____

Activities _____

Occupational Therapy _____

Physical Therapy _____

Social Services _____

Other _____

Diagnosis: _____ Responsible Party: _____

Admitted From: _____

Date: _____ Phone: _____

Team Conference Date: ____/____/____

Restorative Review Date: ____/____/____

AGE	BIRTH DATE		S	M	W	D	RELIGION: ANNOINTED DATE:	HOSPITAL AFFILIATION		DIET	
ROOM	NAME							PHYSICIAN		PHONE #	LEVEL OF CARE

236

Nursing

Physician

Social Services

Dietary

Therapies

Community Resources

Family

Plan of Discharge Recommended at Admission? ☐ Yes ☐ No

Reason:

237

*be dismissed as poor in the average institution and that
hospital staff have a good deal to learn if they are ever to do
a good job in providing long-term care services [p. 109].*

Staffing

During the start-up phase of the program, the resident care coordinator was assigned three to five residents and was responsible for their primary nursing care as well as scheduled afternoon activities. Gradually, as the program became more familiar to the staff, the resident care coordinator was able to pick up acute-care patients to even out the patient assignment. Afternoon activities were then taken over by an activities coordinator. Finding a person who is qualified for this position, yet only desires part-time (two hours per day) employment can be challenging. The occupational therapist can oversee the care plans of whoever fills this position (i.e., a nurse or social worker) if the activities coordinator is not trained for this type of work. Besides having a concept of teamwork, the activities coordinator must be able to assess the residents' diversional activity needs and their prior activity or hobby interests. Planning group or individualized activities for the residents and implementing these plans are all in the scope of the activities coordinator's responsibilities.

Juggling the needs of residents and acute-care patients simultaneously became the next challenge for the nursing staff. Acute-care patients are likely to demand the nurse's attention promptly, but for relatively shorter periods of time. The residents seemed to demand longer visits, but without urgency. It, therefore, made sense to assign one nurse to several residents and several stable acute-care patients. Some nurses did not like an "all resident" assignment, but some preferred this, if there were at least four or five residents.

Nursing assistants who were interested in working with the residents became extremely important. They were able to provide the continuity needed in the residents' activities of daily living (ADLs) while the nurse coordinated the team approach to the resident's care. As the nursing shortage took hold of the hospital, more nursing assistants were hired to support the shrinking professional staff. The idea of "primary partners" was implemented so that both the nurse and the nursing assistant were assigned patients for whom they had previously cared. This was especially important with the extended care of the residents. The nurses were able to become familiar with the assessment and care-providing skills of each nursing assistant and to assign responsibilities accordingly.

Team Approach

The Resident Care Program increased the feeling of teamwork among the nursing, social service, dietary, physical therapy, home health, and medical staff. The team solidified and worked hard toward the goal of discharge for the residents. The challenges of health care in a rural area are especially apparent when discharge plans are being formulated. For example, is the home heated by a wood-burning stove, and is someone tending the fire during the resident's hospitalization so the water pipes will not freeze and crack? In the spring some roads and driveways become impassable because of mud. Therefore, the question must be raised of who will be able to get the resident from the hospital to his or her home. Before one resident was discharged, the physical therapist, nurse, and the resident went to the home to assess any barriers to the resident's independence there. The social worker and nurse visited another resident at home who had left the hospital against medical advice and persuaded him to return (after a home-cooked meal).

Discharge planning for the residents seemed to require much of the team's effort. Perhaps that was because the residents' stays were longer than those of acute-care patients, and this extra time afforded more anticipation of discharge problems. Alternatively, the team may have been better able to recognize the assets of all its members given the framework of the Resident Care Program. Kovner and Richardson (1987) recognized that "increased communication and cooperation, which is necessary for all staff to fulfill their professional responsibility for the resident, engendered a new mutual professional respect among the staff" (p. 36).

Several new team members were recruited for the Resident Care Program. Speech and occupational therapists were hired on a part-time contract basis to provide their services to the residents and acute-care patients as well as outpatients as needed. A part-time activities coordinator was also hired to provide a daily activity for the residents. Although these ancillary therapies are common-place in metropolitan and rehabilitation hospitals, their addition to the services of a small rural hospital was noteworthy. The care of the elderly is greatly improved by the services of a broad inter-disciplinary team.

Another important team member is the utilization review nurse. This member's role is to guide the team in understanding Medicare regulations which specify the criteria for reimbursement based on level of care. Acute-care patients' charts are reviewed daily by the utilization review nurse to determine if there has been a change in level of care that would preclude Medicare reimburse-ment. The physician, resident care coordinator, and social worker are then notified of a potential need for a patient's admission to the Resident Care Program. After the resident's admission, the chart is followed by the utilization review nurse to identify level changes from skilled to intermediate nursing care. Potential problems re-garding reimbursement are avoided with the utilization review nurse working with the team.

No team is complete without the input of the residents and/or their families. Family conferences were frequently scheduled be-fore the patient's admission to resident care from acute care. The options were presented and information about the Resident Care Program was provided to the patient and family by the social worker, resident care coordinator, and/or the doctor. After the resident's admission, the team's plan of care was presented to the resident and/or family. Family input was also solicited regarding discharge planning. As the time for discharge approached, the home health nurse contacted the resident and family. Residents were encouraged to take day trips home with their families prior to discharge to troubleshoot for unanticipated problems.

One new situation was encountered during a younger resi-dent's admission interview with the resident care coordinator. He wanted to know if it could be arranged for him to get married to his girlfriend as soon as possible. The team and the couple met and looked into the availability of the conference room for a wedding and reception. Plans were soon being discussed for a pre-wedding champagne dinner for the couple and the logistics of a one-night honeymoon. Since the resident had complicated wound management and functional deficits from Guillain-Barre Syndrome, the honeymoon was the most challenging to plan. The wedding, reception, and honeymoon went smoothly and certainly will be remembered for some time by the staff as well as the newlyweds. The resident's wife became an important part of all care planning and she was instrumental in his early discharge because of her newly acquired skills in wound and continence management.

The team's efforts with the families of terminally ill residents have been generally greatly appreciated and rewarding for all involved. The Resident Care Program has filled a gap for families who have been physically unable to care for a dying family member at home and for patients for whom a nursing home admission has been seen as unwarranted in the few remaining days or weeks of their lives. One dying resident's 90-year-old wife, for example, visited every day dressed in matching suit, hat, and gloves. Her dignity and apparent lifelong love for her spouse inspired the staff. After her husband's death, the team pursued getting Maude involved in an adult development center where her grief eventually eased and her latent talents in poetry and art began to fill the void in her life.

Sometimes a plan for terminal care needs to be updated, as the team discovered while caring for a woman who was in Vermont for the summer and had taken seriously ill. When exploratory surgery revealed inoperable cancer, the plan was to admit this patient to the Resident Care Program because her death appeared imminent. Several days after her admission the resident became quite lucid and was very interested in all the financial arrangements of her care. Since she was receiving only custodial care, which is not covered by Medicare, she wanted to be transferred to a nursing home that was less expensive. The only available bed in the nursing home that she preferred was on the second floor and she had to demonstrate that she could walk upstairs. Her care plan was quickly updated to meet this need. After her discharge in late summer to the nursing home, she was able to arrange live-in nursing care in her home in Florida. The team was surprised and delighted to receive a Christmas card from our "terminal care" resident in Florida that year. She died shortly afterward but happily in the place where she was most comfortable.

RESULTS AFTER ONE YEAR

Many of the nurses' perceptions about the residents prior to the start-up of the program proved to be unfounded. The perception that the residents would be poor rehabilitation candidates was perhaps the most unfounded as 55 percent of the residents returned to their homes (Table 11–1). The staff also had not expected the residents' length of stay to be relatively short; 16 days on average, with 24 percent of the residents staying for only eight days (Table 11–2). Shaughnessy (1985) and Shaughnessy and Schlenker (1986) use the term "short-term long-term care" to describe the residents' care and length of stay. They cite research findings that suggest swing bed patients across the country have substantially shorter stays and greater rehabilitation potential than nursing home patients.

The nursing staff also was challenged with a new type of client because of the Resident Care Program. Several residents transferred from other larger acute-care settings to complete their rehabilitation closer to home. This brought the two residents under 65 years old, a 19-year-old male with Guillain-Barre Syndrome and a 59-year-old female with Syringomyelia (Table 11–2). Since these diseases are not common to a small rural community hospital, a review of nursing research and literature on the care of these residents was needed.

CONCLUSION

The benefits of swing bed programs have been well documented. Kovner and Richardson (cited in Wiener, 1987) list them as follows:

> *1) an increase in hospital staff sensitivity to the needs of the elderly; 2) an increase in availability of new services to all patients; 3) teaching staff new ways of working*

Table 11-1

Swing Bed Patients: Admissions and Discharges

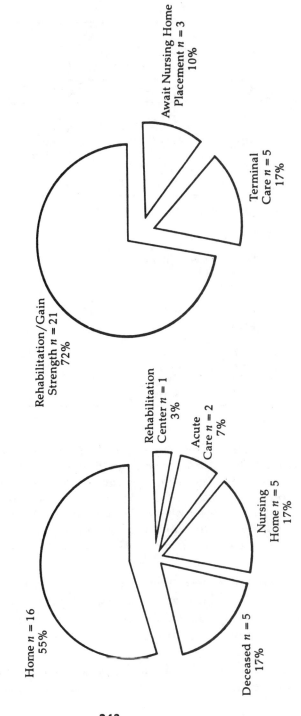

Where discharged to
(n = 29)

Reason for Admission
(n = 29)

Rehabilitation/Gain
Strength *n* = 21
72%

Await Nursing Home
Placement *n* = 3
10%

Terminal
Care *n* = 5
17%

Home *n* = 16
55%

Rehabilitation
Center *n* = 1
3%

Acute
Care *n* = 2
7%

Nursing
Home *n* = 5
17%

Deceased *n* = 5
17%

Table 11–2
First Year Statistics ($n = 29$)

Age (Years)		Length of Stay (Days)	
Range:	19–91	Range:	6–43
Mean:	81	Mean:	16
Mode:	79 (3) 81 (3)	Mode:	8 (17)
Medium:	81	Medium:	14

Diagnosis

Back pain	4
Diverticulitis	4
CVA	4
Cancer	3
Fractured extremities	3
Fractured hip	2
Pneumonia	2
Ulcer	1
Guillain-Barre Syndrome	1
Renal failure	1
G-tube placement	1
Syringomyelia	1
Cardiomyopathy	1
COPD	1
Alzheimer's disease	1

together; 4) a springboard for hospitals to diversify, particularly into other services for the elderly; 5) improved hospital finances through increased occupancy, higher revenues, better utilization of staff, more referrals, and improved physician recruitment; and 6) better care for patients by facilitating recovery near home, where the family can be closely involved with the patient's care [p. 7].

The experience described in this chapter concurs with each of these cited benefits with the possible exceptions of improved physician recruitment and encouragement for hospital diversification which are hard to link to the impact of the Resident Care Program alone.

Nurses' attitudes about the program and flexibility in meeting the residents' needs are key to the success of swing beds.

Information about what to expect, as well as inservice education on the elderly patient and providing short-term long-term care, are extremely important during the start-up phase and intermittently thereafter. Strong nursing administrative support is essential for the success of the program. This support comes from an understanding of the program in terms of staffing needs, ability of the team to comply with complex Medicare regulations for long-term care facilities, and financial incentives for having a swing bed program. Clear support from nursing administration is then transferred to all levels of the nursing staff, from middle management to the unit secretary.

It is equally important for the nurse coordinator to have a positive view of his or her position and the value of the program. Incentives might be needed to entice a qualified nurse from preferred responsibilities with acute-care patients if an experienced long-term care nurse is unavailable. Because the nurse coordinator must interact with a team that works mostly daytime weekday hours, a similar schedule may provide the necessary incentive to keep the position filled. Opportunities for salary increases via a clinical ladder framework can also make the position appealing.

Finally, because there are many swing bed programs throughout the country and more are likely to be started up, the nurses involved would benefit greatly from more nursing literature and research on the subject. A newsletter to exchange resources for staff education, ideas on staffing, case histories, and research studies might be well received. Nurses have met the challenges of caring for the swing bed patient for almost 20 years—it's time to share insights and successes.

REFERENCES

Fulmer, T., Ashley, J., & Reilly, C. (1986). Geriatric nursing in acute settings. *The Annual Review of Gerontology and Geriatrics, 6,* 27–80.

Kovncr, A., & Richardson, H. (1987). The Robert Wood Johnson Demonstration Project. In J. M. Weiner (Ed.), *Swing beds: Assessing flexible health care in rural communities.*

Malone-Rising, D. (1987). *Elder services in Lamoille County, Vermont.* Unpublished manuscript.

Shaughnessy, P. (1985). The use of swing beds in rural hospitals. *Inquiry, 22,* 303–315.

Shaughnessy, P., & Schlenker, R. (1986). Hospital swing-bed care in the United States. *Health Services Research 21* (4), 447–498.

Shaughnessy, P., Schlenker, R. E., & Kramer, A. (1990). Quality of long-term care in nursing homes and swing-bed hospitals. *Health Services Research, 25* (1), 65–96.

Smits, H. L. (1987). Quality of care. In J. M. Weiner (Ed.), *Swing beds: Assessing flexible health care in rural communities* (pp. 105–119). Washington, D.C.: The Brooking Institution.

Wiener, J. M. (1987). Policy issues. In J. M. Weiner (Ed.), *Swing beds: Assessing flexible health care in rural communities* (pp. 13–12). Washington, D.C.: The Brooking Institution.

12

The Nurse Administrator in the Rural Hospital: Selected Issues, Challenges, and Rewards

Karen R. Johnson
Marilyn Barba

Many of the current issues the nursing profession is facing have a different meaning when examined in relation to nursing practice in the rural hospital. Much of what has been written or studied in the nursing profession has been in the context of how it relates to the urban setting. There is scant nursing literature that discusses the problems and challenges of practicing nursing in a rural hospital. There is almost no information on the role of the nurse administrator in rural hospitals. The characteristics of rural hospitals, however, cause them to react and respond to the current and rapidly occurring changes differently than do their urban hospital counterparts. This chapter will review some of the current issues and their effects on nursing practice and the role of the nurse administrator in rural hospitals. Rewards and challenges for the nurse administrator of the rural hospital will be discussed.

For this chapter, the term rural refers to those hospitals of 50 beds or fewer. These hospitals lie in non-metropolitan areas.

RURAL SETTING INFLUENCES ON NURSING PRACTICE
AND NURSE ADMINISTRATORS

While there are several characteristics that rural areas have in common, there are also differences which make it difficult to generalize about rural hospitals nationally. Rural hospitals reflect a rich diversity in health service organizations. Each hospital is uniquely suited to its own community. A hospital develops from the community needs and shares the goals and specialness of the community which it serves. The Governing Council of the American Hospital Association (1990) has identified that health care has substantial variety, where "each region of the country, each state, each locale has built a complement of health services unique to it, with deep roots in the culture and self-image of the community" (p. 9). This is particularly so for rural hospitals. This first characteristic is what contributes to the differences among rural hospitals. Each hospital develops from the community and is held in high regard by its community members. Anything that threatens the hospital or health services of the community threatens the existence of the community itself. Patient confidentiality takes on a new meaning for nurses in the rural setting. Nursing personnel see former patients on a regular basis in stores, at the post office, at church, and at restaurants. They may be asked questions about the condition of patients by well-meaning friends. They may have to care for their own family members in an emergency situation. They will have to share sorrow with people they know well. Their professional lives and responsibilities do not end when they leave the hospital doors, because they are members of that same community. Their role is respected and given significance by the community (Jimmerson, 1988).

There are several characteristics of rural communities, rural health care services, and those living in such areas that have an impact on nursing practices. First, rural communities have higher concentrations of children under the age of 18, and they have higher infant mortality rates. Second, there are higher levels of poverty due to the lower personal income levels of rural communities. Third, the people who live in rural communities are more likely to be uninsured than are their urban counterparts. Fourth, rural communities have relatively more elderly people. In 1967, 9.6 percent of the rural population was greater than 65 years of age, by 1987 that figure had grown to 12 percent. This is an important factor because the elderly are hospitalized more frequently than younger people, and they are more likely to have an increased level of disability or morbidity when they are ill (*Secretary's Commission on Nursing,* 1988). This elderly population also reports higher death rates from hypertension and heart disease. The health costs of this population are usually paid for by the Medicare/Medicaid DRG Prospective Payment systems.

Finally, rural populations suffer from high rates of serious respiratory diseases, such as farmer's lung and silo-filler's disease. They also experience certain cancers and pesticide toxicities. These are not the types of diseases seen frequently in urban hospitals. In addition, they report higher rates of mental health problems.

Rural populations pose different challenges because of the nature of their work-related illnesses. Besides there being a greater likelihood that they work in hazardous or unhealthy places, agricultural work has been identified as the most dangerous type of work in the nation. While over 5 million farm families and farm workers live in rural areas and amount to only 3 percent of the work force, they have over 14 percent of the work-related deaths. A large number of children die or are injured in agricultural accidents yearly (Wakefield, 1990). One can see that quality emergency services are essential in the health care systems in rural areas. Many rural areas, however, do not have access to the 911 emergency dialing system. While some emergency services are provided by emergency medical technicians (EMTs), volunteers provide much of the rural emergency care. The volunteers may not be as highly trained as the EMTs in the urban setting. For example, the volunteers may not be able to defibrillate patients or start IVs. The volunteers are providing basic emergency treatment and may not be involved in advanced life-support services. This often means that patients may arrive at the emergency room of the rural hospitals in unstable, critical conditions.

RURAL HEALTH CARE ECONOMIC IMPACT

Rural hospitals have not been immune to the changes occurring in health care delivery systems caused by such factors as the Medicare DRG Prospective Payment Systems (PPS), Health Maintenance Organizations (HMOs), Preferred Provider Organizations (PPOs), decreased lengths of stay (LOS), and increased acuity levels of patients. In fact, they have experienced the impact of these economic changes more severely than have their urban counterparts.

Changes in the rural economic environment and within the hospitals themselves have contributed to the closure of 161 rural hospitals between 1980 and 1987. There has also been a 7 percent decline in full-time employees within the remaining institutions The changes in the Medicare and Medicaid systems of payment for health care to the hospitals has influenced the economic situation. The economic downturn occurring in the rural communities where the hospitals are located also has had an impact on the negative economic climate (*Secretary's Commission on Nursing,* 1988).

Before 1983, hospitals were reimbursed for patient care in a retrospective cost-based method. The cost of the patient's care was determined after the patient was discharged and the bill was submitted to Medicare. In general, the more the hospital spent, the more it could collect. The incentive for the hospital was to provide as many services as possible for as long as possible. With the signing of the Social Security Amendment in October 1983, the entire system changed. The Medicare DRG Prospective Payment System was initiated. This system provides predetermined fixed rates for certain groups of illnesses. The purpose of this system is to reduce the cost of care and decrease the hospital length of stay of patients. Its ultimate goal is to reduce government spending for health care services (Lowenstein, 1990).

The PPS has resulted in a decrease in the profits in most rural hospitals, while there has been an enormous increase in rural hospital expenses. These increases result from higher prices of hospital goods and services, including wages. The intensity of hospital care and services that are provided to each patient also add to the increased costs (Davis, 1985).

One of the main problems that rural hospitals face with the current PPS is that they have not been able to collect from the federal government at the same rate as their urban counterparts. The larger hospitals receive more money from the government for the same services ("Policymakers Struggle to Define Essential Access," 1990). "In the fourth year of the prospective pricing system, nearly 60 percent of rural hospitals did not break even. Overall payments to rural hospitals failed to cover costs" (p. 38). This means that rural hospitals are closing at higher rates than are urban hospitals. Since 1980, 263 rural hospitals have closed. It is projected that 600 of the nation's 2,700 rural hospitals will close in the next few years. While the discrepancy in reimbursement between rural and urban hospitals will end by 1995, the differences in reimbursement will continue to hurt the rural hospital for the next few years (Wakefield, 1990).

The following discussion illustrates the impact of the prospective payment system on a rural state. Medicare in the state of New Hampshire, which is highly rural in nature, makes up over 40 percent of all hospital business. The New Hampshire hospital marketshare has increased only 22.5 percent while the prospective payment system has increased only 9.5 percent. There has been a 13 percent profit margin loss for hospitals within this state since the initiation of the PPS in 1983 (New Hampshire Hospital Association, 1988).

The American Hospital Association during the last decade has begun to recognize that a difference between small rural hospitals and larger hospitals exists. The association has helped the rural hospital administrators to lobby for equality in prospective payment legislation and essential access legislation ("Policymakers Struggle to Define Essential Access," 1990). The role being played by the federal government in rural health care matters is becoming increasingly important. There will be federal mandates for funding of rural health services, rural health service research, and support for education of professionals from underserved areas. Rural hospitals represent a major example of such an underserved area.

Rural health care needs, issues, and solutions have been largely overlooked in a nation that highly values technology, medical centers, and the medical cures of common urban health problems. Wakefield (1990) is not alone in warning that the health care services for growing numbers of our rural population are being threatened with extinction. The 101st Congress has had over 25 bills introduced to address some of the rural health care delivery problems that have been identified.

In an effort to deal with the economic threats, about half of the eligible rural hospitals have taken advantage of swing bed services to generate needed revenue. (See Chapter 11 for related discussion.)

The use of swing beds in rural hospitals means that the nurses have to provide two levels of nursing care. This is often done on the same floor or within the same building. Nursing care of a long-term patient is different from the care given to an acutely ill patient. The caregiver, who is usually an acute-care nurse, will have to know how to care for two different types of patients—those with acute-care needs and others with long-term care needs. The nurses must perfect their skills in developing interdisciplinary assessments. They must refine their discharge planning skills and develop new skills in assessing the chronically ill patient's needs. They must also be able to carry out a long-term care plan (Grimaldi, 1988).

Reduction in the profits that hospitals have experienced since the PPS was instituted has resulted in increased competition among hospitals for patients. A similar competition occurs for professional personnel. The profit reductions have caused hospitals to cut budgets, freeze salaries, or lay off personnel. The nurse has not been the one who has had to face being without a job. The nurse lives in the rural community, however, and the people who do lose their jobs are friends, neighbors, and relatives (Fuszard, Slocum, & Wiggers, 1990a).

With most rural hospitals having a negative profit margin, they have not had the funding to compete with their urban counterparts for professional personnel, including registered nurses. The rural hospital has experienced the same increased demand for nursing care that most larger hospitals have experienced even though inpatient days in the acute-care general hospital have fallen. There were 50 million fewer inpatient days in 1986 than there were in 1981. The average hospital occupancy rates had dropped 63.4 percent (Aiken & Mullinix, 1990). This was especially true in small rural hospitals with fewer than 50 beds, where the average occupancy rate in 1984 was only 34 percent (Henry & Moody, 1986). The nurse administrator is confronted with the need to find resourceful staffing patterns that will provide the flexibility needed to respond to the fluctuating occupancy rates. One cannot pay several days of salary to a staff nurse who is not needed for direct care to patients. Nurse administrators do not have the budget to use staff nurses' "free" time for special projects.

One approach to dealing with both decreasing occupancy rates and nursing staff shortages is for the hospital to close beds temporarily or to suspend specific services. The impact of closing beds is greater in the rural hospital than in the larger urban hospital. For instance, there is a 50 percent decrease in the hospital's ability to provide intensive care if one of its two intensive care unit beds must be closed. It is an expensive proposition and hurts the hospital's image in the community even though it is done for patient safety (Aiken & Mullinix, 1990).

NURSING WORKFORCE ISSUES

Even with the decrease in occupancy rates, the ratio of nurses to patients has increased significantly nationally. In 1972, hospitals employed a ratio of 50 registered nurses to every 100 patients. By 1986, this ratio had increased by 82 percent, with 91 nurses employed for every 100 patients nationwide (Aiken & Mullinix, 1990). Projections for the year 2000 are that there will be an almost 1:1 ratio of registered nurse to patient (Curtin, 1990).

The demand for registered nurses remains greater than the supply in many communities, even though there are now 2.1 million nurses in the country. Between 1977 and 1984, the number of employed nurses increased by 55 percent compared to a population growth of only 8 percent. Over 80 percent of all registered nurses are working, an unusually high number when compared to other predominantly female professions (Aiken & Mullinix, 1990).

The nursing shortage in the rural communities is more acute than in the urban hospitals. The number of small hospitals reporting a greater than 15 percent vacancy rate is growing faster than the number of urban hospitals reporting the same 15 percent unfilled position rate (*Secretary's Commission on Nursing,* 1988).

In 1984, a national sample survey of registered nurses reported that 18 percent of all registered nurses lived in rural communities. Fourteen percent of these nurses commuted to urban areas to work. In contrast, only 2 percent of urban nurses commuted to rural areas for work. The registered nurses who work in rural hospitals are more likely to be older, less educated, and more likely to work part-time. Their knowledge is more generalized and their practice areas may differ from those of their urban counterparts. These nurses may have to function independently in several different areas within the hospital. They have fewer resources than the nurses in urban hospitals (*Secretary's Commission on Nursing,* 1988). The need to monitor patients closely and use ever increasingly sophisticated technology has increased the need for registered nurses in all hospitals. The supply of nurses is unable to meet the demand. Interestingly, rural areas with 24 percent of the population have only 18 percent of the nurses (*Nursing,* 1989).

A shortage of nurses in a rural hospital produces many of the same problems as in a larger urban hospital. Rural hospitals have fewer options for dealing with the shortage, however. The hospital often does not have the financial resources required to actively and successfully recruit nurses. According to Jones (1990), it costs a hospital between $6,800 and $17,000 to replace a registered nurse. The average cost of turnover is $10,000. These costs may be disproportionately high in the rural system in which resources are very limited. A further difficulty is that salary and benefit packages are not monetarily large enough to attract nurses from other areas.

Another difficulty in recruiting and retention may have to do with the type of relationship the nurse administrator establishes with the hospital administrator. The hospital administrator's perceptions of supply and demand in relation to nursing staff may well color the recruitment and retention efforts of the nursing department.

> *. . . hospital administrators tend to assume that there are a finite number of nurses in any given community and that*

wage competition among hospitals will be costly and will not resolve community shortages. The majority of nurses, if they want to work, must accept the terms offered by hospitals [Aiken & Mullinix, 1990, p. 240].

The availability, dependability, and length of time nurses are in the work force are critical in the rural health care setting. The decrease in ancillary personnel has increased the work load for the registered nurses when they are already burdened with patients who are more acutely ill than before. The fear of losing their jobs, due to the threat of closure of their institution, has also caused increased tension among nurses practicing in rural areas. They know that they cannot go down the street or often even to the next town to find employment if the hospital closes (Fuszard, Slocum, & Wiggers, 1990b).

When a unit is staffed with only one or two registered nurses, the loss of one nurse can be critical. Many of the resources that may be available to a larger institution may not be applicable to the smaller rural hospital. Agency nurses are used frequently by urban hospitals in periods of staff shortages. They may not be an available option for many of the rural hospitals because of the distance that the agency nurses would have to travel. Their high salary level is also problematic for rural hospitals. Since there is already a shortage of registered nurses in the rural hospital, the hospital may not have access to its own per diem pool of licensed personnel. The institution-designed per diem pool is a strategy often used by larger urban hospitals to deal with changing staffing needs.

The hospital may have to use overtime to fill in the vacant nursing positions. Many of the nurses who work in rural hospitals work on a part-time basis. They are older and may neither desire the overtime nor be physically able to work the extra hours. It may take as many as three part-time nurses to fill one full-time vacancy. Most nurses who work in rural hospitals do so because the hospital is in their community. It is too far for them to commute to other hospitals for work. It is also too far for urban nurses to commute to the rural hospitals for work without some type of reward system which the hospital cannot afford (*Secretary's Commission on Nursing,* 1988).

Nurse administrators have difficulty in recruiting nurses who want to focus their practice on professional nursing. Most of the nurses working in rural hospitals do so part-time. Concern for their own families is a primary focus of their attention. As one practicing nurse administrator of a rural hospital stated, "The rural nurse is more interested in the quality of care given to patients than to professional nursing issues" (B. K. Gernhardt, personal communication, January 31, 1991). The part-time nurses are there for the patient and the patient's needs, but less so for the system's needs. They attend local workshops and meetings, but not if held at a distance from their own community.

In addition, efforts to recruit professional practitioners are hampered by low salaries. Nurse administrators are unable to adjust these salaries within the tight resources of the institution.

"Demands upon the nurse in the rural acute-care setting differ from the nurse in a large metropolitan hospital largely in the scope of knowledge and skills needed to provide quality patient care" (Henry & Moody, 1986, p. 38). These differences occur in the scope of activities found throughout the nursing department organization—from the nurse administrator to the staff nurse. The nurses are often required to wear many different hats because of the variety in expectations held. There are only a few nurses working at any one time, with few ancillary staff, and limited resources. The makeup of the rural hospital nursing department consists of more licensed practical nurses and other unlicensed caregivers than one finds in the urban hospital. This composition is primarily a function of the number and type of potential personnel available in the rural setting, often resulting in a staff mix that is not as desirable as a nurse administrator would like to have. Because of the staff mix, the rural nurse administrator may be a proponent of having the licensed practical nurse assume increased responsibilities. Nurse administrators of rural hospitals are often among the leaders in voicing the need to expand the scope of nursing practice for the licensed practical nurse, not because it is desirable for the quality of care, but because it reflects the reality of the staff mix available in the community.

Rural nurses find themselves functioning more independently than do nurses in other practice settings, and yet they are very dependent on their fellow co-workers. Since staffing in a rural hospital is usually stable, the staff knows each others' capabilities and limitations. They are very much like a family, and a camaraderie develops among them. Nursing may be the only department in the hospital working 24 hours a day, seven days a week. This may mean there are no secretarial, housekeeping, dietary, maintenance, medical records, or pharmacy personnel in the hospital after regular business hours. The hospital administrator and the x-ray, respiratory, and laboratory technicians are usually on call during the off shifts. The nurses are the ones who run the hospital's business in the off hours. They do their own work and pick up many of these other jobs. When help is needed, they are the ones who are responsible for coordinating the patient's care by calling other department personnel into the hospital to provide needed services. Some nonessential testing may be postponed until the next day because specific caregivers are not in the hospital around the clock (Jezierski, 1988; Dimon, 1988).

Recently, large urban hospitals have used cross-training of nursing staff as an important strategy to ensure coverage of patient needs. Cross-training is of benefit to the hospital since it allows hospitals to respond more quickly to census changes. When cross-training occurs in urban hospitals, it is usually in an area related to the nurse's primary specialty area of practice. For example, ICU nurses may cross-train for a transplant unit or burn unit. Nurses on a surgical specialty unit will cross-train for other surgical specialty units.

Rural hospitals have used cross-training for years without calling it that. Nurses in rural hospitals have always been expected to function independently in two or more clinical areas.

Specialization in nursing practice, which is prevalent in larger institutions, is neither possible nor desirable in rural ones. While the rural nurse may have generalized clinical knowledge and technical skills, an excellence in clinical decision making is also required. The rural hospital nurse is often the only one who is there for the critically ill patient until a doctor arrives (Jimmerson, 1988).

The rural hospital needs to employ the nurse as a generalist, able to work in several different specialties in the hospital. In larger urban hospitals, the nurse can focus on one specialty and learn that practice well. In a rural hospital, the nurse may be hired for a specific clinical area, but must be able to go wherever needed in the hospital. It is difficult to prepare a nurse to function effectively in all areas of the hospital.

Continuing education and keeping nursing skills updated are challenges that rural nursing constantly faces. Education is an expensive commodity that many small hospitals cannot afford to offer. Yet it is also an asset the rural hospital cannot be without. The low volume of patients seen in rural settings does not present the nurse with enough experiences to keep skills current. Nursing clinical effectiveness can hardly afford to be hampered in today's demanding medical and legal environment. Rural hospitals may need to become inventive in finding ways to keep their staff clinically current. This may mean holding continuing educational programs in a consortium with other rural hospitals. It may mean going to the community to raise the funds for educational purposes. It may mean developing exchange programs with larger hospitals to support and give nurses different experiences (Donatelli, 1988).

Another issue relates to maintaining the skills of the nurse who is working in a specialty unit. How does one maintain a level of specialty practice when the number of patients requiring that level of care is so small? For example, where and how often should a maternity nurse attend professional educational development activities in order to maintain his or her current level of skill? How much education is needed? How can one justify the expense of maintaining skill level through continuing education, workshops, and short courses when the size of the service and the number of staff are so small? How can one maintain expertise in the treatment of major trauma when the hospital deals with an average of one trauma case per month? These questions reflect expectations that are self-imposed by nursing staff and nurse administrators. They are imposed also by outside regulatory agencies.

A secondary skill maintenance issue for staff nurses relates to the feasibility of providing continuing education on topics for which there will be little if any opportunity to use the "new knowledge" in the clinical area. The staff believe they need such knowledge for "maintaining motivation," improving morale, or for professional self-development. The decision not to use scarce resources for this type of continuing education is easier for the nurse administrator to make in this situation. The issues of keeping the nursing staff motivated and interested, however, must be addressed.

THE NURSE ADMINISTRATOR ROLE

The nursing administrator in a rural hospital must be a "jack-of-all-trades." As excellent generalists, nurse administrators "must be able to practice and demonstrate clinically sound nursing, be well informed in several specialties and perform well as managers" (Henry & Moody, 1986, p. 38). Nurse administrators may have less educational preparation for their positions than do their urban counterparts.

The demands and expectations of the nurse administrator in the rural hospital are varied and complex. Henry and Moody (1986) describe the characteristics and major activities of a group of ten Florida rural hospital nurse administrators. They reported in their survey that these nurse administrators were satisfied with their salaries. They also found that while working an average of just under 60 hours per week, three of the directors of nursing of those rural hospitals held second jobs to make ends meet.

At a recent conference of state presidents of the Emergency Nurses Association, a nurse administrator from a northeast state described her experience in trading places with a city nurse for two weeks. She visited everyone in the city hospital who did the same activities she did in the rural hospital. It took her seven days and 12 separate interviews to talk with the 12 people who did her job (Sheehy, 1988, p. 264).

Public relations skills are important aspects of the rural nurse administrator's responsibilities. One must collaborate with the medical staff to develop positive relationships that will facilitate necessary changes. One also works closely with the medical staff to coordinate patient care. The nurse administrator often will work closely with the women's auxiliary and may help volunteers set up a display in the lobby of the hospital or type flyers announcing an educational experience for the community. The nurse administrator has to communicate well with the leaders in the community, as well as the public, because the public has a vested interest in the hospital. The hospital belongs to the community. "In a large hospital technology impresses, moderate care suffices; but in a small hospital highly personal care is a must" (Henry & Moody, 1986, p. 39). The patients admitted to the hospital may be friends, relatives, or neighbors, which makes rural nursing extremely personal (Henry & Moody, 1986).

Many nursing administrators in small hospitals expect to spend time giving direct patient care. They may cover a number of different clinical services. Besides direct care, the nurse administrator is often responsible for more than just the nursing department. The responsibilities may include purchasing, admissions, housekeeping, and other patient care services such as x-ray or physical therapy. He or she may be responsible for attached nursing homes. The positive aspect of this responsibility is that the nurse administrator knows what is going on throughout the institution. The administrator knows all the employees and their capabilities. A disadvantage to such responsibility is that it is difficult to narrow one's focus to any one area of patient care.

While much of the nurse administrator's emphasis is on the day-to-day operations of the hospital, it is not limited to this focus. He or she is also involved in organizational long-range and financial planning activities (Henry & Moody, 1986). As a result of the broad range of responsibilities, the nurse administrator serves on multiple committees in the hospital as well as in the community.

The nurse administrator is often second in command to the hospital administrator and provides institution-wide leadership at times of the hospital administrator's absence. The nurse administrator must then deal with issues not under his or her direct responsibility, but the responsibility of the executive administration. The types of resources taken for granted in larger urban hospitals are not as readily available to the nurse administrator in the rural hospital. For example, secretarial services may include only part-time coverage. Often, the nurse administrator functions as her own secretary.

Physician availability may only be by phone. In some of the larger rural hospitals there may be one physician always available in the hospital. Staff nurses in rural hospitals may be the ones to begin and direct a critical patient's care until a doctor arrives at the hospital. The staff nurse may be the only medically trained person who can accompany the critically ill patient during transfers to a larger institution (Jezierski, 1988).

The nurse and the physician often have a very strong, positive relationship that grows out of mutual respect and need. The physician is dependent on the nurse in the rural hospital and has respect for the nurse's knowledge and skills. John Seavey (personal communication, October 1990) describes the physician as perceiving the nurse in the rural hospital in much the same way that an attending physician perceives a resident or intern. The physician almost views the nurse as an extension of self in patient care decisions. The nurse's knowledge, observational skills, and abilities to assess and communicate patient needs to determine what care is required is valued by the physician.

The availability of specialists or other physicians may be limited. The number of medical personnel involved in the care of each patient is smaller than in the larger urban centers. The doctor and the nurse are forced to work together as a team. If they do not, the job may not get done (Jezierski, 1988).

JOB SATISFACTION FOR NURSE ADMINISTRATORS

Nurse administrators enjoy a number of rewards in their positions of complex responsibility. The nurse administrator gets to see the people in the organization grow and develop knowledge and skills in different areas. As an example, the nurse administrator may see a certified nurse assistant graduate from the local vocational-technical college licensed practical nurse program. That individual may then complete a program leading to registered nurse licensure. One has a sense of family in a rural hospital that large hospitals can often only talk about. The large hospital may try to imitate the idea of family, but the feeling in the large hospital is not the same.

This feeling of family that is so prevalent in the rural hospital applies to patients, staff, and physicians. Nurses are friends with physicians in a social sense, thus establishing very effective relationships with physicians. The physicians hear positive and negative comments from the community and provide this feedback to the nursing staff. Because there are fewer staff in a smaller hospital, there are fewer people to leave. When that turnover does occur, it is felt as a greater loss in the organization because someone has "left the family."

The nurse administrator knows each patient situation in a small hospital. The administrator also hears feedback from the public. The feedback is usually that the nurses are good and that they make a difference in the way patients feel about their care. This gives nurses and nurse administrators job satisfaction because of the opportunities for follow through. One sees the results of one's work.

Perhaps most important, the nurse administrator in the rural hospital has a feeling of accomplishment. Because one sees patients who have recovered back in the community and active, the nurse administrator knows that the nursing care has been a positive force.

CHALLENGES FOR NURSE ADMINISTRATORS

Nurse administrators face several challenges in rural hospital nursing. Directors of nursing who work in rural hospitals have to remain current about what is happening in the profession. They have to examine how professional nursing issues, such as differentiated practice or primary nursing, would affect their abilities to give care. This is particularly true when there are so few colleges available in rural areas to provide a diploma or associate degree graduate the opportunity to earn a baccalaureate or an advanced degree in nursing. The rural nurse should be interested in the educational preparation for nurses. Exposure to the practice of rural hospital nursing is limited for students. Most nursing colleges are affiliated with major medical centers or larger, multi-service hospitals found in urban areas. Students get little if any exposure to rural hospital nursing. Rural hospital nurse administrators need to find ways to make their settings appealing for clinical practice experiences for students from baccalaureate and community college nursing programs. Nursing student enrollments have fallen off or plateaued. With shortages of nurses reported in most settings, many clinical agencies are vying to provide clinical experiences for nursing students.

The rural hospital is at a disadvantage in providing clinical experiences for nursing students for several reasons. First, there are few baccalaureate prepared nurses practicing in the rural hospitals. This lack limits the number of nurses qualified to function in preceptor roles for students. There are even fewer master's prepared nurses available to function in a joint appointment role with a university nursing program. Second, the number of students who can be accommodated for clinical experiences in a rural hospital is usually quite limited because of the number of beds in the setting. It is obvious that two ICU beds, three pediatric beds, and four maternity beds (often not all filled with those particular specialty patients) can provide only limited experiences for a minimal number of students in any one specialty. Accreditation requirements demand faculty be prepared in the specialty they are teaching. Since few student placements would be available in any one specialty in a rural hospital, using rural hospitals for clinical experiences could result in even more expensive undergraduate nursing education. To have one faculty with students in all caregiving settings in the agency would violate the expectation that students were being taught by those educationally prepared in that specialty. Different kinds of arrangements for clinical experiences can be negotiated between educational and service settings. Certainly such exploration can start from the nurse administrator of a rural hospital.

Another challenge for the nurse administrator is to create an environment where nurses will feel empowered. Lang (1987) states that we must "empower nurses to practice in an environment that respects them, values them, offers them a chance to grow personally and professionally. In return, nurses hold answers to the health care problems of today and tomorrow" (p. 11).

The health care delivery future, with its predicted transition of care from institutions to home and community settings raises two questions for nurse administrators. First, will such change further decrease the already dwindling patient population of the rural hospital? Second, can nursing services of rural hospitals begin to focus on caregiving in home and community settings. Rural hospitals already use the "swing bed" concept to shift from acute-care to long-term care beds when the need arises. Nurse administrators with vision will seize the opportunities such changes provide.

Toffler (1990), in his book entitled *Powershift,* predicts the intense and dramatically deep shift to the power that information will hold in the world. This dramatic and deep shift will make those who know how to get, store, retrieve, and use knowledge powerful in future organizations. Nurses will be among these powerful workers. Nurses will be heavily dependent upon informatics as they process information to support care and coordination decisions for patients and families. Will the rural hospital be able to make the shift necessary to use the knowledge of the nurse for the survival of the organization? Can rural hospitals afford the level of computer technology necessary for the effective and efficient functioning of their staffs? Can small rural hospitals afford not to purchase such hardware and software? Will they survive without such support?

Rural hospitals, by using the technology available today, have immediate access to specialists in the tertiary medical center hundreds of miles away. Patient status and clinical data are transmitted for diagnosis and treatment recommendations via computer, interactive television, fax, and telephone. Thus, a similar level of specialty medical care is provided in rural areas that is available from tertiary care centers. Could not nurse administrators from small rural hospitals make use of a similar access to nurse practitioners, clinical nurse specialists, and other patient care resources of larger teaching hospitals by way of similar technology?

Rural hospitals provide settings that continuously challenge the nurse administrator in ways not experienced by his or her urban colleagues. Education for nurses to function in these types of administrative positions is needed. Education experiences rural nurse administrators need to meet the demands of these critical positions have been identified. Rural nurse administrators need to study areas that will provide knowledge of the nature of the changing rural community and the values of the populations. They must learn skills of networking and negotiation to meet the competitive market demands and to provide needed health care services for the different consumer groups. They must know about the financial and resource management of small hospitals (Henry & Moody, 1986). Such education may be hard to come by for the practicing nurse administrator. There are now only six programs offering master's preparation in rural health nursing care (*Nursing,* 1989), but other resources are available. One can obtain management training that may not be a part of a formal educational program. One can also establish support systems with nursing and management programs from state educational institutions. Potentially productive support systems among the nurse administrator's own peer group can be developed within the state or region.

Nurse administrators from rural hospitals often do not find the state or national association for nurse administrators to be particularly helpful to them in dealing with their administrative issues. Nurse executives from the large, multi-service urban or teaching hospitals do not understand the impact that certain decisions the nurse executives would make easily in the urban hospital would have in small hospitals. One can see how decisions related to staffing shortages or decreasing occupancy rates would have different impacts in urban hospitals than in rural hospitals. Likewise, discussions and decisions on differentiated practice or professional models of nursing care delivery may have to be modified. Modifications are necessary because of the realities of the staff mix.

Rural hospitals are expected to meet all of the regulations the large institutions meet. Yet there are no committees to develop policy and procedures books, quality improvement standards, or continuing education programs. Such tasks fall to the nursing administrator to complete. Often the nurse administrator has neither resources of staff who are prepared in education nor clinical specialists who could carry some of these responsibilities. Frequently, the nurse administrator is the most capable individual for doing the special projects that could benefit the entire institution, for example developing an outreach program for cancer patients. To assist with some of these projects, the nurse administrator often calls on the nurse managers or staff nurses who assume responsibility for these important areas in nursing department functioning. These activities expand the responsibilities of the nurse managers and staff nurses. The responsibility often falls to just a few nurses in the setting who have an interest in expanding their responsibilities.

A final challenge for the nurse administrator has to do with what happens to the community if certain services are discontinued or if the entire rural hospital should close. This situation would leave the community without health service coverage. The predictions of increasing rural hospital closings make this a real possibility. Regionalization or networking is a concept that could help the small rural hospital survive (Haglund & Dowling, 1988). Regionalization relates the small hospital to the large hospital in formal ways. Each level of hospital (rural, community, referral) provides the services it does most effectively. Rural hospitals would provide basic services and would serve as places for convalescence and home care following referral to one of the larger hospitals in the region. Unfortunately, there are few examples of successful regionalization, but the concept has potential. Nurse administrators who know their communities, who are politically aware and on top of community issues, can influence decisions affecting the quality and quantity of services available for rural communities. Nurse administrators who look to innovative solutions to rural health service problems can help control costs. They can speak publicly and politically for the health care needs of the community. The nurse administrator, by being active in professional organizations, can keep the rural health care agenda in the public eye.

Rural hospitals and rural hospital nurses face many challenges in the next decade which they will have to meet in order to survive. Many of the issues require that they work together to reach a mutually agreed upon solution. They also can make themselves heard by joining forces. Nurses can be much more involved in the actual hospital business. As they examine their practices they can look at ways they can help control the cost of health care while still maintaining quality. They need to become more aware of governmental policies at both the federal and state levels. This increased awareness will assure that they have a voice on legislation that has an impact on the health care in their communities. They can take an active role in the community to communicate with the public about professional nursing and its contribution to health care delivery (Wright, 1988).

The challenges are many and the demands great for the nurse administrator in the rural hospital. Nurse administrators experience numerous rewards, commitments, and a sense of ownership of the problems. A most important attribute for a nurse administrator to have is flexibility. Flexibility allows the nurse administrator to benefit one or many—nursing, the hospital, the community, or the individual.

SUMMARY

The increasing importance of rural health concerns demands our understanding of the issues that health care providers and recipients in rural areas are facing. These concerns include higher rates of poverty; higher incidence of cancer, lung disease, and other chronic diseases; and higher death rates from hypertension and heart disease. All of this is occurring in an increasingly elderly population. Rural areas also report higher infant mortality rates and mental health problems. To make the problem worse, rural hospitals are closing at higher rates than are urban hospitals.

The field of rural health nursing is an emerging area of concern for the nursing profession. The practice of nursing and nursing administration in the rural hospital shares many of the same characteristics and problems present in the larger urban medical center or community hospital. The impact of these problems on rural health nursing is what differs. The practice of nursing in the rural hospital is becoming distinctive in and of itself. There is even hope among rural nurses that it will become a recognized specialty within the discipline soon.

The need to keep clinical skills current and to provide for competent practice remain critical ones in rural settings. The knowledge of disease processes, nursing issues, governmental legislation, and community needs are vital to professional practice. Nurse administrators need educational support in areas such as economics, the rural community, the poor, the prenatal patient, the elderly, and current legislation affecting the rural hospital. There is a need for exposure to leadership, management, and administrative knowledge and skill development to deal effectively with the unique problems of rural settings. Human relations skills in handling the nursing staff, the health team, and the public are essential.

The practice of nursing at all levels in the rural hospital needs to be studied. Nursing education systems should be encouraged to develop programs to meet the needs of staff and nurse administrators who want to work in rural settings. Finding ways to make these programs accessible in the often isolated rural areas is a challenge for service and education settings alike. Other areas needing research include the rural hospital environment's impact on nursing, nursing administration, and the patient.

As health care systems become more complex, health care itself is becoming more interdependent. There is no single discipline able to meet the diverse needs of patients and families, yet nurse administrators in rural hospitals frequently must provide quality care without access to the many disciplines necessary to meet patient needs. This is evident in the numerous hats that both the nursing staff and the nurse administrator wear to provide necessary care to patients in rural hospitals.

Some nurse administrators and staff nurses choose rural nursing and stay with it; it is a choice of a life-style that allows fulfillment in a challenging nursing career.

REFERENCES

Aiken, L. H., & Mullinix, C. F. (1990). The nurse shortage: Myth or reality? In C. A. Lindeman & M. McAthie (Eds.), *Nursing Trends and Issues* (pp. 238–246). Springhouse, PA: Springhouse Corp.

Curtin, L. (1990, December). Old loyalties in the new organization. *Innovations 90,* Sixth Annual Professional Practice Symposium, Houston, Texas.

Davis, C. K. (1985). An update from HCFA: Effects of Medicare, Medicaid on community hospitals. In M. Beyers (Ed.), *Perspective on prospective payment* (pp. 13–23). Rockville, MD: Aspen Systems Corporation.

Dimon, T. L. (1988). Who is the rural emergency nurse? *Journal of Emergency Nursing, 14*(5), 266–267.

Donatelli, N. S. (1988). Switching places: What we might learn from rural emergency nurses. *Journal of Emergency Nursing, 14*(5), 272–274.

Fuszard, B., Slocum, L. I., & Wiggers, D. E. (1990a). Rural nurses: Part I, Surviving cost containment. *Journal of Nursing Administration, 20*(4), 7–12.

Fuszard, B., Slocum, L. I., & Wiggers, D. E. (1990b). Rural nurses: Part II, Surviving the nurse shortage. *Journal of Nursing Administration, 20*(5), 41–46.

Governing Council American Hospital Association. (1990, March 28). *AHA Section for health care systems,* Chicago: Author.

Grimaldi, P. L. (1988). More hospitals likely to swing beds. *Nursing Management, 19*(3), 24–25.

Haglund, S. L., & Dowling, W. L. (1988). The hospital. In S. J. Williams & P. R. Torrens (Eds.), *Introduction to health services* (pp. 160–211). New York: Delmar Publishers Inc.

Henry, B. M., & Moody, Linda E. (1986). Nursing administration in small rural hospitals. *Journal of Nursing Administration, 16*(7, 8), 37–44.

Jezierski, M. (1988). Rural nursing: The challenge. *Journal of Emergency Nursing, 14*(5), 326–329.

Jimmerson, C. (1988). An evening shift in rural America. *Journal of Emergency Nursing, 14*(5), 265.

Jones, C. B. (1990). Staff nurse turnover costs: Part II, measurements and results. *Journal of Nursing Administration, 20*(5), 27–32.

Lang, N. (1987). Empower the nurse: A time for renewal. In American Nurses' Foundation, Inc. *Nursing practice in the 21st century* (pp. 5–16) Kansas City, MO: ANA.

Lowenstein, A. (1990). Diagnosis related groups: Controlling health care costs. In C. E. Lambert, Jr. & V. A. Lambert, (Eds.), *Perspectives in nursing.* East Norwalk, CT: Appleton & Lange, 333–354.

New Hampshire Hospital Association. (1988). *The facts.* Concord, NH: Author.

Nursing rural America to health. (1989, September). *AACN Issue Bulletin.* Washington, D. C.: Association of Colleges of Nursing.

Policymakers struggle to define essential access. (1990, February 5). *Hospitals,* 38–42.

A rural health services research agenda. (1989). *Health Service Research, 23*(6).

Sheehy, S. B. (1988). Rural emergency nurses: The heart and soul of emergency nursing. *Journal of Emergency Nursing, 14*(5), 263–264.

Secretary's Commission on Nursing. (1988). The shortage of RNs in rural areas. *Secretary's Commission on Nursing* (p. iv–15).

Toffler, A. (1990). *Powershift.* New York: Bantam Books.

Wakefield, M. K. (1990). Health care in rural America: A view from the nation's capital. *Nursing Economics, 8*(2), pp. 83–89.

Wright, J. E. (1988). Changes in federal funding for health services: Effects on nursing. *Nursing Management, 19*(3). 42–46.

Part IV

Research, Governance, Education, and Theory

13

Rural Research:
The Lamoille County Experience

Dorothy Malone-Rising

Mendras (1982) alludes to the difficulties encountered in the conduct of quantitative research in rural communities. Generalization requires a positivist paradigm. However, the increasing tendency toward diversity both within and between communities (Cordes, 1989; Coward, 1979; Gimlin, 1990; Suvar, 1982) makes such generalizations difficult. Determining the most salient issues for investigation within a rural community often requires a qualitative approach.

The Lamoille Area Health Council (LAHC) was organized in Lamoille County, Vermont, in early 1989 to enhance access to comprehensive health and social services for all members of the community. The operational model developed by the council (Figure 13–1), and strongly influenced by the three nurses with membership in the group, called for the council to assess the service needs of the community. This assessment was seen as vital if the group were to make planning recommendations that truly reflected the needs of the community. As the council explored the possibility of conducting a large-scale survey, two decisions were made. First, the participation of health council members and community residents in the project would be solicited and

Figure 13–1
Lamoille Area Health Council Operational Model

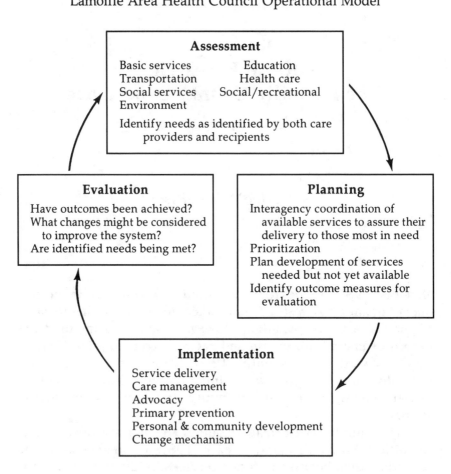

encouraged. We hoped that this collaboration would create a sense of ownership within the council and the community for the project, generating support for the recommendations expected as an outcome of the survey. Second, a design that would provide statistically valid results was desired.

This chapter will explore the process of designing a generalizable, quantitative study using a collaborative, qualitative approach. Issues particular to the conduct of research in rural settings will be discussed as they apply to this project.

THE RESPONSIVE CONSTRUCTIVIST PARADIGM

A positivist paradigm would preclude involvement of those being surveyed in the research process in the name of scientific objectivity. Jasanoff (1989) has stated, however, that "the scientific basis for policy decisions must be genuinely rooted in participatory involvement" (p. 26). For this reason, a methodology that would facilitate collaboration between the providers and consumers of health and social services was sought by the LAHC to guide the development of a survey in Lamoille County. Guba and Lincoln's (1989) responsive constructivist paradigm fosters, indeed demands, such collaboration.

A responsive constructivist methodology is a way of focusing and conducting research (Guba & Lincoln, 1989). The term *responsive* implies an interactive, negotiated process involving all who may have an interest in the research, the *stakeholders. Constructivist* refers to the methodology employed, the efforts to identify and seek understanding of the *claims, concerns,* and *issues* that different stakeholders harbor.

The researcher's task is to assure all possible stakeholders are identified so as to maximize the range of information collected. A process that Guba and Lincoln (1989) call the Hermeneutic Dialectic Circle is employed. Through open-ended interviews salient themes emerge. Interviewing continues "until the information being received either becomes redundant or falls into two or more constructions that remain at odds in some way" (p. 152). The researcher returns to earlier respondents to solicit their reactions to the emerging constructs. The joint construction that ultimately emerges is the end product of the research.

Documents, literature analects, observational data, and the inquirer's own *etic construction* may be introduced into the evolving construction. Guba and Lincoln (1989) acknowledge that this will be viewed by some as a "positivistically repugnant action" (p. 154). Having moved between participants, stakeholders, and respondents, the researcher is likely to have the most informed and sophisticated construction. A true collaboration requires that the researcher validate that construction with the stakeholders. This exclusive access to a more complete set of constructions facilitates the negotiation toward consensus that concludes the constructivist process.

The negotiation toward consensus, or clarification of competing constructs, is a time-consuming process that requires all participants to agree to the "conditions of a productive hermeneutic dialectic" (Guba & Lincoln, 1989, pp. 149–150). These conditions include a willingness to work from a position of integrity, share power, consider alternative constructs as appropriate, and commit the time necessary to complete the process.

The constructivist paradigm in rural community research is empowering for all involved. Roper (1988) talks of local policy-makers and university-based researchers becoming "bound together on an issue" (p. 427) such that both the population being studied and the researcher benefit by a collaborative research relationship. Acknowledging the claims, concerns, and issues of community members makes the product more useful to those it is meant to serve.

Christenson and Garkovich (1985), while acknowledging that "an empirical and quantitative scientific inquiry is (viewed as) more 'valid,' 'desirable,' 'preferable,' or 'scientific' than any other approach to science" (p. 517), have called for an increased use of qualitative methods in rural research. Further support for abandoning a methodology entirely grounded in the positivist paradigm is offered by Falk and Gilbert (1985) in their arguments suggesting that a totally objective, value-free view of the world does not exist in any research, and the pretense of such should be abandoned.

To this end, determining the objectives of the project and the specific research questions, developing the survey tool and the research protocol, and producing the final report with an agenda for action employed hermeneutic dialectic process. In addition, the selection of the sample for the survey, collection, and analysis of data followed conventional quantitative methods. The remainder of this chapter will present details of the Lamoille County experience.

DEVELOPING THE PROJECT

The Setting

Vermont is a small state. Sharing borders with Canada, New Hampshire, Massachusetts, and New York, it is the only New England state without access to the ocean. The population of about 550 thousand places Vermont as 48th in the nation, just ahead of Wyoming and Alaska in rank by population. With 66 percent of all its people living in towns with populations of fewer than 2,500, Vermont is the most rural state in America (U.S. Department of Commerce Bureau of Census, 1985).

Lamoille County (Figure 13–2) is located in the north central portion of the state. It is the only county in Vermont that is not located completely to the east or west of the Green Mountains. The highest peak of this range, Mount Mansfield, lies between two of the larger towns in Lamoille County. The road that connects these towns crosses Smuggler's Notch, which is an unplowed mountain pass during the winter months, usually from October into May. Lamoille County consists of ten towns, ranging in size from Belvidere in the north, with 237 residents, to Morrisville in the southeast with 4,560. The total population of Lamoille County was 17,776 in 1985 (Vermont Department of Health and Human Services, 1986).

Many health and social services in Vermont are organized regionally, using county lines as loose boundaries for catchment areas. Within these service areas a center for service provision evolves. In Lamoille County, Morrisville is this service center. A 50-bed hospital there offers an emergency room, intensive care unit, operating suite, birthing center, and a swing bed program for mostly elderly patients in need of extended health care. Programs for young families, and persons needing assistance because of advanced age, poverty, physical disability, or mental illness, are all coordinated out of offices in Morrisville. Most physicians practice

Figure 13–2
Lamoille County, Vermont

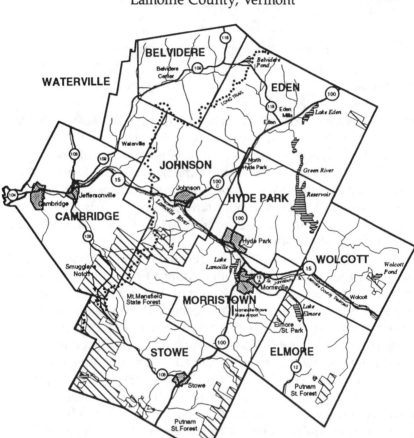

Map prepared by the Lamoille County Planning Commission, 1991. Reprinted with permission.

in Morrisville, with the rest clustered in Cambridge to the west and Stowe to the south. Senior meal sites and well child clinics can be found scattered across the county. The Lamoille Home Health Agency, a Medicare certified provider, brings a variety of skilled and unskilled services to the homes scattered through the hills. The closest tertiary care medical facility is located about 40 miles west of Morrisville at the Medical Center Hospital of Vermont in Burlington.

The History

There is a perception in Washington of a "crisis in the availability and affordability of health care in rural America" (Rovner, 1989). Program location, transportation, per person delivery costs, limited physical facilities, and program staffing are but a few of the issues affecting access to health and social services in rural communities (Coward, 1979). The LAHC was organized in January 1989 to enhance communication in a fragmented health and social service system and to enhance access to comprehensive health services for all members of the community.

The council consists of representatives from the health and social service programs operating in the ten towns of Lamoille County, as well as residents of these communities. While the council was originally organized to facilitate communication in the resolution of interagency problems, it soon became clear that system-wide planning and coordination was needed. The members of the council desired an active role in this planning and coordination process.

As the council was organizing, the Department of Human Services in Vermont announced a major restructuring (State of Vermont, 1989). Administrative oversight for all state programs servicing the elderly and disabled has been consolidated under the new Department of Aging and Disabilities. The restructuring has provided an opportunity to rethink service delivery in Vermont. Regional planning and regional control have been emphasized at the state level as the LAHC sought to develop a structure that fostered cooperation between service providers and communication with community members.

The Project

Typically, policies and programs are viewed as having been designed for urban areas and then applied to rural areas almost as an afterthought (Coelen, 1981). Coward (1979) makes a case for the value of formal and informal needs assessments "to assure that (health and social service) programs are built on real and not assumed needs" (p. 279). Council members decided in March 1989 to conduct such a survey.

My involvement with the LAHC grew from a personal and professional interest in the concept of coordinated community services. As a resident in the county, I seek to ensure the availability of comprehensive, high quality services within my community. As a gerontological nurse practitioner, I bring a unique expertise to the group in light of the continued growth of the elderly population in rural communities (Cordes, 1989). When I joined the council in April 1989 I was invited to join the Survey Planning Committee.

Five council members (two nurses, two social service professionals, and one community member), with regular feedback from the council as a whole, developed a 75-item list of the full range of health and social services that would exist in the comprehensive system envisioned by the council. My earliest involvement as a "negotiator," which Guba and Lincoln (1989) suggest is the major role of the researcher conducting collaborative research, occurred during the development of this survey tool.

Originally a list of 100 items was generated. In the discussions around the final length of the tool, two groups emerged. One group, mostly rural natives, felt that less was more, and that many of the listed services were unnecessary extravagances in their small towns. The other group, consisting primarily of urban transplants, insisted on preserving the list.

Guba and Lincoln (1989) warn that negotiation toward consensus can be a time-consuming process. The negotiator must acknowledge the validity of each participant's position while encouraging flexibility. The process has potential for becoming endlessly cyclical. The researcher must ensure movement toward consensus, maintaining sensitivity toward the divergent views that emerge. After several months of meetings, 25 items were eliminated. An equal number remain, their necessity to be determined by those surveyed (see Appendix 13–A for the complete survey tool).

In September, ten council members (29 percent), representing nine service organizations along with one consumer organization, completed surveys for each of the ten towns in the county, identifying services felt to be available to members of each community. Members were asked to note if any barriers to access were due to lack of finances, lack of transportation, or lack of existence of the service in the area. Surveys were analyzed by the Department of Aging and Disabilities' staff in January 1990. After completion of the survey, council members critiqued the tool, and further adjustments were made.

During this time I was asked to direct the ongoing project. Having been recently introduced to qualitative research methods, I began at this point to keep formal field notes. A notebook binder was organized using headings such as tool development, volunteer researchers, random lists, and research protocol. All field notes were copied to appropriate sections of this notebook. The many notes taken in the previous nine months were filed. Field notes were written before and after each formal and informal meeting for the duration of the project. In addition, notes made during meetings were kept. Continuous review of these notes was required to ensure that salient points were not lost between groups as the project evolved. The field notes, completed surveys, and statistical data generated by this project now fill a file cabinet drawer.

Objectives and Research Questions

Between August 1989 and January 1990, the Survey Committee and the council as a whole worked toward defining specific objectives for the ongoing project. As results from the provider surveys were tabulated, the objectives emerged as follows:

1. Identify service needs as perceived by providers and consumers.
2. Identify differences between providers' and consumers' perceptions.
3. Identify gaps in services as perceived by providers and consumers.

Clearly, a survey of the community was necessary. In light of the council's expressed wish to ensure broad-based community input with scientific validity, the constructivist paradigm was used in planning the quantitative survey.

The specific research questions were developed with ease, probably because of the months of work that had led to the council decision to conduct the survey. The following questions were asked:

1. What is the perceived availability of services?
2. What are the perceived barriers to access?
3. What is the desired scope of service?
4. What are the differences in the perceptions of providers and consumers?
5. To what extent have services been used by members of the community?

Definitions

The use of the term *community* entailed significant discussion among the current stakeholders in the project. Planck (1982) discussed the ambiguity of the term. While the discussion was valued because of the prominent use of the term in the specific questions to be asked of respondents, the group ultimately chose to leave the definition of community up to the individuals participating in the survey.

Definitions for the 75 services listed on the survey were developed and agreed to by members of the council. This list of definitions was used during interviews to ensure consistent interpretation of the survey. All were written in the form of questions to facilitate use during interviews with consumers.

Medical services were easily defined (e.g., *Home care nurse:* Do you have access to a nurse who could come to your home to do such things as monitor health problems, help you care for wounds, and help you learn to take care of yourself after an illness or injury?). Definitions for other services were discussed at length. A local college student jokingly asked if we were referring to dogs or students when he read the statement, "Are *unleashed animals* a problem in your community?" The interested reader may find the complete list of definitions appended to the final report of the survey (Malone-Rising, 1991).

Sample

Stokes and Miller (1985) have characterized sampling as "the weakest aspect of data collection" (p. 546) in the conduct of rural research. In their review of 50 years of empirical research published in the journal *Rural Sociology,* they found a five-fold increase in the use of probability sampling. Still, only 33.9 percent of these studies rely on such samples.

Sample size is a recognized problem in rural research. Stokes and Miller (1985) found 50.6 percent of the studies they reviewed used samples of fewer than 500 subjects. Since its inception, only 9.4 percent of the studies published in *Rural Sociology* drew samples of 2,500 and over. Generalization of findings from research conducted with small samples is limited at best, and recommendations based on such findings must be made cautiously.

A stratified random sample of 5 percent of the households in each of the ten towns of Lamoille County was drawn from the census lists and a list of block rental units generated by council members. Two hundred ninety-nine households were sampled. New names were drawn from each list as necessary to replace households that refused to participate. While our sample contained a larger percentage of homeowners than the population of the county, the sample was generally representative (see Malone-Rising, 1991, for details).

A great deal of publicity preceded the collection of research data. The local newspapers printed press releases that informed the community of the goals of the project and kept them informed of its progress. The radio station also broadcast regular announcements. Postcards were produced that informed a household of their selection for participation. Name tags identifying researchers as Lamoille Health Council Volunteers were made. The police and sheriff's departments and all town clerks received a list of volunteer researcher's names, and community members were regularly reminded of this so as to confirm a researcher's legitimate involvement in the project.

Two other surveys were found to have been conducted in the past decade in Lamoille County; both focused on the needs of the elderly. Interestingly, before the data collection for this project was complete, three other large surveys, including a national census which people in our area found particularly offensive, had been conducted in Lamoille County. In spite of what we came to call "survey saturation," the rate of nonparticipation was low (4 percent). We attribute this high response rate to our care in preparing the community for the survey, and the use of community members as researchers.

Volunteer Researchers

I entered a new phase as project negotiator as we began recruiting surveyors. The council had decided that surveys would be conducted in person, both to ensure accurate completion of the tool and to provide visibility to the work of the health council. Because funding was essentially nonexistent, we decided to recruit volunteers from the community who could be trained to administer the survey, our "volunteer researchers" (Malone-Rising, 1990). We began a search for 30 volunteers willing to devote an estimated 15 hours each to this effort.

Numerous presentations on the project were offered to such groups as Retired Senior Volunteer Program; Retired Teachers; American Association of Retired Persons; and Home Dems, our county extension office women's group. Members of the health council were urged to recruit volunteers. Students taking research courses at both the local college and the university were able to receive some academic credit for their involvement in the project. In spite of our best efforts, only 15 volunteers were recruited for this project, leaving nearly half the surveys to be collected by the project director. Travel costs in conducting the interviews were surely a factor in our inability to recruit volunteers.

Many suggestions were offered at these presentations that were incorporated into the research protocol, which was being developed during the recruiting phase. These potential volunteers, for example, suggested that postcards be mailed to selected households before volunteers made contact. A significant concern for invasion of privacy forced elimination of a demographic question seeking to identify household income level. Instead, a question which reads "Do you have sufficient income to meet necessary expenses" was substituted. A structured research protocol evolved from these discussions (Malone-Rising, 1991).

We experienced the full range of joys and challenges available to those dependent on volunteers. Most of our volunteers were involved with at least one other volunteer activity (80 percent). Much nurturing was required to maintain energy and enthusiasm. Continued support was essential. Recruiting and supporting volunteers became an all-consuming role for me as project director.

Volunteers were oriented to the purpose of the project and the use of the tool. Volunteers practiced with the tool during these sessions. Other topics discussed in orientation sessions included the concepts of confidentiality and informed consent. We also discussed methods for controlling interviews and possible responses to requests for assistance. Regular support was offered through frequent telephone contact. Despite the support and encouragement offered, only one volunteer researcher completed ten surveys.

Data Collection

Before the first community survey was administered, a research protocol was finalized (Malone-Rising, 1991). Instructions to researchers for identifying the "household spokesperson" (a term selected by the researchers to replace the "head of household"), assuring confidentiality, and obtaining consent were defined. Researchers were urged to maintain these aspects of the protocol. Instructions for administering the survey and the definitions of terms completed the protocol.

Methods were employed to ensure the confidentiality of respondents. The volunteer researchers were each given a list of ten households to contact for interviews. Researchers' first act was to renumber the list, using the new number as identification on the survey tool. The renumbered lists were not submitted to the project director with the completed surveys, thus ensuring anonymity.

The consent of participants was obtained twice, first when telephone contact was made to schedule an interview, and again before the survey was administered. Written consents were not obtained. Instead, consent was implied, after an explanation of the right to refuse, by the participant's willingness to respond to the survey.

For each of the 75 items on the survey, subjects were asked the following questions:

1. Is this service available to members of your household if needed?

2. If the service is not available, is this because of high cost, lack of transportation, or because the service is not available in this community?

3. Should this service be available to people in your community?

4. Has any member of your household used this service in the past year?

Demographic data was obtained to allow evaluation of the representatives of the sample. Subjects were asked if they would like to receive a summary of the results. If so, their names and addresses were listed on a separate researcher summary sheet.

RESULTS

Statistical analyses have become increasingly more sophisticated in the 50 years of rural research reviewed by Stokes and Miller (1985). While 39.1 percent of studies published between 1936 and 1945 relied primarily on descriptive statistics for analysis, less than 5 percent rely on this method now. Instead, regression analysis has become the primary method of analyzing rural research data. Tests of statistical significance are cited in about 70 percent of 292 articles published between 1976 and 1985. Stokes and Miller call this disturbing in light of the failure to draw probability samples for many of these studies.

The 75 items of the survey were coded as though each had generated six questions: 1) Is the service available? 2) Is the service not available due to lack of transportation? 3) Is the service not available due to high cost? 4) Is the service just not available in this community? 5) Should the service be available? 6) Did anyone in your household use the service in the last year? Each response was coded as a dichotomous variable. The original survey, as completed by service providers, had not asked whether the service should be available, or about personal use of services. To allow comparison of provider and consumer surveys, questions 5 and 6 were coded as missing variables on provider surveys.

This coding scheme resulted in problems in the analysis of data. The data file was enormous, with 517 items in each of 359 records. The mainframe computer at the university would not display the file. Instead, the file was compressed to 15 lines, both on the screen and in the machine's memory, whenever display was attempted. This required transporting the file between the mainframe and a personal computer for review and revision. Fortunately, the university offers support for unfunded faculty learning the intricacies of computer interfaces.

Detailed results of the statistical analysis conducted with the SPSS-X package are found in the report of the project (Malone-Rising, 1991). Frequencies were tabulated for the sample as a whole as well as for within-town groups. Only five of these groups are of sufficient size to suggest the results are generalizable (Morrisville, $n = 77$; Stowe, $n = 50$; Johnson, $n = 42$, Hyde Park, $n = 39$; Cambridge, $n = 30$). Wolcott ($n = 20$), Eden ($n = 13$), Elmore ($n = 12$), Waterville ($n = 11$), and Belvidere ($n = 4$) were not oversampled to allow a reliable individual analysis.

As a test of consistency, survey data collected by volunteer researchers ($n = 84$) was compared with surveys I collected ($n = 215$). The chi-square (χ^2) analysis was conducted to test for significant differences in the responses to the 450 survey questions (six questions for each of 75 items) between the two groups. As none was found, surveys collected by volunteer researchers were grouped with the other surveys for comparison with provider responses.

Provider and consumer responses to individual items on the survey were compared for significant difference, again using the chi-square (χ^2) analysis. A phi coefficient (φ) was calculated for all values with a $p < .05$ to measure the strength of the relationships identified by the χ^2. Four provider surveys were not included in the survey because of lack of response to over 50 percent of the survey items. As one provider stated, "I only responded to items I knew about." Each provider survey was coded as ten separate surveys, one for each of the ten towns of the county.

DISCUSSION

The focus of this chapter has been the process of conducting quantitative research utilizing a qualitative methodology. Therefore, the discussion of findings for the Lamoille County project will be limited to a review of the specific research questions and a sampling of the results. The interested reader is referred to the complete report for details (Malone-Rising, 1991).

Frequencies calculated for two groups of surveys (providers and consumers) were evaluated to seek answers to the questions about perceived availability of service and barriers to access. Of the 75 items on the survey, 11 were identified as unavailable by 50 percent or more of consumers, including public transportation services ($n = 192$, 64 percent), social rehabilitation programs ($n = 164$, 55 percent), and assistance with treatment decisions ($n = 164$, 55 percent). Numerous housing options were perceived to be unavailable in Lamoille County. Homeless shelters ($n = 243$, 81 percent), formalized homesharing options ($n = 210$, 70 percent), congregate housing services ($n = 172$, 58 percent), and options for independent living with staff support ($n = 153$, 51 percent), were most frequently cited. Medical services were generally felt to be available, with 100 percent of consumers, for example, stating that physician care was available if needed. Frequencies for service utilization, while not a focus of the survey report, may be useful to specific providers in comparing sample responses to utilization data for their specific programs.

Our third research question, related to desired scope of service, was not felt to be adequately answered by our survey. Only consumers who identified barriers to access also stated a particular service should be available. This suggests that the question was not phrased properly to elicit support for continuation of services already perceived to be available. Despite this shortcoming, this question did produce useful data. Several services, all felt to be generally unavailable, were thought needed by a large proportion of respondents. For example, central coordination of services (high visibility assistance), felt unavailable by 77 percent of the sample ($n = 230$), was thought to be a necessary service by 49 percent of the total sample ($n = 146$). The council has viewed this particular finding as significant enough to support efforts to develop a service and information outreach project.

Provider perceptions differed from those of consumers in numerous areas. For example, only 40 percent of providers felt that physician care was available to all members of a community if needed. Statistical analysis demonstrated this difference to be significant ($\chi^2 = 192.44$, $df = 1$, $p = .00000$). The project report lists the statistically significant differences, along with questions raised by these findings.

The perception of availability comparisons has produced two major categories of findings now being discussed by the council. First, educating the public about services known to be available, but perceived as unavailable, is essential. Consumers cannot access services that they do not know exist. Second, providers must carefully consider requests to expand services that consumers feel are already available in sufficient supply. Perhaps the most significant outcome of this survey is the potential influence on future program development in Lamoille County that such findings may produce.

DISSEMINATION OF RESULTS

A 50-page report entitled *A Survey of Health and Social Service Availability in Lamoille County* has been produced (Malone-Rising, 1991). As project director I wrote each draft of the report, which was then circulated to those involved in the project for review. Most of the suggestions offered were directed toward the use of language that would be understandable to all and the production of charts that would clarify findings. The outline for the report is similar to the outline of this chapter, with emphasis on the results instead of the process.

Nearly 100 copies of the full report have been distributed. Recipients include the ten town clerks in Lamoille County, chairs of key state legislative committees (Health and Welfare, Appropriations), the secretary of human services, the governor, and anyone else in the state we felt might use the information for program and policy planning. The distribution of this report is particularly timely as the state legislature spends this summer session considering the state's role in the provision of the full range of human services.

A five-page summary report has been distributed. Respondents who expressed an interest in results ($n = 72$) received this report. Others in the state who might be interested in the full report have received the summary, with a notation that the full report is available for purchase from the council. This summary was printed in the local newspaper to publicize completion of the project.

IMPLICATIONS FOR FUTURE RESEARCH

While the positivist approach to scientific inquiry is the preferred mode, the constructivist paradigm provides a better fit in matters of human inquiry than does the positivist paradigm (Guba & Lincoln, 1989). This idea has been demonstrated in the use of this approach in the conduct of rural community research.

Lareau (1983), finding little consistency in the process of needs assessment as conducted by a random sample of 400 agencies servicing the elderly, has suggested that a comprehensive needs assessment should include a "1) description of the population, 2) description of the problems of the target group, 3) description of available services, 4) description of unmet needs or of service components needed, and 5) list of service priorities" (p. 519). She further suggests that a survey of respondents is the only methodology employed by agencies sampled that provided data applicable, at least in part, to all five areas. Indeed, the survey is the predominate methodology employed in rural sociological research for the past 40 years (Stokes & Miller, 1985). The project conducted by the LAHC has fulfilled all these criteria.

Smith and Carter (1989), in support of the use of interviews in survey research, note the need for such researchers to ensure use of language that is understandable to the general public. They note the need for such activities as convening focus groups, administering pretests, and developing specific interviewer protocols to ensure the suitability of the survey tool. The use of the constructivist paradigm required such activities in the construction of the survey.

If I were to repeat this project, I would first make a concerted effort to fund the research. We were fortunate to have some support, which funded photocopying, some mailings, and refreshments at orientations for volunteer researchers. At the very least, the input and analysis of data has been a time-consuming process that is more efficiently completed by someone more skilled than myself. A current proposal to expand the survey included funding for such an individual.

I have given much thought to the role of the volunteer researcher in this project. Those who became involved contributed a great deal to the success of the project. Many had valuable suggestions that facilitated access to the sample. Recruitment and management of this group, however, was a monumental task. One person should be identified specifically for the recruitment and support of volunteers.

Future surveys must address the underrepresentation of renters versus homeowners in the sample. The original suggestion to conduct a telephone survey was discounted due to a desire for high visibility for the council. However, this method of accessing households would certainly have resulted in a more representative distribution. Telephone, instead of personal, interviews may also have been more attractive to volunteer researchers, who often expressed a reluctance to intruding on neighbors.

In a time when health systems are viewed as fragmented and difficult to access, a collaborative approach to community-based research improves the communication between providers and consumers. Both groups become intimately involved in the research process. The results are a product that is meaningful to those being researched. The involvement of community members in the development and administration of this survey is felt to be the reason for the high rate of participation by respondents. Research directed at determining the perceptions of respondents is enhanced by the involvement of those served in the research process.

REFERENCES

Christenson, J. A., & Garlovich, L. E. (1985). Fifty years of "rural sociology": Status, trends, and impressions. *Rural Sociology, 50*(4), 503–522.

Coelen, S. F. (1981). Public service delivery in rural places. *Rural Development Perspectives, RDP-*4, 20–23.

Cordes, S. M. (1989, December). *The changing rural environment and the relationship between health services and rural development.* Paper presented at the Rural Health Services Research Agenda Conference, San Diego, CA.

Coward, R. T. (1979). Planning community services for the elderly: Implications from research. *The Gerontologist, 19,* 275–282.

Falk, W. W., & Gilbert, J. (1985). Bringing rural sociology back in. *Rural Sociology, 50,* 561–577.

Gimlin, H. (1990). The continuing decline of rural America. *Editorial Research Reports, 1,* 414–425.

Guba, E. G., & Lincoln, Y. S. (1989). *Fourth generation evaluation.* Newbury Park, CA: Sage Publications, Inc.

Jasanoff, S. (1989). Public science for public policy. *Technology Review, 92*(2), 26, 28, 78.

Lareau, L. (1983). Needs assessment of the elderly: Conclusions and methodological approaches. *The Gerontologist, 23,* 518–526.

Malone-Rising, D. (1990, November). *Rural community volunteers as researchers.* Paper presented at the West Virginia Nurses Association's Annual Research Symposium, White Sulfur Springs, WV.

Malone-Rising, D. (1991). *A survey of health and social service availability in Lamoille County.* Morrisville, VT: The Lamoille Area Health Council.

Mendras, H. (1982). Forward. In H. Mendras & I. Mihailescu (Eds.), *Theories and methods in rural community studies* (pp. ix–x). Oxford, England: Pergamon Press.

Planck, U. (1982). Typologies of rural collectivities and the study of social development: Theoretical and methodological aspects. In H. Mendras & I. Mihailescu (Eds.), *Theories and methods in rural community studies* (pp. 33–57). Oxford, England: Pergamon Press.

Roper, R. (1988). Collaborative research and social change: Applied anthropology in action. [Review of *Westview Special Studies in Applied Anthropology*]. *Applied Anthropology, 90,* 427.

Rovner, J. (1989). Coalition seeks to overcome rural health care woes. *Congressional Quarterly, 47,* 695–697.

Smith, T. W., & Carter, W. (1989). Observing "The observer observed": A comment. *Social Problems, 36,* 310–312.

State of Vermont. (1989). *Executive order #70.* Issued for action by Governor M. Kunin, Montpelier, VT.

Stokes, C. S., & Miller, M. K. (1985). A methodological review of fifty years of research in *Rural Sociology. Rural Sociology, 50,* 539–560.

Suvar, S. (1982). The typological method in the study of Yugoslav villages. In H. Mendras & I. Mihailescu (Eds.), *Theories and methods in rural community studies* (pp. 23–32). Oxford, England: Pergamon Press.

U.S. Department of Commerce Bureau of Census. (1985). *Statistical abstract of the United States.* Washington DC: U.S. Government Printing Office.

Vermont Department of Health (March, 1986). Public health statistics bulletin. Waterbury, VT.

Appendix 13–A
Lamoille Area Health Council Survey

Key

1: Service available if needed
T: Service not available due to lack of transportation
$: Service not available because can't afford it
N/A: Service is not available in this area/Don't know if service is available
2: Services that should be available in this area
3: Service used in last year

A. Survey code: _____
B. Town of residence: _____
C. Researcher's name: _____

Services

A. Medical Services	1	T	$	N/A	2	3
1. Home care nurse						
2. Dental care						
3. Physician care						
4. Hospital discharge planning						
5. Outpatient services						
6. Laboratory						
7. Provision of adaptive equipment						
8. Prescription monitor						
9. Alternative therapies						
10. Physical therapy						
11. Speech therapy						
12. Medical care						
1) primary						
2) acute						
13. Drug & alcohol counseling						

B. Developmental Services	1	T	$	N/A	2	3
1. Education						
2. Cultural exposure						
3. Employment opportunities						
4. Volunteerism						
5. Library						
6. Occupational therapy						
7. Participatory art opportunities						
8. Intergenerational learning						
9. Sharing accomplishments						

C. Community Services	1	T	$	N/A	2	3
1. Public transportation services						
2. Religious support						
3. Access of public buildings						
4. Emergency system						
5. Hospice care						
6. Food shelf/commodity distribution						

D. Social/Recreational	1	T	$	N/A	2	3
1. Multi-purpose senior center						
2. Intergenerational opportunities						
3. Parks, picnic tables, benches						
4. Walkways						
5. Clubs						
6. Gym & work out places						
7. Meal sites						

E. Environmental Services	1	T	$	N/A	2	3
1. Rubbish disposal						
2. Air quality						
3. Cross walks						
4. Side walks						
5. Unleashed animals						
6. Ice safety						

F. Social Services	1	T	$	N/A	2	3
1. Mental health counseling						
2. Vermont State Hospital Discharge plans/ options						
3. Dept. Social Welfare financial emergency						
4. Social rehab programs						
5. Court diversion						
6. Health education						
7. Assist with treatment decisions						
8. Death education						

G. Housing Services	1	T	$	N/A	2	3
1. Subsidized housing						
2. Formalized homesharing						
3. Independent living w/staff support						
4. Congregate housing services						
5. Safe homes						

G. Housing Services (Continued)	1	T	$	N/A	2	3
6. Shelters						
7. Community care homes-Level III & IV						
8. Nursing homes Level I & II						
H. In-Home Services	**1**	**T**	**$**	**N/A**	**2**	**3**
1. Personal care						
2. Meal preparation						
3. Meal delivery						
4. Housework						
5. Shopping & errands						
6. Heavy home maintenance & repair						
7. Accessibility adaptation						
8. Respite care						
9. Companionship						
10. Nutrition education						
11. Affordable utilities						
12. Life line/emergency aid						
I. Information & Advocacy Services	**1**	**T**	**$**	**N/A**	**2**	**3**
1. Legal services						
2. Client advocacy						
3. Ombudsman						
4. Guardian ad-litem (court related)						
5. Referral options/care management						
6. Central coordination of services (high visibility assistance)						

DEMOGRAPHICS

Survey Code:_____   Researcher:_____

I'd like to get a little information about the people in the household. We'll use this information to see how well our selection of households really represents the whole population. Again, I need to tell you that this information will be completely confidential. I'm the only one that will know that you answered a survey, and your name will not be on this survey at all. The only people who will see this are the people who will be analyzing it.

1. Can you give me some information about the people living in this household?

	Age	**Sex** M F	**Relationship to** **Spokesperson**	**Occupation**
1.				
2.				
3.				
4.				
5.				
6.				

(Please note additional residents in any available space)

2. Do you own or rent your home?   (check one)   Own   Rent
   How would you describe your home?
   (check one)   Single family house   Duplex
                      Condominium   Townhouse
                      Trailer   Apartment
                      Other (specify)_____

3. Would you say your home is located:
   (check one)   In the village
                      Within 1 (one) mile of the village
                      1 to 5 miles from the village
                      > 5 miles from the village

4. Do you have sufficient income to meet necessary expenses?
   (check one)   Yes   No

5. Do all members of this household have enough health insurance coverage to meet their needs?
   (check one)   Yes   No

14

Shared Governance in a Rural Health Care Setting

Teresa A. B. Lyons

Shared governance at Fairbanks Memorial Hospital is in the process of implementation. Transition and change are occurring. The vision has been established. Realistically that vision will be modified many times as we continue the implementation. However, upon completion of the project, it is my belief that we will have a process designed for Fairbanks Memorial Hospital which enhances the role of the professional nurse and ultimately will result in excellence in patient care.

Donna L. Woodkey
Assistant Administrator of Nursing
Fairbanks Memorial Hospital

This chapter focuses on the activities of the nurses at Fairbanks Memorial Hospital (FMH). It addresses how the control of nursing practice became an issue and how a shared governance structure was implemented in the Department of Nursing.

SETTING

Fairbanks is the central hub for the Interior of Alaska. FMH provides acute health care services for over 100,000 people living north of the Alaskan range. All services are available in this area except cardiac and neuro surgery, neonate intensive care, and residential mental health care. The health issues most frequently encountered in this area are accidental injury, substance abuse, violent trauma, maternal-child health care, and tourist illness or injury. Nurses play integral roles in providing services to people in all these situations. Approximately 250 nurses are employed at FMH, and perhaps another 200 to 300 nurses are employed throughout the community. The population is a cross-cultural mix of Native Alaskans: Inupik, Yupik, and Athabascan; white; Asians; Hispanics; and blacks. The mean age of the community's population is 27.

This country is vast, the environment harsh but exquisite in its raw beauty (Figure 14–1). It is a land that lends itself well to the innovative individualist and the self-motivated survivalist, attitudes also reflected in the nurses of this community.

In the pioneering individualist way, we nurses of FMH have embarked upon a journey to create our own future. We have chosen to implement the philosophy of shared governance throughout the Nursing Department in order to develop our own professional practice model for nursing.

BACKGROUND

FMH is an acute-care facility licensed for 177 beds. The daily average occupancy is 60. It is the only civilian hospital in the community. Some collaboration exists between FMH and nearby Bassett Army Community Hospital.

Like hospitals in the rest of the country, over the past five years there has been a decline in length of stay of our patients and, paradoxically, an increase in acuity. The nurses who practice at FMH are 86 percent registered nurses with 3 percent having master's degrees, 40 percent having baccalaureate degrees, 34

Figure 14–1
Alaska

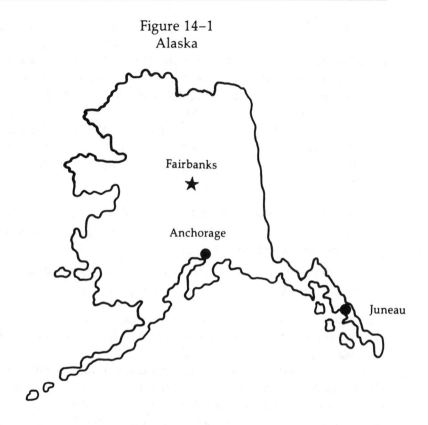

percent having associate degrees, and 9 percent being diploma-
prepared. Forty percent are certified in their specialty areas.
Their mean age is 38. The nurses come from a variety of backgrounds.

In 1986 the factors of cost-containment and increased patient
acuity were experienced in Alaska. These factors were compounded by the 1986 decline in oil revenue resulting in a two-year
economic crisis for the Fairbanks community.

In the bureaucratic tradition of the hospital, decisions were
made by the management which were indicative of the belief that
nurses did not control nursing practice. The nurses became pain-
fully aware of this when productive and progressive nursing units
were closed and the staffs and patient populations were merged

with other units. These decisions were made without involving the nurses who were the most affected. This awareness was furthered as the organization instituted a reduction in force. The decision to implement the reduction in force was made over a weekend and was announced the following Monday. Several employees read about it in the local paper on Saturday.

Motivated by these events, a group of staff nurses began investigating options to ensure that nurses would have control and input into decisions affecting nursing practice. Three options were examined:

1. nursing representation by a national labor union;
2. nursing representation by the American Nurses' Association's collective bargaining unit; and
3. restructuring the Department of Nursing into a shared governance framework.

Much thought was given to the idea of unionization. Unions are certainly a legitimate mechanism for workers in an industrialized society.

A trade union attempted to organize the nurses into a collective bargaining unit. It became clear through conversation with the trade union representatives, that they did not have any understanding of nurses or nursing. We were continually assured that we would be representing ourselves; they would teach us and help us. We were struck by the idea that we would have to *pay* for the permission and the privilege of representing ourselves. The trade union did not "sign up" enough nurses to qualify for a unionization vote.

A second option for unionization was to seek help from the Alaska State Nurses Association. However, it does not have an economic and general welfare unit. The closest state nurses association with such a unit was Washington state. The Washington State Nurses Association (WSNA) was, at this time, being raided by competitors in the national labor business, so we decided that involvement with WSNA was not in our best interest.

Control of nursing practice was the issue upon which we focused. As a group we were not convinced that collective bargaining was compatible with professional responsibility and accountability. We studied the impact of collective bargaining in several situations and found that it has not made gains in control over practice issues. Legally, hospitals are not required to bargain for practice issues under the National Labor Relations Act (DeYoung, 1985). Further, DeYoung reports that there is *no documentation* in the literature or in practice to provide evidence that collective bargaining in nursing has enhanced professionalism; increased recognition of professional status; supported the public service orientation of a profession; created a climate for professional autonomy; or provided for an equitable, voluntary, fully participative professional association (DeYoung, 1985). We decided that by accepting the responsibilities and accountabilities of our social mandate, we would find common ground in the profession and begin to develop a true sense of unity.

After study and discussion, it became apparent that restructuring the Department of Nursing into a shared governance framework would serve our needs better than the alternatives.

A group of staff nurses conducted the research, but nurse managers and the nurse executive also were interested in developing a system and a climate that would benefit nurses and nursing. Economic concerns demand that health care costs be efficiently contained and that quality of care provided to the public remain excellent. With these requirements clear to all of us, we came to sense that we had to overcome the adversarial climate created by our recent experiences in the organization. We realized that we needed to understand what was happening. We needed to change the adversarial climate within the institution that interfered with our providing quality patient care.

In 1988, administrators, managers, and participating staff nurses attended workshops in shared governance. In January 1989, the designing and restructuring of the Department of Nursing began.

CHANGE THEORY

Before initiating the change process at FMH, it was helpful to review the change theory of Kurt Lewin. Lewin describes three phases of change: unfreezing, movement, and refreezing. The change process requires a dynamic model, one that takes the disharmony, chaos, and conflict, and with assessment, planning, implementation, and evaluation, creates the changed environment.

Unfreezing

Step 1 in the unfreezing phase is assessment, that is, identification of the problem, current status of the organization, current expectations of behavior, and formal and informal leadership.

Step 2 in the unfreezing phase is to identify organizational supports and constraints, understand the change event (i.e., what initiated the change process), and identify behavioral and system expectations of the outcome.

Step 3 in the unfreezing phase is to determine the change factors. What are the tools available: personnel, plans, and resources. What is the process: strategies, starting point, educational plan.

Step 4 in the unfreezing process is to build organizational support by developing action groups and developing and disseminating educational materials. Communication is essential. It is in Step 4 that a safe environment must be established to stimulate innovative thought, discussion, and debate, throughout the organization.

Movement

Step 1 in the movement phase is to assess the situation and ask questions. Is the vision clear? Do we know where we are going? Are the tasks of the structure specific? What are the immediate outcomes? How is the power based? It is essential that in the first step of the movement phase, negotiation and communications skills are functioning at excellent levels for all those involved in the change.

Step 2 of the movement phase is the planning step. In this step, it is necessary to identify specific tasks to accomplish, identify goals and actions to achieve the goals, track achievement, and reward immediately. Step 2 is continued as actions are monitored and evaluated and support is established within the organization for the change and for each individual. Support is critical during the change process, not only for the organization but for the individuals initiating the changes. While other organizations have undertaken restructuring and have been successful, it is uncharted territory for each new group.

Refreezing

Step 1 in the refreezing process is change completion. A sense of completion occurs when behaviors have been altered and the new system is functioning.

Step 2 of refreezing brings evidence of change. New values are apparent, the organization validates the change, and past behaviors are no longer apparent (Porter-O'Grady & Finnigan, 1984).

To have a solid understanding of the theory was necessary for the initial planning. As the change process has progressed, it has been useful to re-visit the theory in order to gain perspective and help in objective evaluation of the process.

SHARED GOVERNANCE

Shared governance is a concept based on organizational theory. The models and theorists contributory to the concept of shared governance are the Neoteric Model (Wade, 1960s), the Rational Democracy Model (Abell, 1970s), and the Open Organization System (Mink et al., 1970s) (Porter-O'Grady & Finnigan, 1984). The works of these theorists dovetail with the predictions made by Naisbitt and Aburdene in *Megatrends 2000,* "The most exciting breakthroughs of the 21st century will occur not because of technology but because of an expanding concept of what it is to be human" (Naisbitt & Aburdene, 1990, p. xxiii).

All three theorists describe organizations that are people oriented. The hierarchies they describe are not vertical but lateral, meaning each individual is equal to the other. The structures are loose and move along continua of responsibility, accountability, and authority of the individuals within the organization. These are key to ownership of decision making and contribution to the organization.

Companies of the 21st century must be able to change rapidly, communicate with excellence, and be flexible and receptive to the marketplace in which they operate (Drucker, 1989).

Porter-O'Grady and Finnigan describe shared governance in nursing:

> *It is upon these theoretical bases that the concept of shared governance in nursing is based. In an effort to restructure the organization to make it supportive of professional nursing activities, it is necessary to have some legitimate theoretical underpinning for providing a unique thinking process for unfolding professional nursing practice. It must be different from what has been experienced in the past. Neoteric, rational democratic authority, and open organizational approaches, all provide a general base for moving toward a more humanistic structure that operates more effectively in human-intensive settings such as hospitals [1984, p. 56].*

We took the concept of shared governance, worked with it, and molded it to fit our own environment and culture. We have defined it for the Department of Nursing at FMH. Shared governance is an organizational design built upon the philosophy that all members of the organization have positive value and have the right and the responsibility to contribute to the decision-making processes that directly affect the setting in which they practice. It is understood that not all organizational decisions will be to the liking of everyone. Shared governance is a concept based within the theory of futurists. It is not participative management (Porter-O'Grady, 1990).

OUTCOMES OF A SHARED GOVERNANCE STRUCTURE

The following list of outcomes has been developed from a review of current literature and a retrospective review of our experience in Fairbanks.

- Shared governance moves nurses from subservient to autonomous roles by giving them authority over practice decisions.

- Shared governance enhances the contributions of nurses in the changing health care system.

- Shared governance allows trusting relationships to be built in an environment of openness, self-disclosure, and integrity.

- Shared governance establishes a framework that allows for communications to be clarified and reduces uncertainty by giving staff nurses direct access to information and to persons who can clarify the information.

- Shared governance promotes quality performance and attitudes by providing a framework of systems that support professional behavior.

- Shared governance results in high productivity, low absenteeism, and low turnover by creating an environment where job satisfaction is high.

- Shared governance reflects the value and promotes advancement of the individual and the profession.

As the turn of the century approaches, change is becoming the constant rather than the variable. In the health care industry, we are grabbling with issues that require significant changes: too much technology; too much cost; too little time, money, and resources. Nursing is a member of this dynamic industry. Nursing is affected by many of these issues: there are too few nurses and we are, perhaps, the best cost containment managers. Out of the debates and disagreements, one fact about nurses is emerging: we are mediators in the "high-tech" vs. "high touch" debates. Nurses are accountable, responsible, and autonomous in rendering nursing care to patients/clients. Shared governance in nursing establishes firmly that nursing care is the focus of nursing; therefore, nurses must control their own practice.

In Fairbanks, we began the process of preparing to define our professional future. In order to further our education, we studied organizational theories of bureaucracy and professional values.

Study of the bureaucratic structure (Figure 14–2) reveals a hierarchy of vertical communication. The degree of authority in a bureaucracy is dependent upon the level within the hierarchy. Bureaucracy reflects the values of the Industrial Age in its orientation to control and productivity. Bureaucracy is an autocratic structure.

An autocratic structure contradicts professional values, autonomy, and knowledge-based practice. Figure 14–3 lists the potential areas of conflict that emerge when professional values are placed in a bureaucratic framework.

Nursing is a highly skilled profession requiring judgment, education, and technical expertise. To provide optimal patient care, nurses need to work freely within the organizational structure, to make decisions and contribute to the collaborative processes. Nurses must ask for and receive the resources they need to provide patient care. Those resources may be dressing supplies, special equipment, education, or more staff. Nurses must be part of the collaboration with other health care professionals to provide the very best for the patients. Nurses are the key communicators and gatekeepers for patients. Patient care is more than the eight- or 12-hour shift of the individual nurse. Planning patient care is long range. Methods used in planning a patient's care are based in the scientific body of knowledge that is specific to nursing.

In reviewing the behavior characteristics of nonprofessionals and professionals (Figure 14–4), it becomes clear that dissonance

Figure 14–2
Nursing Organization within the Corporate Structure

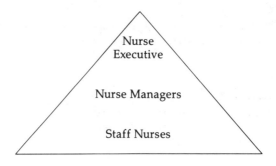

Figure 14–3
Organizational Performance Characteristics

Characteristics	Nonprofessional	Professional
Structure	Tight control High degree structure	Low structure
Distribution of influence	Low total influence Centered at top	Even distribution of influence
Superior–subordinate relations	Directive Low freedom	Participation High degree of freedom
Colleague relations	High coordination Few differences	Diffuse relations Low coordination Many differences
Time orientation	Immediate, short term	Long range
Goal orientation	Technical, high task	Professional Scientific High interaction
Management style	Task centered High control	Task and relationship orientation

Reprinted from *Shared Governance for Nursing* by T. Porter-O'Grady and S. Finnigan with permission of Aspen Publishers, Inc., © 1984.

will and must occur for those who recognize the inherent professional characteristics of nursing, yet practice in settings better suited for nonprofessional behavior. It is equally apparent, therefore, that change can and must occur.

PLANNED CHANGE TO SHARED GOVERNANCE

Change in an organizational structure must be founded on a change in behavior. Changing the organizational chart is simple. It is more difficult for people to change their behaviors.

A few questions must be answered before structural changes can be implemented. First, one must find out what the organization is: What is the mission of the hospital? Why does the hospital

Figure 14-4
Sources of Dissonance Between Bureaucratic Organization
and Professional Practice

Dissonance

Bureaucratic Organization		Professional Practice
Ordered	. .	. . . . Consultive
Hierarchial	. .	. . . . Collaborative
Controlled	. .	. . . . Knowledge based
Vertical	. .	. . . . . . Lateral communication
Authoritative	. .	. . . . Judgment rendering
Structured	. .	. . . . Developmental
Administrative	. .	. . . . Standard centered
Pyramidal	. .	. . . . Measurable
Policy governed	. .	. . . . Interdependent

Dissonance

Reprinted from *Shared Governance for Nursing* by T. Porter-O'Grady and S. Finnigan with permission of Aspen Publishers, Inc., © 1984.

exist? Who makes up the governing board of the hospital? How are the decisions made at the governing board level?

The nurse must ask: what is my mission as a nurse? Why do I practice nursing? Is my personal mission in harmony with the mission of this institution? Initiating change requires commitment from individuals involved to learn more about themselves and the institution in which they practice. If there is consensus between the institutional values and the individual's values, there is at least a beginning. If there is not consensus, then the nurse must decide to stay within the institution or go. Choosing to stay, one must accept the consequences of conflicting values or investigate mechanisms to begin a change process. Initiating change can be risky for the individual. The worst outcome is that one will be fired; the best is that positive change will occur.

We must create for ourselves a work environment that will allow us to innovatively deal with the issues within the realm of nursing care. To implement a shared governance framework, everything in the work setting must be viewed as a patient care issue (Figure 14-5). In establishing a structure that supports professional practice and requires professional behavior, communica-

Figure 14–5
Partnership in Care

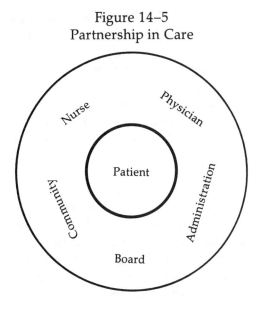

tions must be free flowing and a spirit of "share the knowledge" must prevail. A shared governance structure is centered around the patient.

SHARED GOVERNANCE IN NURSING

The concept of shared governance developed in the theorists' realm and was introduced in the early 1980s in nursing. Porter-O'Grady and Finnigan published a book, *Shared Governance for Nursing: A Creative Approach to Professional Accountability,* in 1984. A review of the literature published since 1980 indicates sporadic references, ranging from none to two or three per year until 1986, when interest in the topic accelerated. A National Shared Governance Conference is hosted annually by three of the first organizations to restructure their nursing departments according to the shared governance concept. Those three organizations are Rose Medical in Denver, St. Michaels in Milwaukee, and St. Joseph's in Atlanta. These hospitals are large organizations located in urban centers. The process of bringing the concepts of shared governance into a rural health care setting is discussed below.

The first component of bringing shared governance to a nursing unit is to always put the patient at the forefront of the thought process. Remembering to put the patient first helps to keep one's perspective. Putting the patient first sounds easy; doing it requires some reorientation. Nurses must keep in mind that the patient is a person with a family and a life beyond the walls of the hospital or clinic. Patients' lives are affected by more than our daily routine. Talking with patients and their families fosters a patient-centered point of view.

In order to implement change, communication skills and group dynamic workshops are in order for nurses and others who have the power to initiate change. All involved in the change process need to hone their communication skills because communication is the key to success. Shared governance hinges on professional behavior. Nurses must learn how to communicate with each other and with others in order to describe what the work of nursing is. Communicating clearly, honestly, and concisely will foster an understanding of the resources required for nurses to be effective.

Many barriers must be taken down before we can design a structure that will support the work of nursing. The barriers are those that we have built over time as a result of the bureaucratic chain of command, socialization of nursing as a feminine profession, and natural resistance to change. It is essential to explore the idea that "nursing is business" to replace the concept of nursing as a "personal" activity.

Socialization of women in the United States has been fraught with contradictions. Janice K. Lanier writes,

> *Despite the women's movement, political advances, and a growing public appreciation of the capabilities of women, the dichotomy of role expectations versus reality that has plagued women for centuries exists yet today. Only when women can function as individuals first and women second will they be able to contribute fully to the betterment of society [DeYoung, 1985, pp. 166–167].*

Ninety-seven percent of the nursing profession is made up of women. The challenge to nurses is to first develop their individual identity, and then translate their individual strengths to develop their professional identities.

Involvement in a changing organization is personally and professionally challenging. It is the individual people of the organization who establish and maintain the changes. Shared governance is a concept that is exhibited through the behavior of individuals. Barriers to change are created by people. To resolve barriers, behavioral changes are necessary at the individual level.

Recognition of initial barriers is essential to appropriate planning. In Fairbanks, we initiated several work sessions that dealt with communication skills of women, women working with women, professional practice, small-group dynamics, organizational culture, and change. These interactive workshops were designed to help us identify our own behaviors and skills and to give staff nurses, managers, administrators, and support personnel equal access to skills and education that would allow us to communicate as openly and honestly as possible. We began to recognize our commonalities, strengths, and needs. Change in any area of an organization has a ripple effect. It was, and continues to be, important that we attempt to work together positively so that we can collectively offer the highest quality of health care to our patients.

To avoid alienating the medical community, several short presentations were initially made to the Medical Executive Committee. Increased visibility of staff nurses on various hospital-wide committees and a purposeful effort to keep the physicians informed about the developments of the shared governance structure at FMH have decreased, if not eliminated, physician resistance. It is important to note that we did not ask for permission or even a vote of confidence from the medical community. It is our belief that control of nursing practice is solely the responsibility of nurses.

THE CHANGE PROCESS AT FAIRBANKS

The staff nurses of FMH initiated the education program about the concepts of shared governance. During this time the hospital and nursing administrators at FMH were changing on a fairly regular basis. As a result of this frequent turnover, nurse managers had their hands full trying to keep up with day-to-day operations.

In 1988, administration began to stabilize. The new nurse executive supported the concept of shared governance. Staff nurses in our organization were educated in, and supportive of, the concept of shared governance, as was the nurse executive. The nurse managers were neither for nor against the change.

The nurse manager's role in a shared governance framework differs from the traditional role. Nurse managers are often the ones who feel most threatened by shared governance. The perception that the nurse manager's position is no longer required is a misconception. Nurse managers can be barriers to the implementation of shared governance if they believe themselves to be threatened by it. Role clarification and definition are useful in averting this misconception. Issues of authority, power, and prestige must be freely discussed among all levels of nursing personnel.

The roles of staff nurses and nurse managers take on new dimensions under a shared governance structure. Staff nurses are the managers of patient care. Nurse managers are the managers of resources to support the nurses in providing patient care. Staff nurses are the core of patient care in nursing. Nurse managers provide the resources to nurses so that they can render quality patient care. What is different under a shared governance system? Nurse managers *do not* manage nurses. Nurses, in meeting the demands of professional practice, evaluate each other through quality assurance and peer review. Nurse managers are not responsible for setting standards regarding patient care. Staff nurses are responsible for standards of care.

Our decision for change at FMH was made with consensus from the four levels of the bureaucracy: staff nurses, nurse managers, the nurse executive, and the hospital administrator.

Within our organizational structure, a communication forum, the Nursing Affairs Committee, was chaired by the nurse executive. As a result of a suggestion from the staff nurses, this committee was restructured into the Nursing Affairs Council (NAC). The members are staff nurses representing each nursing unit. The chair is elected from the members, by the members. Formal bylaws were developed and approved by the council, nurse managers, and the nurse executive. NAC's purpose is to facilitate communications between administration, management, and staff. The council was reorganized into its current form in 1987 and was instrumental in pursuing the concepts of shared governance.

NAC accepted the responsibility for developing the shared governance program at FMH. The first action was to learn about who we were as an organization. The members of the council spent time with the hospital administrator reviewing and discussing the mission of FMH and the strategic plan of the organization. The NAC then established the shared governance subcommittees. Initially there were four. The Conceptual Framework Committee was to develop a nursing philosophy and write bylaws that would reflect a shared governance framework. The Nursing Models Committee was to research and recommend a nursing model that reflected the culture of nursing as practiced at FMH. The Education Committee was to take the work of the above committees and develop educational packages for the marketing committee. The Marketing Committee was to sell the new ideas and concepts, via education, to the rest of the staff nurses, nurse managers, and all others interested.

In retrospect, the education and marketing committees should have been one because they each had information the other needed. The activities of the two committees reinforced the need for excellent communication skills. The two committees seemed to be getting in each others' way. Finally, a discussion was initiated about what was wrong. The solution was to merge the committees. It took a bit of work to get through the personal issues around who was going to chair the committee, and what the status of the individual members would be. This is a committee of staff nurses, and no one is immune to the emotions brought on by change.

We found a few clichés to be helpful.

If it is broken, fix it.
Don't beat a dead horse.
Business is business.

These clichés became a shorthand that helped build group solidarity.

When embarking on a journey such as restructuring an organization, everyone's ideas are needed. That everyone is of value is the cornerstone of shared governance. We are all responsible for keeping each other honest. Letting go of the power and status issues is not easy, but necessary for change to occur.

CHARACTERISTICS OF THE NURSES AT FMH

There is no recipe for implementing shared governance. Some essential components must exist in order for an organization to function in a professional practice framework (i.e., shared governance). The approach to change comes from within the culture of each organization. It is essential to understand the culture and values within the organization. Many organizations are made up of people differing in age, education, religion, cultural origin, and language. The approach to change must be tailored to each individual organization. The key to success is keeping the focus on the patient and providing quality care.

The average age of the nurses at FMH is 38. A large number come from the Midwest. The educational background of the nurses is predominantly associate degree or diploma, and the ethnic background is largely white.

These factors have several implications. We need to emphasize professional behavior and set up systems to reward professionalism. Many of the nurses at FMH have technical backgrounds. In designing their future, many nurses seek to expand their educational foundations, to become more open minded, and to examine global concepts. Discussions of theory and concepts must be rooted in everyday language with concrete examples. "What does all this mean on the 7:00–3:00 shift?" Communications at FMH can be direct; language and cultural orientation within the Nursing Department are not issues.

Without sensitivity to who the nurses are, however, the changes desired will not be effective. The very people who are at the core of the change will resist if the sensitivity to "who we are" is lacking.

At least 20 percent of the staff nurses must be supportive of the change. There must be visible safe means for the other 80 percent to be involved or have input into the decisions being made. Approximately 20 percent of the nurses will resist all change. Everyone is important, but 100 percent consensus is unrealistic and unnecessary. The remaining 60 percent of nurses are the "show me" group. This is the group on which permanence of the change depends. The "show me" nurses are interested in finding out if shared governance is just another fad. They want to see how strong the commitment is and how it will affect patient care. Access to participation is vital.

Solutions and new ideas must be encouraged in all phases of restructuring.

> *If you always do what you always did,*
> *you will always get what you always got.*
>
> Paul Radde

There has been tremendous response to this quote, from uncomfortable silence to downright disgust. In time, though, our nurses began to risk "doing it differently." Letters of suggestion have come forward. Fresh volunteers appeared to take on new projects associated with changing the nursing environment at FMH. With each risk it is important to acknowledge the risk, the person, and the idea.

The increase in wages that nursing has seen around the country has been accompanied by an increase in part-time employment. Part-time nurses value patient care, but are usually less interested in organizational goals. "I'll work on a committee if they pay me" is a typical comment. Initiating change requires commitment of time, resources, and money. The organization is the overall beneficiary of these changes.

To demonstrate the value of committee work, each member nurse of the shared governance subcommittees was allocated eight hours a month for meetings in 1990. In 1991 *every nurse on the staff* has been budgeted four hours a month for meeting time. Productivity is expected. Action plans and time lines have been drafted, presented, and approved by NAC. Scheduling time for staff nurses to participate in designing the professional practice of nursing within an organization must be supported by resources, money, and creative staffing.

COMPONENTS OF OPERATIONAL DESIGN

If we want nursing practice to be controlled by nurses, then the structure must show that the power, authority, accountability, and responsibility are at the level of the bedside nurse. We established a structure in which the seat of power is in the individual nursing unit. Unit-based shared governance establishes that the individual nursing units have the authority to operate their own units.

Five components are identified by Porter-O'Grady (1984) that must be included in the operational design for a professional practice model that is based on the concepts of shared governance: practice, education, quality assurance and peer relations, and governance.

Terminology is very important. *Council,* the term used to describe the structural components, denotes a representative group with decision-making authority as defined by the bylaws of the shared governance structure. *Membership* of all of the councils is composed of 95 percent staff nurses and 5 percent nurse managers. The nurse executive is a member ex officio of the department-wide councils. The *Practice Council* is the heart of nursing. Its responsibilities are related to issues of nursing care provided to patients. It is in this council that standards of care are developed, discussed, and adopted. The *Education Council* supports the practice of nursing. This council has the responsibility and accountability for providing educational opportunities for professional development and patient education. The *Quality Assurance and Peer Relations Council* measures and monitors the practice of nursing. The focus of this council is to relate research, creation of new knowledge, and staff development directly to practice. Accountability for measuring the minimum standard of practice is at the peer level. This council is responsible for taking any needed corrective action. The *Governance Council* coordinates with the other councils to ensure flow of communications. This council could be called a coordinating or house council if the title "governance council" is found to be offensive. This coordinating council is the keeper of the bylaws and developer of the strategic plans for the organization of the Nursing Department. It is chaired by a staff nurse. The nurse executive is a voting member of this council at the department level.

UNIT-BASED AND DEPARTMENT-WIDE STRUCTURES

Professional behavior begins with the individual. A professional environment must be established throughout the organization. Communication is critical. Nursing and nurses do not exist within a vacuum; therefore, mechanisms for coordination and communication must be defined.

In Fairbanks, the vision of our structure, a design based on our culture and organizational climate, looks like this:

Unit-Based Councils

Each unit will establish a council to address practice, education, quality assurance and peer review, and governance. The units are not limited to these issues. Some units have addressed other issues (e.g., future directions, research and marketing, human resources).

Clinical Councils

Each unit will be a member of a clinical council. These councils are composed of representatives from like units (e.g., Labor and Delivery, Nursery, Pediatrics, Maternal-Child). These councils meet quarterly and are essential communication forums for developing budgets, sharing resources, sharing information, and resolving problems.

Department-Wide Councils

Department-wide councils coordinate practice, education, quality assurance and peer review, and governance. Also, a Management Council is made up of the nurse managers, nurse executive, and the chair of the Governance Council (who is a staff nurse). These councils facilitate the unit-based councils. If a unit has an issue that it is unable to resolve, it can elect to send the issue to the appropriate council or the governance council. When an issue is sent forth, the unit clearly communicates the expectation, "solve this issue" or "send us some recommendations on how to resolve this issue."

DRAWBACKS TO IMPLEMENTING A
SHARED GOVERNANCE STRUCTURE

The time, effort, and energy required are the drawbacks to implementing a shared governance program. Change takes time, careful planning, and high energy. A common complaint is "there is so much meeting time."

Many of the time commitments will decrease once the communications and group dynamic skills are refined. Changing an organization from a stiff bureaucracy to a free-formed professional practice model requires patience and perserverance.

Unwillingness to assume accountability is a drawback of wanting the goodies but not the liability. Nursing is a profession; in accepting this statement it is important to understand that the word, profession, comes from the Latin root of *profitere,* which translates to "to promise publicly." Leah Curtin writes:

> *The profession of nursing has made certain promises to the public, and these promises make up our contract with society. Specifically, nurses have promised (1) to help the ill regain their health, (2) to help the healthy maintain their health, (3) to help those who cannot be cured to realize their potential, and (4) to help the dying to live as fully as possible until their deaths [DeYoung, 1985, p. 149].*

To practice with autonomy demands that accountability (liability) be equally applied. A drawback of our profession is that the educational preparation can be so varied. Many practicing nurses are not aware of the social mandates they are honor bound and legally obligated to uphold.

A final drawback that may be perceived in a shared governance organization is the amount of time it takes to get a final decision. Gaining consensus is time consuming, especially in groups that have had limited decision-making power in the past. In Fairbanks, however, we have seen implementation time and resistance to change diminish dramatically. This makes sense because, if all those involved participate in the design and selection of a new project, there should be an element of ownership. Acceptance and implementation, therefore, should be more smoothly achieved.

CHALLENGES

Education

Time, energy, and resources must be put into providing every member of the organization with the same level of understanding of the concept. In a nursing department, all nurses need access to a Nursing Code of Ethics and Social Mandates, standards of professional behavior, a review of bureaucracy, and a short definition of shared governance.

Communication

It is essential that *all* members of the organization be educated in the skills of communication and group dynamics. The challenge then becomes to reinforce the desired behaviors and to resolve conflicts caused by covert communication. Avoidance is not acceptable. Challenge and confrontation are risky and uncomfortable. To maintain an environment that feels safe for the free flow of ideas, covert communications must be addressed quickly and openly.

Power

Because role definitions of staff nurses and nurse managers become ambiguous under a shared governance structure, discussions must be initiated about power. Nurse managers can hinder the growth of the staff nurses by creating an emotionally unsafe environment, withholding information necessary to make sound decisions, and rescuing staff nurses when things are not running smoothly. The nurse manager is a powerful individual in the authority-based structure of a bureaucracy. When discussion occurs about "flattening out" the organization, the concern is that, perhaps, nurse managers will be "flattened out" completely. Roles are different and responsibilities change in a true shared governance structure. A nurse manager does not necessarily need to be a nurse; the nurse manager becomes a resource manager. The best person for the job of nurse manager would be a nurse who has an education in business management. The work of nursing is the business of nursing. Shared governance allows nurses to define what the business is.

Staff nurses must be aware of the personal and professional power that is theirs by virtue of their education and expertise. Accompanying that power comes the responsibility for the control of nursing practice (DeYoung, 1985).

Militancy is a type of power, but it is not useful in defining new organizational structures. Militancy is counterproductive to developing a climate safe for innovation and growth.

Consensus is useful for developing organizational harmony. Consensus does not mean that everyone is in total agreement. It means that everyone accepts the final decisions of the group. It means that everyone is publicly committed to standing by the decisions made by the group. This should not imply that discussion cannot continue within the context of "free flow of communication."

The responsibility that comes with power is to discuss it openly and to clarify appropriate places for it to be exercised. Getting individuals to openly discuss their feelings, concerns, and fears about power is a challenge unto itself. Persistence is generally effective. The most important element is developing an environment that is safe.

COMMENTARIES

The following commentaries were solicited from staff members of FMH. Each person was asked to respond to a series of questions. They have not had an opportunity to read this chapter. Each person questioned has been involved in the development of shared governance at FMH.

Assistant Administrator of Nursing

Implementing shared governance must be a well defined and planned process. Implementation is enhanced if the chief executive officer of the organization works in tandem and supports the nurse executive and staff in the decision to pursue shared governance. At FMH, we are currently in transition to a total shared governance process. A three- to five-year process, this transition has not been without pain and difficulty. However, meeting the challenges far outweighs the probabilities of what might have occurred if we had not pursued shared governance here.

"What are our choices? Should we go union or should we look at shared governance?" These were the questions that were being discussed by the nursing staff at FMH on my first day of employment with the hospital. Approximately 60 percent of the nurses were in a meeting conducted by staff nurses that day. The topics of discussion were needing someone to speak for them, lack of respect for each other and management, general dissatisfaction with the clinical practice environment, and having no input into the decisions that affected their professional practice of nursing. It was of interest that the issues of staff intolerance, having enough staff, and salary were not part of the discussion. As a nurse executive new to the facility, I was somewhat concerned by this meeting. However, it provided an opportunity to work with the staff and to facilitate future discussions.

The staff nurses inquired of my knowledge of shared governance and the degree to which I would be willing to explore the concept for our nursing organization. On the other side of the organization my colleagues questioned: "Isn't there a danger in relinquishing management responsibility? How can we approach this concept which may be trendy, especially in a remote rural area of interior Alaska? What happens if shared governance fails? Do we have the professional staff to implement such a process? Will you, as the nurse executive, commit to seeing the project through? What will this accomplish for the patient?"

I shared my thoughts with both my colleagues and the staff. The patient will be affected by shared governance:

- *The professional nurse will assume accountability for the clinical care provided to patients.*
- *The concept of patient care will expand for the nurse because our shared governance process includes not*

only practice, but also quality assurance, education, and financial responsibility.

- *Nurses will be concerned and responsible for ensuring the competency of their peers and the quality of care provided to the patient.*
- *Collaboration between the physician and nurse will be facilitated.*

"When physicians and nurses work together optimally, relationships are positive, and disagreements are collaboratively resolved to the benefit of the patient, and patient care flows smoothly" (Prescott & Bowen, 1985).

Staff implementation of shared governance would

- *increase the satisfaction of the professional nurse;*
- *provide nurses with greater control over their professional destiny;*
- *facilitate the nurses' development as clinical decision-makers; and*
- *provide an opportunity for nurse managers to grow and develop as facilitators of the process.*

As the nurse executive, my primary objectives were to

- *provide an environment that would foster the development of a shared governance process;*
- *create an organizational culture that would support shared governance;*
- *provide resources necessary to accomplish the transition to shared governance;*
- *provide education through coaching and formal programs for the nurse managers in their role change; and*
- *provide an environment in which it is safe to "try on" new behaviors.*

The transition of an organization to shared governance takes at least three to five years. Taking short cuts initially will only lengthen the process and may cause deterioration not only in the progress of the transition, but in relationships. As a strong advocate and practitioner of participative management, I believed the transition could be shortened. I learned quickly, however, that I was harming the process I strongly believed in by attempting to implement the process hastily.

It is easy for the nurse executive to focus attention on assisting the staff in developing the process and neglect the development and role change of the nurse manager. I found that it was important to design a developmental plan for each nurse manager. This plan included an introduction to shared governance, the role of the nurse manager in a shared governance organization, and a plan for facilitating the process. Some managers adjusted quickly. Others have decided that they cannot work within a shared governance organization.

In summary, the following are suggestions for others who may wish to consider implementing shared governance within their respective organizations:

- *Develop a process that is designed for your organization. Examine multiple models but do what is best for your organization.*
- *An organization of any size can develop a shared governance process.*
- *Commitment of the nurse executive is critical.*
- *The nurse managers require deliberate focus and support during the transitional process.*
- *The transition to a shared governance structure is a three- to five-year process.*
- *Support of the hospital administrator is beneficial.*

Shared governance at FMH is in the process of implementation. Transition and change are occurring. The vision has been established. Realistically, that vision will be modified many times as we continue the implementation. However, upon completion of the project, I believe that the process designed for FMH will enhance the role of the professional nurse and ultimately result in excellence in patient care.

Donna L. Woodkey

Hospital Administrator

Question: *When the concept of shared governance was accepted by the Nursing Affairs Council, nurse managers, and the administrators in 1988, what changes did you hope would be accomplished for nursing and patient care?*

Answer: *I found it to be a challenge to entertain the concept of shared governance in 1988. I was aware of the increase within the nursing industry of concern for their [nurses'] economic value to be noticed. I believed that the health care industry needed to create a work place that was more satisfying and rewarding for professional nurses. I was interested in being involved in a process that would increase the participation of the nurses in decisions that affect their practice and their profession.*

Question: *In 1991, what changes have occurred as the implementation of shared governance has begun?*

Answer: *Now that shared governance has been partially implemented, there are a number of staff nurses actively involved in the process. I think that there have been fundamental changes. Nurses are encouraged and expected to be involved in the care delivery system at this facility. Nurses are expressing that they are accomplishing needed changes. They are further expressing that they have been involved in the decision-making process that has resulted in these changes. I have observed nurses taking control of their own practice. I have also seen evidence of and increased collaboration between the medical and nursing staffs.*

Question: *What has been your involvement in developing the concept of shared governance?*

Answer: *It has been necessary to have a director of nursing who believes in the concept and is willing to put the time and effort into it. I was involved in selecting a new director of nursing who was a team player and who would and could work hand-in-hand with the professional staff.*

I have been involved in securing the resources for meeting and training time for many of the nurses. I believe that it is essential that there be a broad degree of knowledge throughout the facility about the concepts of shared governance.

I believe it is important to have upper management support for the basic concept. In the early stage of development, it was necessary to provide for additional meetings giving the work force time to work on the development of the shared governance process.

Question: *What do you believe the eventual outcome will be when the restructuring to a shared governance organization is complete?*

Answer: *I believe the outcomes will be: 1) Nursing will take complete control of the disciplinary process of their peers. 2) Nurses will be actively involved in the resource management of those areas that affect their practice. 3) Nurses will set in place an organizational structure consistent with the mission, strategic plan, goals, and objectives of the organization for which they work. 4) Salaries, working conditions, and benefit programs necessary to hire and retain professional staff will fall into place once the shared governance philosophy is implemented.*

Question: *What words of wisdom or solace would you offer to others considering the challenge of restructuring?*

Answer: *My advice would be to have confidence in a highly professional group, the nurses of your organization. The desire by professional nurses to be involved in the decision-making process related to the patient care process has been overlooked. Those considering the concepts of shared governance must put trust and faith in this highly professional group of people.*

Shared governance is a key that will help in gaining a perspective on nursing and specific outcomes that are a major challenge of our time. Nursing outcomes must be integrated throughout the entire workings of the hospital. There must be a clear relationship between the services delivered and the issues of cost and quality in today's health care environment. Cost containment and quality of care are primary issues in our organization. Shared governance will focus on outcomes and the ability to operate within the resources available to provide excellence in patient care to our community.

James H. Gingerich

Nurse Manager, Maternal-Child Health Services

Question: *In 1988 what did you think shared governance would mean for nurses at Fairbanks Memorial Hospital?*

Answer: *I had a little knowledge of shared governance. My sister is a nurse practicing in a hospital in the East that functions with unit-based shared governance. She has always spoken highly of it. I believed that shared governance would offer us more control over our nursing practice.*

Question: *In 1991, what changes have you observed with partial implementation of shared governance?*

Answer: *With the initiation of the unit-based councils, I am beginning to see positive changes. I believe that patient outcomes are better. The staff nurses in the maternal-child health units are establishing standards of practice that are higher than the minimum standards.*

Question: *What has been most useful in implementing shared governance?*

Answer: *I have done lots of reading. Many of the staff nurses are directly involved in the design and implementation of shared governance. The establishment of unit-based councils has been the most useful event for most of the nurses. Councils including staff nurses make the whole function of shared governance real.*

Question: *What have been some of the drawbacks of shared governance?*

Answer: *It seems to take a long time to get decisions made. It is expensive to initially get the new structure implemented.*

Question: *What has happened to the implementation time of new projects?*

Answer: *There seems to be a decrease in the implementation time of new ideas and projects once the decisions have been made. There also seems to be a higher compliance and acceptance of the changes.*

Question: *Is shared governance a fad?*

Answer: *I don't believe it is. I believe it is here to stay. I also think it is something that continues to grow and develop as the professionals evolve. I want it to stay.*

Question: *What words of wisdom would you share for others that may consider restructuring to a shared governance organization?*

Answer: *Take short breaks of time off to refocus and reorient. I found reading and educating myself in group process, interpersonal communication, and management skills to be helpful.*

Donna Wade

Nurse Manager, Critical Care Services

Question: *In 1988, what did you think about the concept of shared governance.*

Answer: *It scared me. I felt threatened. I did not understand how I would be involved as a nurse manager. I didn't think that staff nurses could do it.*

Question: *In 1991, what do you think about shared governance?*

Answer: *I believe in the shared governance concept. I believe that it is good for nursing. I found out that the staff nurses could do many things. I do see that not everyone is comfortable with it.*

Question: *What are the benefits of shared governance?*

Answer: *I believe there is an increased appreciation for both the staff nurses and the nurse managers.*

I really enjoy that the staff are involved in the peer evaluation process. I believe that evaluation by peers adds validity to the process.

Question: *Is shared governance a fad?*

Answer: *I certainly hope not. No, I don't believe it is.*

Question: *What words of wisdom would you share with others who are considering a shared governance organization?*

Answer: *I would encourage managers to learn as much about the concept as possible. I believe a strong budgetary commitment is necessary to begin the learning process.*

I would urge people to attend the National Shared Governance Conferences.

I found writing my goals to be helpful.

I also found that a solid self-examination of who I was

and what kind of manager I really was has been invaluable in coming to understand that I have choices.

Lynda Jenks

Staff Nurse, Post Anesthesia Care Unit

Question: *In 1988, what did you think shared governance was?*

Answer: *I thought it was a tool to gain job satisfaction.*

I get job satisfaction by having authority in how my job gets done.

Question: *In 1991, what is happening with this idea of shared governance?*

Answer: *I believe many of the staff nurses are grasping the concepts better. I believe some are going to accept it and others are going to reject it. Those in the middle will probably just follow.*

I believe that shared governance is a method built on a concept, whereby the staff nurses control all aspects of their clinical practice and accept the responsibility for that control.

I also think that shared governance is hard to grasp. It's tough to touch it, smell it, wear it, or even see it. It's kind of like religion. You've got to believe it. It's a system of beliefs based on a set of values that are put into practice.

Question: *What will be the outcome of the implementation of shared governance?*

Answer: *I believe a system will be put in place that will support the control of nursing practice by nurses.*

I think it will also improve the delivery of nursing, ensuring quality care, competence, and will ultimately enhance my job satisfaction.

Question: *Is shared governance a fad?*

Answer: *Absolutely not! At least not for professional nurses.*

Question: *What words of wisdom would you offer to others who are considering a shared governance system?*

Answer: *I found giving myself time to learn and try new ideas and behaviors to be very useful. I believe trying to move too fast, both individually and as an organization, only serves to cause confusion, frustration, and an increased resistance to the change.*

Attending group dynamic and communication workshops has really helped me as we have developed our system here.

Alyce Weckwerth

SUMMARY

Shared governance is a concept for organizational design that embraces and values the contributions of the individual. It is based on behaviors that are attuned to professions. Nursing is a profession that is by and large practiced in organizations of a bureaucratic design.

As the industrialized age gives way to the information age of the 21st century, organizations must restructure in order to remain viable. The health care industry of the United States is not exempt. Nurses, as members of the industry, have the opportunity to participate in designing the health care delivery system of the future. In order to effectively contribute to the profession, nurses must define and articulate fully the business of nursing. Shared governance is an organizational concept enabling the professional to control practice and allowing for productive contribution to the profession and the institution.

Shared governance is a win-win concept that provides fulfillment for the individual professional. The framework is particularly suited to organizations centered around providing human services, such as health care. Nurses and organizations providing health care services in rural environments can benefit from and successfully design and implement professional practice models based on the concepts of shared governance.

REFERENCES

DeYoung, L. (1985). *Dynamics of nursing*. Princeton: C.V. Mosby Company.

Drucker, P. F. (1989). *The new realities.* San Francisco: Harper & Row Publishers.

Naisbitt, J., & Aburdene, P. (1990). *Megatrends 2000.* New York: Avon Books.

Porter-O'Grady, T. (1990). *Reorganization of nursing practice; Creating the corporate venture.* Rockville, MD: Aspen Publishers, Inc.

Porter-O'Grady, T., & Finnigan, S. (1984). *Shared governance for nursing: A creative approach to professional accountability.* Rockville, MD: Aspen Publishers, Inc.

Prescott, P., & Bowen, S. (1985). Physician/nurse relationship. *Annals of Internal Medicine, 103,* 127–133.

15

Implementing Rural Preceptorships in Baccalaureate Nursing Education

Candace Corrigan

Rural preceptorships in baccalaureate nursing can address an array of interdependent issues in both nursing education and rural health. Nursing education seeks alternative and innovative clinical education opportunities in the growing non-acute domain using expert clinical role models and advanced clinical experiences for RN students. Rural regions seek clinical consultation, the dynamic exchange of ideas fostered by interactions with students and faculty, and to recruit health professionals.

In this chapter, the design and implementation of a rural registered nurse preceptorship program will be discussed from the perspective of the nursing faculty member coordinating this community nursing clinical program. This goal will be accomplished by presenting approaches to establishing and maintaining the necessary cooperative relationships, the need for and contents of a preceptorship manual, sample contracts and evaluation documents, and preceptor and preceptee evaluative comments.

PRECEPTORSHIPS IN NURSING EDUCATION

What Is Preceptorship Study?

The preceptorship program, considered in this chapter, is a study/practice experience designed to offer a flexible, specialized, and independent learning opportunity to RN baccalaureate nursing students. With a few changes, it could easily serve the generic student. Students work individually with their faculty instructor in identifying a clinical site and making the necessary arrangements for the preceptorship. In addition to meeting the general course objectives for the Community Health Nursing Clinical Practicum, preceptees seek to meet additional objectives for the Rural Community Health Preceptorship.

Preceptorships hold special advantages for students. Not only do students gain the opportunity to work with a clinically expert nurse in a specialized setting, but they receive role socialization and mentoring from an active practitioner. Preceptors are the individuals best prepared to select an appropriate caseload for the student, assist the student in interdisciplinary collaboration with the health team and collateral services, and orient the student to specialized community resources. Preceptees learn invaluable practical knowledge and skills from their preceptors. Students benefit from a one-to-one relationship that offers them immediate feedback and individualized attention; these promote student feelings of competence and confidence. The preceptorship program provides students with unique educational opportunities—rural and culturally diverse experiences are highly valued and, at this time, rare in nursing education.

The preceptor, in turn, receives valuable professional stimulation both from the student and from association with the faculty and the university. Although working with students requires time and energy, preceptors report that working with preceptees affords them opportunities or incentives to hone their knowledge and skills, to seek further education, and to practice as leaders and teachers.

Agencies also benefit from the preceptorship program. They no longer feel estranged from academe; they have direct input into the structuring and implementing of clinical education. The presence of students and faculty is a resource to the agency in terms of humanpower, sharing of information, and problem-solving. Preceptees also return to agencies as licensed providers, thereby helping to alleviate problems of maldistribution, isolation, and staff retention.

An Historical Perspective

No doubt, throughout the history of our nursing profession, every nurse can identify individuals whose clinical excellence and close association as mentors or preceptors provided seminal experiences and served as important role models. For many years, nursing faculty have recognized that formalizing and promoting these relationships will

- produce more confident, acculturated, and skilled BSN graduates (Goldenberg, 1987; Itano, Warren, & Ishida, 1987; Shamian & Lemieux, 1984; Lee, 1988; Dobbs, 1988; Chickerella & Lutz, 1981; Thomas, 1986);
- increase variety and flexibility in clinical experiences (Ferris, 1980);
- introduce rural health issues and channel health professionals into rural employment (Stuart-Siddall, 1987; Arlton, 1984; Predhomme, 1985; Stuart-Burchardt, 1982; Koehler, Broome, Clayton, & Morse, 1988);
- augment existing rural health services (Wiese, Howard, & Stephens, 1979) and resocialize degree-seeking RNs (Viar, 1988; Marcus, Swint, Valadez, Ward, & Williams, 1988);
- recruit minority students into the health professions by providing experience working with rural minority clients (Baldwin, Baldwin, Edinberg, & Rowley, 1980);
- compensate for growing research demands on faculty that preclude practice-based clinical expertise necessary for clinical teaching (Myrick, 1988);
- reduce students' experience of clinical-related stress (Turkoski, 1987);

- offer RN students an advanced, accessible, and/or specialized clinical experience (Carroll & Artman, 1988; Lethbridge, 1988); and

- enhance students' collaborative and multidisciplinary skills (Edinberg, Dodson, & Veach, 1978).

Formal preceptorship programs take many shapes; a few of the most remarkable provide valuable models. For example, in response to the RN baccalaureate student who typically works full-time, attends school part-time, takes care of children, and travels many miles, the University of New Hampshire implemented a self-directed, independent study, clinical program (Lethbridge, 1988). Course objectives were met in rural settings in cooperation with local clinical preceptors and university faculty.

The University of New Mexico conducted a five-year demonstration project that sent 230 senior nursing, medicine, and pharmacy students to rural areas to gain experiential learning and multidisciplinary collaborative skills and, secondarily, to augment existing health services (Wiese et al., 1979). They developed clinics and organized and offered previously unavailable services. Well-received by the communities and local health professionals, many preceptees went on to careers in community, rural, and/or primary health care.

A similar program was implemented at the University of Nevada to introduce American Indian students to health careers via interdisciplinary student teams precepted in remote unserved reservation sites (Baldwin et al., 1980; Edinberg et al., 1978). These teams of Indian and non-Indian nursing, pharmacy, premedical, health education, social services, predentistry, nutrition, and special education students received a weeklong orientation prior to a two-week clinical experience conducting screening and health education programs and making referrals. Direct outcomes included requests for student teams to provide additional services in other communities or programs, continued use of health services after the teams left the communities, increased enrollment in health professions by Indian students, and an increased preceptee commitment to rural practice and primary care upon graduation.

Responding to the need for providers in rural areas, the University of Northern Colorado implemented a one-quarter senior rural nursing practicum (Arlton, 1984). Following four weeks of intensive preparation, the students were precepted in a variety of rural health agencies for a six-week period. Students developed a new sense of professional competence and community. Preceptors grew in self-confidence, clinical knowledge and awareness of rationale, and teaching skills. Graduates with the rural experience accepted rural employment at a rate of 33 percent as compared to 4 percent of the graduates who elected not to take the rural practicum.

In a similar program, California State University at Sonoma offers a junior-level spring course, "Developing Contracts for Preceptorship Study," in preparation for the senior year (Freed & Dean, 1976). In identifying an agency and preparing a contract, the nursing student develops expertise in such domains as negotiating entry, selecting a faculty advisor and preceptor, setting goals and writing objectives, peer critique, and evaluation tools and strategies.

Collaborative Roles

Successful preceptorships are founded on a collaborative interdependent relationship between the preceptor, the student preceptee, and the nursing faculty member. It is through this collaboration that the many benefits inherent in each role are realized.

The Role of the Preceptor. The preceptor is a clinically expert role model. Identified by the student, the faculty, or the agency, the preceptor has the skills and qualifications needed by the student to fulfill the preceptorship. The preceptor collaborates with the student and the faculty in determining the objectives and goals, the implementation, and the evaluation of the student's experience. This collaboration may be accomplished via on-site visits, teleconferences, preceptor-preceptee conferences, and correspondence.

The preceptor as a role model and mentor is the most significant person in the student's clinical experience. The preceptor guides and enhances the meeting of clinical objectives by providing resources, information, guidance, and feedback. In addition to receiving the "Preceptor Manual" (Corrigan, 1988), novice preceptors benefit from an orientation to their role that includes the following (Ferguson & Hauf, 1973a, 1973b; Arlton, 1984):

> *an overview of the nursing program, specific course, and*
>   *preceptorship objectives;*
> *legal and professional concerns;*
> *clinical teaching and evaluation strategies;*
> *roles/responsibilities of the preceptor, student, faculty;*
> *preceptor role development;*
> *audio-visual and other media; and*
> *the counseling process.*

Preceptors working with the University of Montana earned six credit hours of graduate (or undergraduate) credit by completing three workshops, interim assignments, and precepting community health clinical students (Ferguson & Hauf, 1973a, 1973b).

The Role of the Student.   The student takes a central role in designing and orchestrating the preceptorship. The student may identify the setting and the preceptor. Collaborating closely with the faculty and preceptor, the student meets all of the general and specific clinical objectives within the context of the specialized practice setting. While the student works most closely with the preceptor, he or she will also communicate with the faculty on a regular pre-established schedule.

The clinical practice role of the student will vary with the context and the content of the preceptorship. Staffing clinics; home visiting; inservice education; designing, implementing, and evaluating programs; intramural and extramural practice; and management practice are all appropriate to student preceptorship.

The Role of the Nursing Faculty.   The faculty advisor is a member of the university faculty with a special expertise in community health and responsibility for the student's clinical education (including meeting the clinical objectives). The faculty assists the students to understand and implement the preceptorship.

As a liaison, the faculty advisor collaborates with agencies, preceptors, students, and communities to implement the preceptorship program. This collaboration may include orienting agencies and preceptors to the preceptorship program and serving as a resource to the agency. While direct clinical supervision lies with the preceptor, the faculty advisor will make regular on-site visits and be available by telephone.

The faculty advisor monitors documentation pertinent to the preceptorship. This documentation includes student logs and written work, contracts, conference notes, and evaluations. While the faculty advisor has primary responsibility for the student's grade, evaluation of the student's performance will be made in collaboration with the preceptor and the student. The faculty advisor coordinates the preceptee's and preceptor's evaluation of the preceptorship process.

Direct benefits of this consultative role are enriched relationships with clinical colleagues that often give rise to collaborative practice, applied research opportunities, and further consultation not related to student supervision. While preceptors may undertake graduate education, faculty may pursue part-time or seasonal clinical practice with the agency; together, they may seek funding to implement programs or conduct research.

THE RURAL REGISTERED NURSE PRECEPTORSHIP

Cultural and Physical Aspects

The northern Arizona region is wholly rural. While dotted with many communities, the largest, Flagstaff, is home to only 50 thousand. One is as struck by its remoteness as its scenic beauty. The region is the traditional home of the Southern and San Juan Paiutes, a hunting and gathering people; the Hopis, a sedentary farming and trading people; and the Navahos, later arrivers who came to trade and herd sheep. First visited by Europeans during the Spanish conquests, northern Arizona also became home to Anglo traders and ranchers in the 18th century and to a large Chinese and black population who came along with the railroad.

In the west, the region is dissected by the Grand Canyon, dropping two thousand feet to the desert-like river bottom where the climate parallels that of Phoenix and Tucson, hundreds of miles to the south. In contrast, the Flagstaff area, in the midst of the world's largest Ponderosa Pine forest, sits at the foot of the 12,000-foot, snow-capped San Francisco Peaks and boasts downhill skiing in April. In the east, the ancient pueblo villages loom at the top of sweeping mesas where traditional life, regulated by seasonal ceremonies, is still practiced without electricity or running water. The entire region is held sacred by the indigenous people and the ethos is one of harmony and synchrony with nature and the ebb and flow of the seasons and human life. No distinction is made between the sacred and the secular.

The warm sun and blue skies belie the harshness of the climate and the poverty of resources and health experienced by many rural people. Of special note are diabetes and diabetes-induced renal failure and hypertension, substance abuse, accidental and violence-related injuries and deaths, poor maternal-infant health, and malnutrition. Exacerbating these problems are the long distances between the scattered population and the treatment centers and a scarcity of human and material resources.

The Rural Preceptorship Program grew out of the growing mutual interests and needs of regional rural health agencies and a baccalaureate RN clinical program. It was hoped that a collaborative effort fostering alternative educational opportunities for baccalaureate nursing students would also help meet agencies' needs for recruitment and retention of health professionals and access to the educational and consultative expertise of university faculty. Registered nurses were the likely beneficiaries of the first preceptorships because they were licensed professionals in their own right and required minimal direct supervision. This program was ideal for them because it offered a unique and independent experience that focused on a specific population or needed skills, recognized and built on current knowledge and competencies, and provided clinical flexibility in their already full lives.

Early work on the program was funded by NAAHEC, the Northern Arizona Area Health Education Center. In its role as a resource to rural health agencies and to accomplish its goal of recruitment of health professionals to underserved areas, NAAHEC and the faculty identified the following objectives:

1. contacting clinical agencies and arranging preceptorships;
2. identifying challenging clinical opportunities for RN students;
3. developing course objectives and goals for RNs;
4. refining and coordinating the meshing of the community and community mental health components of the clinical course;
5. developing long-range plans in rural areas that would ultimately accommodate generic nursing students; and
6. assisting with health professional recruitment while working with the clinical agencies.

NAAHEC supported clinical site development, research into the preceptorship model, curriculum development, and the preparation of the preceptorship manual.

Implementing the Program

Recruiting Preceptors. Expert nurses are easily recruited to the task of precepting students. More than willing to add this time- and energy-consuming role to their already full schedules, they are pleased to have their clinical excellence acknowledged by their agency and the university. They welcome the intellectual stimulation and challenge of precepting, calling it "a shot in the arm" and "fun."

The faculty coordinator made the initial agency contacts by telephone with administrators or directors of nursing. Following a brief introduction to the concept of preceptorship study and the benefits to agency and student, these individuals were pleased to refer the faculty coordinator to likely preceptor candidates (in one instance, the student identified a preceptor and initiated the contact). Telephone contact with prospective preceptors furthered the dialogue about preceptor-student fit. Appointments for the faculty coordinator and preceptors (and occasionally an administrator) to meet for planning the implementation were made. These telephone contacts were immediately followed with mailings of course materials, preceptorship objectives, descriptions of preceptorship study, and the collaborative roles of preceptor, student, and faculty. Initial meetings between faculty coordinator and preceptors included introductions to other staff, tours of the facilities, exploration of clinical opportunities, and establishing a working relationship. Often, because of the distances involved, this was the only meeting prior to the student's arrival. While it was a faculty intention to meet with preceptor and student at least once in the field, it was more likely that the next time the faculty met with the preceptor was to undertake evaluation of the experience, make adjustments, and plan for the next student. In the interim, faculty and preceptor collaborated weekly by telephone.

Agencies and preceptors remained fluid resources and the faculty-preceptor relationships, dynamic. As time passed, other preceptors came forward by word-of-mouth; or an agency, suffering from staff turnover and the strains of training new staff, might take a "semester off" without students. The faculty would make additional trips to the agency to provide clinical consultation or make a research presentation. Likewise, preceptors, in town on business, would connect with the faculty for a campus visit, to share a meal, or meet informally.

Once the program was in place, the most important function of the faculty coordinator was facilitation. Being available by phone for consultation; checking in with preceptors; and providing teaching materials, clinical resources, constructive critique, support, and encouragement were vitally important to the continued success of the preceptorship relationship. This could not be overdone. Agency personnel were willing to participate only as long as they experienced faculty support in their preceptor role and easy access to faculty consultation and back-up.

Types of Experiences.   Rural clinical sites are likely to offer valuable opportunities for cross-cultural practice whether it be with poor migrant groups, American Indians, minimally literate, or mountain people. Most populations will be unserved or underserved by the existing health care system and often alienated from it. Rural preceptorships challenge students to provide holistic care and advocacy within the constraints of complex economic, political, and cultural factors.

In these contexts, RN preceptees functioned as home health and community health nurses, traveling with a driver/interpreter, by four-wheel drive vehicle, to such remote locations that often only three home visits could be accomplished in a single day. Preceptees set up screenings and health fairs, participated in the case management of high risk perinatal and pediatric clients and their families, and provided relief and insights into the care of "difficult clients," ones about whom other staff nurses were feeling hopeless. Students took on special projects. For example, one preceptee worked with a group home for the developmentally disabled, creating an independent and consultative role that included providing physical assessments of all the residents, staff inservices, case management, and updated care plans and Kardexes.

Rural Community Health Nursing Preceptorship Objectives. In addition to the general objectives required of all community health students, those participating in the preceptorship program addressed the following objectives:

1. Identify specific health needs of rural populations.
2. Discuss the role of the Indian Health Service in providing health services.
3. Identify cultural beliefs that are significant to rural populations (American Indian and otherwise).
4. Describe nursing interventions in a rural setting and compare to the urban setting interventions.
5. Identify areas of independence, interdependence, and dependence in rural nursing practice.
6. Identify factors that inhibit/enhance professional practice in rural settings.
7. Describe the interdisciplinary collaborative qualities of rural health care services and delivery.
8. Demonstrate knowledge of the organization of the practice setting and its impact on the scope of nursing practice.
9. Utilize effective problem-solving and self-management in planning, implementing, and evaluating the preceptorship.

10. Describe the bio-psycho-cultural characteristics of the unique client population identified by the preceptorship.

11. Demonstrate behavior which is characteristic of movement toward self-actualization.

These objectives address the unique qualities and opportunities afforded by rural preceptorship clinical practice. They support a preceptor-student relationship that promotes the analysis of new roles and collaborative professional relationships, the integration of more sophisticated insights into the complexities of rural health (and non-rural for that matter), and the practice of a more advanced, interdependent, and holistic practice.

The Preceptorship Manual. The preceptorship manual is a resource for all participants in the preceptorship program. It includes a description of preceptorship education and the concomitant roles of those involved; the clinical objectives for community health practice in the rural setting (as well as those course objectives and outlines related to the theory portion of community health); the mechanisms for evaluating the role performances of the participants; a comprehensive bibliography of the existing literature in this area; and sample publications for the reader's quick reference. The following is a list of the manual's contents:

> *Introduction and Overview*
> *What Is Preceptorship Study?*
> *The Role of the Preceptor*
> *The Role of the Student*
> *The Role of the Nursing Faculty*
> *Clinical Objectives*
> *Rural Nursing Preceptorship Objectives*
> *Evaluation*
>   *Student Performance Evaluation*
>   *Preceptor Evaluation of Preceptorship Experience*
>   *Student Evaluation of Preceptor*
>   *Student/Preceptor Evaluation of Faculty*
>   *Faculty Evaluation of Preceptor*
> *Bibliography*

Appendices
  Community Health Nursing Theory Syllabus
  Community Health Clinical Syllabus
  Student Clinical Evaluation
  Faculty Evaluation
  College of Nursing/Health Agency Agreement
  Selected Readings (from the bibliography)

Each preceptor and appropriate agency administrator receives a copy of the manual. Students receive one for the duration of their participation in the program.

Contracts.   A brief comment about contracts seems helpful here. Certainly, if the College of Nursing does not have an existing contract with the clinical agency, this should be initiated. While the standard contract used by most nursing programs is adequate to cover preceptorship study, the agency may request additional agreements. This was not our experience.

The most salient agency concerns seem to center around liability (both for personal injury and malpractice) and the evaluation of student performance. A lengthy preceptorship contract developed by students as part of their preparation (Freed & Dean, 1976) is a valuable tool and guide to their learning (Appendix 15–A).

Evaluation

Evaluation was both formal and informal. Informal evaluation took the form of dialogue between faculty, students, and preceptors and a written log, submitted weekly by the student to the community health faculty. Compiled in a thin, standard-sized spiral-bound notebook, the log included the following:

- narrative and discussion of the week's experiences;
- research abstracts related to clinical problems (two-week minimum);
- discussion of preceptorship objectives and how they are being met;

- messages and queries to faculty; and
- responses to faculty comments from the previous week.

Preceptee, faculty advisor, preceptor, and the program were formally evaluated as the preceptorship experience came to a close. The student/preceptee's clinical grade was dependent on general course criteria as well as on those objectives specific to the rural preceptorship. The preceptor completed a written evaluation of the preceptee's clinical performance (Appendix 15–B) and the preceptorship program (Appendix 15–C). Faculty and preceptor role performances and the program were evaluated by the student (Appendices C, D, and E) and the preceptor received an evaluation from the faculty (Appendix 15–F).

Preceptor Assessments.   Preceptor enthusiasm for this program was reflected in their consistent efforts to hire their preceptees into staff positions upon graduation. Twenty percent of those students completing rural preceptorships have accepted such employment. Typical preceptor comments offered during evaluation include the following:

> *Jane's ICU experience is definitely a valuable asset [to us].*
>
> *An added benefit to us was improved communication between the hospital and our agency [because the preceptee worked there].*
>
> *We found [her] very helpful in updating our staff's knowledge regarding nursing procedures.*
>
> *We are short-staffed, she decreased the burden of this for us.*
>
> *[The preceptee] provided an influx of new ideas and ways of doing things . . . . Got us thinking again.*
>
> *It's a lot of fun for us! Send us more.*

Preceptors were quick to identify benefits to students:

> *Students learned how difficult compliance can be in the home setting and the need for support of caregiver [family member].*

> *Students were given assignments and worked very inde-*
> *pendently . . . which is required of the PHN [public health*
> *nurse].*

They were just as quick to point out ways in which the programs could be strengthened:

> *Too little time [7 weeks] . . . to spend with families . . . to*
> *build rapport . . . to comprehend all our clinics and other*
> *community services.*
>
> *Make it a whole semester.*

Student Assessments. Student insights complemented preceptor assessments. The following are students' statements about their preceptors:

> *She was never too busy to give assistance or information or*
> *listen. If she didn't know something she took the time to*
> *find it . . . .*
>
> *[I was] very much [a part of the staff]. The primary nurses*
> *were frequently in touch with me, asking questions, and*
> *referring to my charting, reviewing concerns, and progress*
> *of clients.*
>
> *She worked very hard to find families that would accept me*
> *as part of their health team/support system.*
>
> *We planned experiences together to coordinate with client*
> *families, but work was completed independently.*
>
> *They were very helpful when my clients were non-compliant.*

Students' comments reflected that the program exceeded their expectations:

> *So much to be done for these families . . . so much to learn.*
>
> *[The preceptorship was a] much more interesting way of*
> *learning about Public Health and services available in the*
> *community by working through with the staff, by contract-*
> *ing and being responsible for my own work, and keeping*
> *the contract (a good learning experience!).*

Students offered valuable insight into strategies for improving the program. Like the preceptors, they learned that seven weeks is a woefully short community health experience. Other critiques were offered:

> *Set [a] responsible backup person for referral of problems if [my preceptor is] unavailable . . . .*
>
> *Although I would have enjoyed a more varied experience, I put a lot of time into 2–3 types of patients [gaining specific expertise].*
>
> *I would have liked to travel with them [the agency nurses] more often (seeing various clients) if staffing were better.*

Given the flexibility and nascent qualities of the program, it is easy to integrate this constructive and insightful feedback into program design. Combined with faculty evaluation, suggestions are offered below.

RECOMMENDATIONS

Recommendations focus on preceptor training, student contract development, protecting the special role of the student, and developing a faculty role that would accommodate the demands of coordinating preceptorship study. Faculty need additional time to train and support preceptors and to conduct the evaluation process necessary to facilitate the refinement and growth of the program toward the ultimate inclusion of generic baccalaureate students.

Formal orientation/training to the preceptor role would alleviate the anxiety and uncertainty experienced by most new preceptors. Held on campus and offered in conjunction with a clinically based workshop, this orientation would go far to introduce the preceptor to the academic setting, other faculty, and college resources and provide a tangible acknowledgement of preceptor contributions in the form of a workshop on a salient issue, or new and advanced clinical skill valuable to rural practitioners. Such an orientation, combined with socialization with other preceptors and expert clinicians, nourishes a network that is valuable to the rurally isolated professional.

Developing a preceptorship contract would be useful to the student both in identifying the specific qualities and goals of the desired clinical experience and in establishing a working relationship with the agency and preceptor. The program would be strengthened by fostering preceptee independence in this domain.

Several evaluative comments focused on the extent to which students, especially registered nurses, can relieve the strain in understaffed agencies. While student resources are an incentive to the agency to accept them, their role as learners must be protected at least to the extent that they are able to meet their clinical objectives.

Lastly, nursing faculty developing such programs experience role strain as they integrate these new responsibilities, the need to travel more, and new demands on their time with their existing role as faculty for generic students on campus and in local community agencies. A more realistic role might be one that combines preceptorship program responsibilities with the recruiting, advising, and counseling of all registered nurses. This combined role would foster the implementation of preceptorships throughout the RN clinical curriculum.

CONCLUSION

The Rural Nursing Preceptorship Program exceeded our goals and expectations. Students had excellent clinical experiences that provided them with advanced practice opportunities, mentors, and role models. They grew in their understanding of and interest in rural health issues and practice. Cooperation between the College of Nursing and rural agencies was initiated or enhanced; collegiality and friendships bloomed, resources flowed more freely, rural nurses' interest in graduate education was piqued, and clinical research opportunities multiplied. For students, faculty, and preceptors, rural preceptorships proved to be a challenging, exciting, and pleasing new approach to practice.

REFERENCES

Arlton, D. (1984). The rural nursing practicum project. *Nursing Outlook, 32,* (4), 204–206.

Baldwin, D. C., Baldwin, M. A., Edinberg, M. A., & Rowley, B. D. (1980). A model for recruitment and service—the University of Nevada's summer preceptorships in Indian communities. *Public Health Report, 95*(1), 19–22.

Carroll, T. L., & Artman, S. (1988, February). Fitting RN students into a traditional program: Secrets for success. *Nursing and Health Care,* 89–91.

Chickerella, B. G., & Lutz, W. J. (1981). Professional nurturance: Preceptorships for undergraduate nursing students. *American Journal of Nursing, 81*(1), 107–109.

Corrigan, C. L. (1988). *Preceptorship manual: Rural community health nursing.* Flagstaff: Northern Arizona Area Health Education Center, Inc.

Dobbs, K. K. (1988). The senior preceptorship as a method for anticipatory socialization of baccalaureate nursing students. *Journal of Nursing Education, 27*(4), 167–171.

Edinberg, M. A., Dodson, S. E., & Veach, T. L. (1978). A preliminary study of student learning in interdisciplinary health teams. *Journal of Medical Education, 53*(8), 667–671.

Ferguson, M., & Hauf, B. (1973a). The preceptor role: Implementing student experience in community nursing, part 1. *The Journal of Continuing Education in Nursing, 4*(1), 12–16.

Ferguson, M., & Hauf, B. (1973b). The preceptor role: Implementing student experience in community nursing, part 2. *The Journal of Continuing Education in Nursing, 4*(5), 14–16.

Ferris, L. (1980). Cardiac preceptor model: Access to learning by nurses in rural communities. *The Journal of Continuing Education in Nursing, 11*(1), 19–23.

Freed, L., & Dean, H. (1976). *N396: Developing contracts for preceptorship study.* Course syllabus, California State College/Sonoma, Department of Nursing, Sonoma, California.

Goldenberg, D. (1987). Preceptorship: A one-to-one relationship with a triple "P" rating (preceptor, preceptee, patient). *Nursing Forum, 23*(1), 10–15.

Itano, J. K., Warren, J. J., & Ishida, D. N. (1987). A comparison of role conceptions and role deprivation of baccalaureate students in nursing participating in a preceptorship or a traditional clinical program. *Journal of Nursing Education, 26*(2), 69–73.

Koehler, C., Broome, M., Clayton, G., & Morse, J. (1988). Rural preceptorship program for baccalaureate students. *Nurse Educator, 13*(2), 5–6.

Lee, S. (1988, September). How to turn a student into a colleague. *RN*, 20, 22,

Lethbridge, D. J. (1988). Independent study: A strategy for providing baccalaureate education for RNs in rural settings. *Journal of Nursing Education, 27*(4), 183–185.

Marcus, M. T., Swint, K., Valadez, A. M., Ward, K., & Williams, R. (1988, September). Community care practicums ready RN students for new levels of practice. *Nursing and Health Care,* 377–380.

Myrick, F. (1988). Preceptorship—Is it the answer to the problems in clinical teaching? *Journal of Nursing Education, 27*(3), 136–138.

Predhomme, J. (1985). Bringing baccalaureate nursing education to the rural setting. *Journal of Nursing Education, 24*(3), 123–125.

Shamian, J., & Lemieux, S. (1984). An evaluation of the preceptor model versus the formal teaching model. *Journal of Continuing Education in Nursing, 15*(3), 86–89.

Stuart-Burchardt, S. (1982). Rural nursing. *American Journal of Nursing, 82*(4), 616–18.

Stuart-Siddall, S. (1987). Rural clinical nurse placement center alternative. *Prairie Rose, 56*(1), 13.

Thomas, J. (1986). Preceptorship program in a rural hospital. *Kansas Nurse, 61*(2), 4–5.

Turkoski, B. (1987). Reducing stress in nursing students' clinical learning experience. *Journal of Nursing Education, 26*(8), 335–337.

Viar, V. (1988). Research preceptorship for degree-seeking RNs: A strategy for resocialization. *Journal of Nursing Education, 27*(7), 329–331.

Wiese, W. H., Howard, C. A., & Stephens, J. A. (1979). Augmentation of clinical services in rural areas by health sciences students. *Journal of Medical Education, 54*(12), 917–924.

Appendix 15–A
Preceptorship Contract

Name: _____ Soc. Security No. _____

Preceptorship Title: _____

Advisor: _____

Preceptor:
    Name: _____

    Agency: _____

    Address: _____

    Agency Administrator: _____

Beginning Date: _____ Completion Date: _____

Existing Contract with Agency?

Previous Experience Related to This Preceptorship:

Purposes or Aims:

Objectives:

Activities:

Support to Be Provided by—
    Faculty Advisor:

    Preceptor:

Results Projected:

Methods of Evaluation:

Does This Contract Require Special Resources or Carry Special Implications? If yes, please explain or attach.

Student's Signature _____ Date _____

Advisor's Signature _____ Date _____

Preceptor's Signature _____ Date _____

Adapted from Freed and Dean, 1976.

Appendix 15–B
Preceptor's Evaluation of the Student/Preceptee

Student's Name ———————————— Placement Dates ————

1. What are your observations about:
   a. The student's strengths—

   b. Areas for further student attention/improvement—

2. If you had a job opening for which this student was qualified, would you employ this individual: Yes ——— No ———
   Why:

3. Additional comments:

Name of the evaluator: ————————————————————

Agency: ———————————————— Date: ————

Appendix 15–C
Preceptor's Evaluation of the Preceptorship Program

1. What are your observations about the Preceptorship Program:

2. What are the most positive features of the experience:

3. What are the least positive features of the experience:

4. What are your recommendations to improve this program:

5. Additional comments:

Your Name: _____   Your Agency: _____

Date: _____

Appendix 15–D
Student's Evaluation of Preceptor

1. **The preceptor as a role model:**

   a. How many times did the preceptor meet with you and did he/she allow you an exchange of feedback?

   b. Did you sense that there was open communication and trust between you and your preceptor?

   c. Did your preceptor offer you support? How?

2. **The preceptor as a resource person:**

   a. Willingness to share expertise?

   b. Demonstration of procedures as appropriate?

   c. Assistance in finding resources?

   d. Clarity of demonstrations and explanations? Did you give your preceptor feedback?

3. **The preceptor as a designer of instruction:**

   a. Discuss your preceptor in respect to orientation to the facility.

      Introduction to staff?

      Discussion of mutual expectations?

      To the community?

   b. Did you feel accepted? Part of the staff?

   c. Was your preceptor able to provide useful and meaningful experiences for you to meet your objectives?

   d. Did you plan your educational experiences together or independently?

   e. Was there optimal use of your time?

   f. Did you participate in ongoing evaluation of your performance? Was this satisfactory?

4. **The preceptor as a supervisor:**

   a. Did your preceptor provide appropriate supervision?

   b. Did you have weekly conferences? Were they satisfactory?

 c. Did he/she impose his/her viewpoint on you?

 d. Did he/she encourage self-expression, individuality, self-initiation, and self-evaluation? How?

5. **Describe ways in which your preceptor excelled:**

6. **Describe ways in which your preceptor can improve:**

Student: _____ Preceptor: _____ Date: _____

Adapted from Stuart-Siddall and Haberlin, 1983.

Appendix 15–E
Evaluation of the Faculty Advisor

1. What were the faculty advisor's strengths?

2. How could the faculty advisor be of greater assistance to you in your preceptor role?

3. Other comments about working with the faculty advisor:

4. Other comments about the preceptorship program:

Faculty Advisor: _____

Your Name: _____ Date: _____

Appendix 15–F
Faculty Evaluation of the Preceptor

1. Preceptor's strengths:

2. Areas for continued attention:

3. Additional comments:

Preceptor: _____

Evaluating Faculty: _____ Date: _____

16

Distance Learning: New Partnerships for Nursing in Rural Areas

Lorraine M. Clarke
Judith A. Cohen

Educational technology has made it possible to create distance education within a rural state. The case study discussed in this chapter presents a description of the characteristics of a rural state, the circumstances which determined a need for nursing education, and an account of the interagency collaboration which produced distance education. The experience of making a transition from traditional to distance education and using an educational technology, interactive television, is the focus of the case study.

The demographics and characteristics of rural life influence the types of nursing services needed and the utilization of nursing resources, both in the hospital and the community. Rural areas have higher concentrations of elderly and children under 18, higher levels of poverty, and a higher percentage of medically uninsured individuals (U.S. Department of Health and Human Services, 1988). Registered nurses play key roles in the provision of cost-effective health care in rural settings. Although settings and the scope of practice vary, this nursing role involves greater independence and a need for more generalized knowledge (Lassiter, 1985; Stuart-Siddall & Haberlin, 1985). Given the relative lack of other health professionals in rural areas, nurses' roles often encompass a broad range of responsibilities and skills.

Opportunities to begin or continue formal nursing education are limited for individuals living in rural areas. These individuals are often married and have children, or they are single parents and heads of households who are not able to take advantage of programs that require extended periods away from family and/or work. Maximizing educational opportunities and providing nursing educational outreach programs through distance education can be effective in expanding the overall pool of registered nurses in rural areas.

Vermont is a rural state, small in both size and population. The 1984 population estimates place the state's population at 530,000. Only Alaska and Wyoming have fewer residents. Vermont's population density, however, is over 55 people per square mile, compared to 1.7 in Wyoming (Vermont Department of Health, 1987). Located in the northwestern corner of New England, Vermont is approximately 180 miles long from the Canadian border to Massachusetts and 86 miles across at its widest point.

East-west travel, although only a short distance, is severely constrained by the mountain chain that forms the spine of the state. There are only a handful of gaps that cross the Green Mountains. Most east-west travel must pass these gaps, which in winter can be treacherous. The bulk of the population has settled in the lower areas on the east and up and down the west-side corridor. Most Vermonters (about 70 percent) live in rural areas or small communities with fewer than 2,000 residents (Vermont Department of Health, 1987). The distribution of Vermont's population (1986) is represented in Figure 16–1.

Vermont's geography has fostered three of the state's major industries: skiing, tourism, and agriculture. Vermont has some large electronic firms in Burlington, granite quarries in Barre and Proctor, and machine tool plants along the Connecticut River. Mirroring the U. S. economy, Vermont's job growth has been in the health services, employing 4 percent of the non-farm labor force (Vermont Department of Health, 1987).

The demand for registered nurses within Vermont exceeds the supply. In 1987 there were 7,461 nurses in the state—5,462

Figure 16–1
1986 Vermont Population

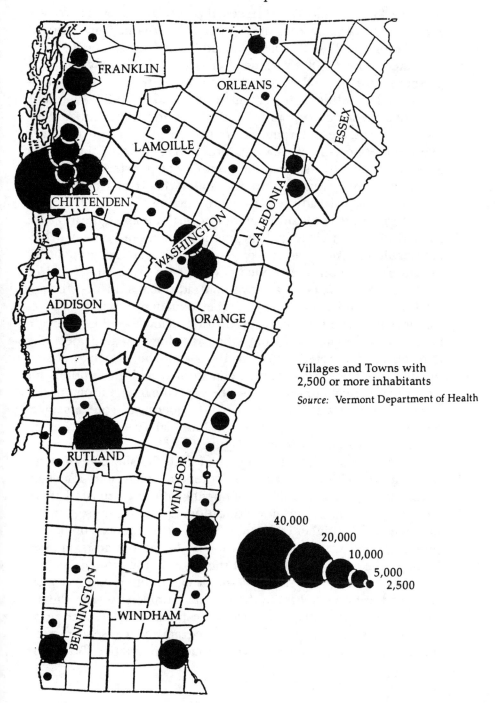

Villages and Towns with
2,500 or more inhabitants

Source: Vermont Department of Health

40,000
20,000
10,000
5,000
2,500

registered nurses and 1,969 licensed practical nurses. There was a mean RN vacancy rate of 7 percent (Vermont State Nurses' Association, 1987). The need for additional nurses by 1995 is projected to be 1,600 (Vermont Department of Employment and Training, 1987), yet the number of graduates from Vermont nursing schools declined 38 percent from 1986 to 1987 (Vermont Student Assistance Corporation, 1988). In addition, many of Vermont's nurses are older and are expected to retire in ten years (Vermont State Nurses' Association, 1987). One of the largest applicant pools to increase the numbers of registered nurses in Vermont comes from within the state, the licensed practical nurses, a group already committed to nursing.

Opportunities to continue their formal nursing education are limited for rural nurses such as practical nurses in Vermont. They are unable to take advantage of programs that are geographically distant or that require extended periods away from family and/or work. It is also this population of nontraditional students who are established residents of Vermont. They remain in Vermont to practice as registered nurses upon graduation. They, therefore, provide an excellent population from which to draw to help meet the demand for registered nurses in the state. The associate degree nursing programs are attractive educational mobility options for licensed practical nurses because they provide recognition of prior learning and an attainable path to RN licensure. Four associate degree programs accredited by the National League for Nursing (NLN) are located in Vermont (Figure 16–2).

The State of Vermont, concerned with the shortage of registered nurses within the state, its potential deleterious affect on health care, the inaccessibility of nursing education in rural areas, and limited resources for new educational programs raised public policy issues for higher education. These issues focused on how to provide 1. *access* to higher education for licensed practical nurses living in the southeastern part of the state, 2. the same *quality* of courses that the University of Vermont had to offer, and 3. *equality,* or educational access to the one state university. The University of Vermont School of Nursing responded by delivering an outreach associate degree nursing program to licensed practical nurses in southeast Vermont via Vermont Interactive Television

Figure 16–2
Hospital and Nursing Education Programs in Vermont

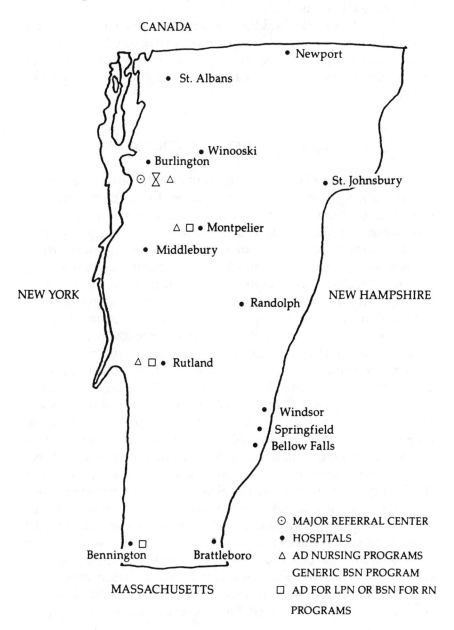

(VIT). VIT is an educational technology which brought the teacher and learner face to face and allowed interaction between them over long distances.

This chapter examines the concept of distance education and its development. It includes theories of distance education, a description of educational technology, and a case study drawn from one faculty's experiences of delivering a nursing program through interactive television.

CONCEPT OF DISTANCE EDUCATION

Distance education is a generic term that traditionally was limited to the teaching/learning strategies referred to as correspondence education in Great Britain, home and/or independent study in the United States, and external studies in Australia (Keegan, 1990). In 1982, however, the term *distance education* became more broadly defined to reflect the evolution of educational technologies.

Historically, *home study,* a term mainly used in the United States, is confined to describing further education in vocational or technical institutions rather than in higher educational institutions. Independent study in the American context was conceptualized as a "range of teaching/learning activities that sometimes go by separate names: correspondence study, open education, radio-television teaching, individualized learning" (Wedemeyer, 1977, p. 2115). Independent study is often used as a term for distance education programs of higher learning. This term commonly denotes independence from an educational institution which is not the case in distance education. The Australian term, external studies, describes education that is external to, but not separate from, the faculty of the educational institution. There are two groups of students: one on campus and one off-campus. The same faculty teach both groups using the same examinations and degree. The word *correspondence* is felt to be associated solely with the written word, whereas other forms of media such as audiotapes, radio, telephone, computer, and television communication supplement the written word in what is now termed distance education. It is this recognition of the need for a broader conceptualization of providing education at a distance that led to the adoption of the label *distance education.* Consequently, the International Council for Correspondence Education changed its name to the International Council for Distance Education (Garrison, 1989). The name change reflected the significant changes in the delivery of education at a distance that had been occurring since 1971. These included the inception of the Open University in Great Britain and its adoption of educational technology with respect to hardware and design processes (Keegan, 1990); the establishment of ten distance teaching universities similar to the Open University (Holmberg, 1986); the development of new communication technology (Bates, 1982); and improved instructional materials (Holmberg, 1981).

The adoption of the term *distance education* brought together both the teaching and learning elements of this field of education (Keegan, 1990). It not only indicated the distance between the teacher and learner which characterizes this form of education, but it also encompassed two operating systems: distance teaching and distance learning.

Moore (1973) emphasized the importance of communication between teacher and learner but also suggested that there were instructional methods that were appropriate to distance education. He described distance teaching as:

> *All those teaching methods in which, because of the physical separation of learners and teachers, the interactive (stimulation, exploration, questioning, guidance) as well as the preactive phase of teaching (selecting objectives, planning curriculum and instructional strategies), is conducted through print, mechanical, or electronic devices [p. 669].*

Thus, distance teaching describes the institutional role in the process, whereas distance learning is the process as seen from the student perspective. Figure 16–3 describes the relationship of distance education to distance learning and teaching.
Holmberg (1977) defines distance education as:

> *the various forms of study at all levels which are not under the continuous, immediate supervision of tutors present*

Figure 16–3
Relationship of Distance Education to
Distance Teaching and Learning

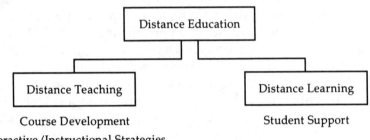

Course Development   Student Support
Interactive/Instructional Strategies

Adapted from *Foundations of Distance Education* (p. 32) by D. Keegan, 1990. London: Routledge. Reprinted by permission.

with their students in lecture rooms or on the same premises, but which, nevertheless, benefit from the planning, guidance, and tuition of a tutorial organization [p. 9].

Holmberg's definition, like Moore's, identifies the separation of teacher and learner. In contrast to Moore, who emphasizes the dialogue and communication between teacher and learner, Holmberg focuses on the educational organization which structures learning materials and links them to facilitate effective learning by students.

Peters's definition of distance education as cited by Keegan (1990) focuses on the "use of technical media, the mass education of students at a distance, and the industrialization of the teaching process" (Keegan, 1990, p. 36). He saw distance teaching/ education as a new form of industrialized and technological education where the interpersonal face-to-face communication commonly found in direct, conventional education is replaced by an apersonal, electronic communication created by technology/ industrialization. Peters (1973) defines distance teaching/ distance education or *Ferunterricht* as:

A method of imparting knowledge, skills, and attitudes which is rationalized by the application of division of labor and organizational principles as well as by the extensive

*use of technical media, especially for the purpose of repro-
ducing high quality teaching material which makes it possible to instruct great numbers of students at the same time
wherever they live. It is an industrialized form of teaching
and learning [p. 206].*

In an attempt to synthesize a descriptive definition from previous
research, Keegan (1990) conceptualized distance education as a
form of education characterized by the following:

1. *the quasi-permanent separation of teacher and learner
   throughout the length of the learning process (this distinguishes it from conventional face-to-face education);*
2. *the influence of an educational organization both in the
   planning and separation of learning materials and in the
   provision of student support services (this distinguishes
   it from private study and teach-yourself programs);*
3. *the use of technical media—print, audio, video, or
   computer—to unite teacher and learner and carry the
   content of the course;*
4. *the provision of two-way communication so that the
   student may benefit from or even initiate dialogue
   (this distinguishes it from other uses of technology in
   education); and*
5. *the quasi-permanent absence of the learning group
   throughout the length of the learning process so that
   people are usually taught as individuals and not in
   groups, with the possibility of occasional meetings for
   both didactic and socialization purposes [p. 44].*

THEORIES OF DISTANCE EDUCATION

As research has evolved and defined the field of distance education
and its characteristics, the need to develop a theoretical structure
which would embrace this whole field and guide its further development and recognition has been urged by researchers in the field
(Moore, 1973; Wedemeyer, 1974). The theoretical positions
formulated fall into three categories: 1. theories of autonomy/

independence, 2. theories of industrialization, and 3. theories of interaction/communication.

Theories of Autonomy/Independence

The theories of autonomy/independence evolved in the late 1960s based on research of Delling (German) and Wedemeyer and Moore (American). According to Keegan (1983), Delling (1975, 1976) tends to reduce the role of the teacher and the educational organization to a minimum and emphasizes the autonomy and independence of the learner. The role of the educational organization is to facilitate the learning (at the wish of the learners) that they cannot do for themselves, with the ultimate goal of the learners becoming autonomous. When autonomy is achieved, the role of the educational organization is to provide student support services, library facilities, information, and documentation. Keegan (1990) states, "Delling seems to want to place distance education outside the field of educational theory. He sees it falling within the range of communication processes and to be characterized by industrialized mechanisms which carry on its artificial dialogue and two-way communication processes" (p. 54). His emphasis then is on distance learning rather than distance teaching.

According to Garrison (1989), Wedemeyer presents another theoretical approach that emphasizes independence and reflects his humanistic philosophy and belief in a democratic social ideal. He believed that every individual should have the opportunity to learn despite socioeconomic status, health, or geographic location. Independent study did not imply independence from the teacher but a shift in emphasis from the educational process, prepackaged content, and isolated learning to the learner and learning activities (Garrison, 1989). This approach, then, represents a shift away from the teacher-centered approach which determines educational needs of students to a learner-centered approach, which values self-pacing, individualized learning activities and methods, and freedom in goal selection. The independent learner assumes responsibility for the overall control of the learning process.

Wedemeyer stresses the value of the teacher in independent study/distance education. The interactive tutorial relationship between the teacher and learner is key to the success of distance education.

Moore (1973) believes that independent study should be defined not only by distance but by autonomy. He classifies educational programs utilizing these two variables of distance and autonomy. There are programs with more autonomy and dialogue (provision for two-way communication) and programs with less. They can vary in distance. The goal is to match the program to the learner so that the learner can exercise the maximum of autonomy or self-directedness and growth. Moore also measures programs according to their responsiveness to individual student needs. He labels this *structure*. Thus, Moore believes it is important to measure the responsiveness of teaching programs to the student's capabilities, goals, needs (structure) and to determine whether the communication medium permits two-way communication (dialogue). Table 16–1 summarizes these types of distance teaching programs.

Moore (1983) defines autonomy as "the extent to which the learner in an educational program is able to determine the selection of objectives, resources and procedures, and the evaluation design" (p. 82). To the learner who is autonomous and needs little direction, the teacher's role is that of respondent, not director. The educational organization becomes a facilitative one. There are learners, however, who need more direction in formulating objectives, identifying sources of information, and measuring achievements. It, therefore, becomes important to match the autonomy dimension of educational programs to the needs of the student. According to Keegan (1990), Moore believes that independent study is "any educational program in which the learning program occurs separately in time and place from the teaching program, and in which the learner has an influence equal to the teacher's determining learning goals, resources, and evaluation decisions" (p. 69). There is no value judgment associated with the terms autonomy and distance.

Theory of Industrialization

Much of the early work in distance education was done by Peters (1973) between the early 1960s and 1970s. He analyzed distance

Table 16–1
Types of Distance Teaching Programs
(S = Structure   D = Dialogue)

	Type	Program Types	Examples
Most distance	–D–S	1. Programs with no dialogue and no structure	Independent reading-study programs of self-directed study
	–D+S	2. Programs with no dialogue but with structure	Programs in which the communication method is radio, television
	+D+S	3. Programs with dialogue and structure	Typically programs using the correspondence or interactive method
Least distance	+D–S	4. Programs with dialogue and no structure	A Rogerian type of tutorial program

Source: Foundations of Distance Education (p. 65) by D. Keegan, 1990. London: Routledge. Reprinted by permission.

teaching systems and identified that analysis of distance teaching from the conventional instructional theory was unproductive. He identified that because distance education was structured so differently from the conventional direct, face-to-face education, another theoretical model was needed in order to build systems. He proposed new categories taken from economic and industrial theory for the analysis of distance education. He identified that the evolution of correspondence or distance education and the industrialization of society were intrinsically linked. Peters further stated that the mass production and distribution of learning materials, as well as the logistics of administering and coordinating the activities of dispersed populations of teachers and learners involved the application of principles drawn from industry. The division of labor relative to technologies associated with the development and production of learning materials is characteristic of distance education. The skills of operations/production management are needed to ensure proper development and timely delivery of services to students. Peters's conclusion is that there is a fundamental distinction between direct conventional, face-to-face education based on interpersonal communication and indirect or redirected education.

Figure 16–4
Relationship of Distance Education to
Other Forms of Indirect Eductation

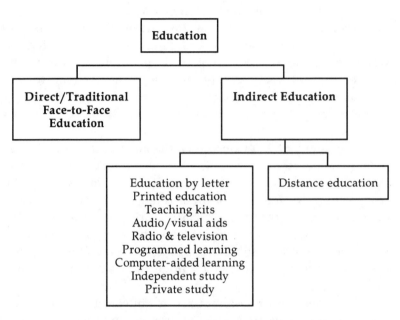

Source: Foundations of Distance Education (p. 22) by D. Keegan, 1990. London: Routledge. Reprinted by permission.

Figure 16–4, developed from Peters's ideas, diagrams the relationship of distance education to other forms of indirect education.

Although these other mediated forms of education are similar in some respects to distance education, they lack one or more of the essential components of distance education. For example, education by letter or printed material such as pamphlets or teach-yourself manuals may lack the structuring of an educational organization characteristic of distance education. Any of the remaining mediated forms of education may lack the required two-way communication characteristic of distance education.

Theories of Interaction/Communication

The theorists who have focused on interaction and communication being central to distance education are Baath (1982), Holmberg (1977), and Sewart (1978, 1987).

Baath has been associated with coining the concept, *two-way communication,* in correspondence education. Throughout the 1970s, he undertook a series of projects on the different forms of two-way communication in distance education. He researched the potential of facilitating interaction within the materials via exercises, questions, and self-assessment exams. He identified the central role of the teacher in providing communication with the learner through mail, computer, telephone, or face to face. He saw the role of the teacher as not only correcting errors or evaluating student progress but also as especially in promoting study motivation.

Holmberg (1977) describes distance education as a guided didactic conversation. Study in distance education is self-study but this does not mean isolation from the teacher. Students benefit from a course developed for them and from interaction with teachers and support from the educational organization. It is the relationship between the learner and the supporting educational organization which Holmberg characterizes as didactic conversation. Distance education as a guided didactic conversation is depicted in Figure 16–5.

Holmberg has recommended a conversational style for distance learning materials and two-way communication to increase the connectedness between the teacher and learner, thereby increasing motivation, comprehension, and pleasure. This conversation can either be real or simulated.

According to Keegan (1990), Holmberg's humanistic philosophy is prevalent in his views of student autonomy and independence, and his emphasis on didactic conversation. Individual learning is of primary importance and "distance education is considered to be particularly suitable for individual learning because it is usually based on personal work by individual students more or less independent from the direct guidance of tutors" (p. 88).

Sewart (1978) has characterized his theory of distance education as a continuity of concern for students learning at a distance. He identifies that the situations and needs of students learning at a distance differ from those of students in conventional, face-to-face education. Differences stem from the absence of quick feedback and support of a peer group, and the lack of a framework

Figure 16–5
Distance Education as a Guided Didactic Coversation

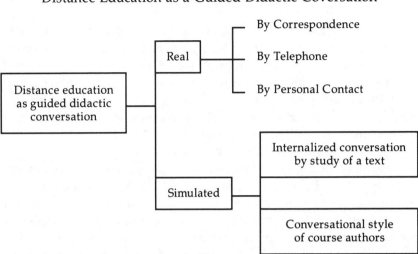

Source: Foundations of Distance Education (p. 89) by D. Keegan, 1990. London: Routledge. Reprinted by permission.

of study (Sewart, 1981). The needs of distance learning students require an interactive mode not supplied by the learning materials. They require an intermediary role to bridge the gap between the individual and the teaching package. According to Keegan (1990), Sewart concludes that "the introduction of the human element is the only way to adapt a distance system to individual needs" (p. 97). The distance education institution is responsible for advising and supporting as well as providing the teaching package and contributing to a decrease in the attrition of distance learning students.

EDUCATIONAL TECHNOLOGY

Educational technology, although essential to the success of distance education, is not synonymous with distance education. Keegan (1990) distinguishes between educational technology in conventional and distance education by stating: "In educational technology, the technology is usually a supplement to the teacher; in distance education, it is usually a substitute for the teacher" (p. 25).

Educational technology in conventional education is usually found in classrooms or lecture halls and can be in the form of print, audiotape, videotape, or computer-based instruction. When used as a one-way communication to supplement teacher instruction, the technology is not included in the concept of distance education. Because educational technology in conventional education is a supplement to the teacher, the cost of teaching increases.

The technology of distance education may decrease the cost of teaching because of more efficient use of existing resources (faculty, no additional buildings or institutions needed) and increased student enrollment. The technology of distance education that is seen as a substitute for the teacher and enhances two-way communication can include print-based correspondence; audio-tapes used for transmission of information; interactive communication between teacher and learner; computer-based interactive software or graphics-based telecommunication systems; and video-based technology such as satellite, teleconferences, fiber optics, or compressed video. The latter facilitates interactive full motion or near full motion video conferencing, as well as the more traditional cable television or microwave technology.

SUMMARY

Three theoretical structures—the autonomy/independence of the learner; the development and production of learning materials based on a model of industrialization; and interaction/communication between teacher and learner are the dominant concepts of distance education. Each perspective differentiates distance education from traditional face-to-face learning. The individual's responsibility in the learning process, dissemination of the products of education, and connectedness between the teacher and learner over space are the hallmarks of distance education. Educational technology is a vehicle for actualizing the theory of distance education.

DESCRIPTION OF THE OUTREACH PROGRAM

In September 1988, the Southern Vermont Education Center (SVEC) was established in Springfield, Vermont, and funded through the state legislature. It is currently staffed by a director, two coordinators, and an administrative assistant. Also housed at the SVEC site is a Vermont Interactive Television studio. The center's purpose is to provide access for the residents of the southeastern part of the state to educational courses offered through Vermont state colleges (Castleton, Lyndon, Johnson, Vermont Technical College, Community College of Vermont), and the University of Vermont (the only state university). The southeastern part of Vermont is especially underserved with respect to higher education. There are no state colleges in this area. The SVEC is seen as a way to provide this access to the already existing state educational institutions without having to build another institution.

The first initiative between the University of Vermont (UVM) and SVEC created a linkage between the associate degree nursing program and general education courses in the state college system. The objective of the initiative was to provide access to nursing education for licensed practical nurses in the southeastern part of the state where no programs existed. Licensed practical nurses were selected as a population to serve because of the existing shortage of registered nurses, support from employers, and the existence of UVM's educational track for practical nurses.

Collaboration between staff of the SVEC and the faculty of the nursing program began with recruitment of students. SVEC took responsibility for securing the availability of comparable general education courses required for the associate degree nursing program. Courses not offered by area colleges were added (e.g., anatomy and physiology). New courses were designed using input from the respective departments at the university. During the instructional phase, SVEC provided support by ordering textbooks, distributing course materials, and providing space for student records. This collaborative effort with SVEC provided a structure whereby practical nurses may complete the associate degree curriculum within their own local area without having to commute daily to the Burlington area or spend extended periods away from employment or home.

Vermont Interactive Television

VIT was begun in response to several problems which confronted the Vermont state colleges system, and the state as a whole. There was the problem of delivering education to remote sites. Faculty members found themselves driving long distances at night, often in mountainous terrain in the dead of winter. The immediate alternatives to this situation were not entirely acceptable. Adjunct faculty were and are used but present potential problems concerning the delivery of education when used on a large-scale basis. These problems stem from lack of familiarity with the curriculum, student needs, and increased educational costs. Videotaped lectures would allow only minimal interactivity with the primary instructor (Thompson, 1989a).

At the same time, questions were being raised on a state level. Questions focused on the quality of education in Vermont; the inequality of access to education because of geographic location; the increasing need for job training; the need for graduate level courses for teachers, engineers, and other disciplines; the need (or viability) of sharing educational resources; and the impact of all of these factors on economic development (Thompson, 1989a). The solution to these problems, and the one to which the state committed itself, was the evolution of an interactive television system. This system allowed for distance education.

VIT is a two-way audio and video link (compressed video) with Vermont Technical College in Randolph Center (the original station), North Country Area Vocational Center in Newport, the Southern Vermont Center of the Vermont State College in Springfield, Lyndon State College in Lyndonville, and the New York/New England Telephone Building in Burlington. It is expected that the system will continue to slowly expand with proposed linkages to Rutland and Bennington. The present and proposed linkages in VIT are depicted in Figure 16–6.

Compressed video was selected because the transmission medium, over telephone lines, is almost universally available and

Figure 16–6
Vermont Interactive Television Sites

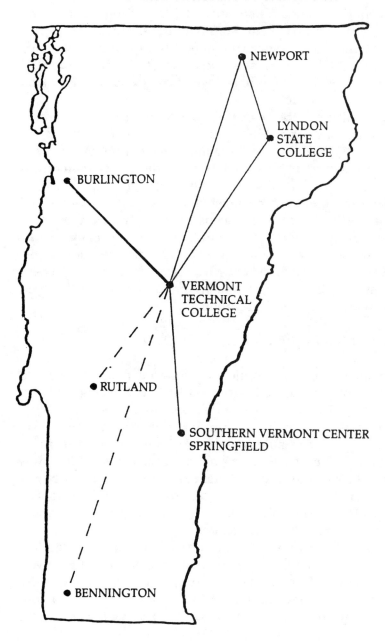

is environmentally acceptable to the state (as opposed to the high towers necessitated by microwave links). It is similar to regular video except that it has a frame rate of 12 to 15 frames per second compared to the normal rate of 30 frames per second. The result is that movement is not tracked as smoothly as full-motion video (Thompson, 1989b). Progress in the development of the technology has been rapid and compressed video comparable to television transmission is available.

One faculty member can teach students in all four remote sites. For this project, the Burlington site and one remote site (in Springfield, VT) was initially used and a second remote site was added. This is a major achievement because the university requires eight to ten students in a course or it is cancelled. It would be possible to have three students in one location, two in another, and four in another location. Such a scenario virtually guarantees educational mobility to practical nurses and others in remote areas. Since VIT was already a resource in the state, the evolution of this medium as a primary method of providing access to the University of Vermont's associate degree nursing program without the need for daily commuting was a natural one.

Implementation of the Project

The implementation of the project focused on enhancing the two components of distance education—distance learning and distance teaching. Distance learning was facilitated through advisement of students, evaluation of prior learning, student orientation to the educational technology, and the development of learning opportunities. The second component, distance teaching, was facilitated through the establishment of a relationship between faculty in the associate degree nursing program, the SVEC coordinator, the VIT coordinator, development of the clinical site, and faculty orientation to the technology.

Given the availability of the resources such as SVEC and VIT to carry an outreach nursing program to a remote site, the University of Vermont performed a needs assessment to determine 1. the level of interest of practical nurses in southeast Vermont to continue their education if they had access to an associate degree nursing program, and 2. clinical agency support for practical nurses to continue their education.

General information sessions were publicized by SVEC and conducted by the faculty of the University of Vermont. Information about the curriculum and how the courses would be offered via VIT was provided. In these sessions, there was a clear commitment from the practical nurses to begin general education course work through Community College of Vermont.

There were also meetings between the University of Vermont and clinical agencies within southeast Vermont. The agencies expressed support for the project in hopes of increasing the numbers of needed registered nurses. They identified institutional incentives such as stipends, full tuition, liberal release time and scheduling to attend classes to support their employees in this effort.

Advisement

On-going advisement and communication with the students was a priority. The project director and co-project director assisted individuals to return to school and/or be admitted to the University of Vermont through pre-admission advising structured by the needs of the individual student. Previous academic credentials were reviewed. A plan of course work was established which provided guidance for reentry or study skills and admission requirements for the adult learner (high school diploma or its equivalency which included two years of algebra and biology). Course selection advisement considered work schedules, family responsibilities, and previous academic experience. For practical nurses who met UVM admission requirements, advisement was provided for the general education course work required in the curriculum (nutrition, human development, anatomy and physiology, English, sociology, two electives), at the course load level desired by the learner.

Evaluation of Prior Learning

Transcripts of previous education along with course syllabi and descriptions were sent by the coordinator for nursing at SVEC or by the individual student to the University of Vermont for evaluation by the Office of Transfer Affairs. The Office of Transfer Affairs compares the course(s) to the content, nature, and intensity of courses taught at the university. According to university policy, transfer credit will be granted if the course has two-thirds comparability to those offered at University of Vermont, was offered at an accredited institution of higher learning, and a grade of C or above was achieved.

Courses in which students were enrolled in other institutions of higher learning are monitored by the Office of Transfer Affairs for quality and depth. Comparability listings of courses offered by all the state colleges already accepted for transfer credit were continuously updated and disseminated to SVEC. Equity was assured through the same admission standards being applied to these students as the on-campus associate degree nursing students. Once admission was granted, the students were eligible for advanced placement on ten credits of nursing through teacher-made examinations. Students received advisement and preparation study guides for the advanced placement examinations which were administered in the vicinity of SVEC. Once the practical nurse successfully passed the examination, advisement was also given about the summer mobility track (bridging process of two to three academic credits given in the summer before the second year clinical nursing courses).

Student Orientation to the Technology

Students were introduced to the system by the site coordinator. They were given a tour of the classroom, advised of the locations of the cameras (overhead camera, camera #2 placed in the back of the classroom to cover the instructor at the front of the room; camera #3 placed at the front of the room to show the faces of the students in the classroom) and the locations of the television monitors. There was one table microphone for every two to three students, and they were instructed to always use a microphone before making comments or asking questions. Students were also encouraged to provide feedback to the technician, site coordinator, or teacher about what was working and not working.

Development of Learning Opportunities

Students communicated with the personnel at SVEC or directly with the University of Vermont School of Nursing via letters, telephone, or, at times, via VIT.

A scheduled time for communication over the interactive network was initiated by students. Students determined that a half-hour session every two weeks was needed to give them an opportunity to converse with a faculty member. This time has been used to discuss any new event, such as pre-registration for the next semester, or problems encountered in the course. For example, students requested that exams not be given on a day that they had clinical laboratory experience. Students felt that commuting between home, the clinical site, and the classroom site necessitated getting up early and, consequently, they were being tested when they were tired. The examination schedule was adjusted. These communications have been instrumental in immediately adjusting the learning environment in response to unanticipated problems.

Development of the Clinical Site

The development of a clinical site near the southeastern part of the state was also a priority. It was paramount that students from southern Vermont would be assured of an academic and clinical program equal to that of the on-campus students. The Medical Center Hospital of Vermont is the facility used for clinical placements for students on campus. It is a full service, 500-bed tertiary care facility—the only one in the state. It serves as a major referral center for Vermont and upstate New York. Clinical experiences at this facility provided a level of acuity, complexity, and diversity unachievable at other clinical sites in the state. A clinical agency that was similar in character, size, and educational opportunities was essential for students who live in southeast Vermont, because the distance for commuting was prohibitive. A clinical site at Dartmouth-Hitchcock Medical Center was developed for these students for their clinical experiences in their second year. Dartmouth-Hitchcock Medical Center is located in Hanover, New

Hampshire, only 35 miles from Springfield, Vermont, the site of SVEC and VIT. The University of Vermont hired a clinical faculty member who lived in southern Vermont to provide clinical supervision at Dartmouth. She had credentials equal to those of faculty on campus and held a New Hampshire nursing license. Ongoing negotiations with the director of nursing education assure appropriate clinical units for the experiences.

Faculty Orientation

Because teaching via interactive television was a new experience for the faculty, an orientation program was provided. The faculty who taught on campus were identical to those teaching to the remote site; therefore, all faculty participated in the distance education program.

Faculty were introduced to the site coordinator, technician, and to the studio arrangement. The studio is located in the New York/New England Telephone Building, two miles from campus. Instructional adaptations and techniques that were necessitated by the use of this technology were explained. For example, because of an overhead camera, the instructor can display a picture from a book or printed materials without the use of transparencies or the chalkboard. The image of what is being written by the instructor or being highlighted from printed material can be combined with the image of the presenter talking about it. Local and remote students, both looking at television monitors, see the same thing. This overhead camera also allows the presenter to face the students at all times, thereby increasing the likelihood of interactivity. Perhaps the major task for the faculty was to learn to interact with the students not physically present. Having the technician shoot tight compositions of the students helped the faculty member make good eye contact with the students on the monitor from the remote site. This facilitated identification of facial expressions and other forms of nonverbal communications upon which teachers depend for feedback.

Faculty were instructed that if they did use the chalkboard, or developed printed materials for use with the overhead camera, to write several short lines rather than one long line. Video has an aspect ratio of 4:3 (four units wide and three units high) so that anything written is seen within a border of these proportions (Thompson, 1989b).

Faculty were instructed that they could walk or pace while teaching if that was a habit but that because of video's limited resolution and the fact that people at remote sites are watching comparatively small screens, it was desirable to shoot tight compositions (Thompson, 1989b). Again, this limited movement would increase the opportunity for close-ups and good eye contact.

The orientation included a discussion of potential audio transmission problems. For example, the microphones on tables in front of the students may not pick up a question or comment. It may, therefore, be necessary for the instructor to repeat the comment or question for the benefit of the students at the remote sites. Feedback noise from the microphones or voices in the classroom could be a problem; the technician would need to control the volume. It might also be necessary for the instructor to remind a student, whether in the classroom or at the remote site, to use the microphone to ask questions.

Faculty were urged to solicit feedback from the technicians and students about what works well and what does not. This feedback may include comments about the clarity of audio or video transmission as well as color contrasts to enhance television viewing (the teacher should avoid wearing white).

Faculty who had used a similar system were given opportunities to share their experiences. This sharing facilitated discussion about faculty's nervousness or fears about using the system. It highlighted the advantages and potential that interactive television can offer. Discussion focused on how to help decrease the intimidation factor of this new medium for students. Faculty were advised to have students interact immediately by introducing themselves, asking questions, or sharing their concerns about the medium.

Finally, the faculty were given time to practice with the media. Seeing themselves on camera, becoming comfortable with looking at the television monitor for the remote site, and learning to use different instructional media on interactive television (i.e., slides, videotape) were helpful. The emphasis was always on using this new medium to increase interactivity in teaching and to engage the learner. The initial department faculty meeting of the year was held on the interactive network to allow time for instructors to become comfortable with the technology and to include remote site clinical faculty in the meeting.

EVALUATION OF THE PROJECT

Evaluation will assess distance education from the perspective of using an educational technology, interactive television, and the process of teaching/learning.

Classes have been delivered over VIT for one summer session and one academic semester. The first class at the remote site graduated with their on-campus classmates in May 1991. Formative evaluation of the interactive television system will be from the perspectives of the faculty and the students. White (1989) offers suggestions for evaluating learning when interactive television is part of the education.

- Does TV enhance or trivialize the material?
- Are some students more motivated because of TV?
- Does the medium alter the message?
- Does the learning environment in which the teacher and learner are separated affect learning?

In the Vermont project, student satisfaction will be evaluated by administering the LPN Student Satisfaction Scale to all students and comparing the remote site students to those on campus. In addition, course evaluations, including examining the use of this technology, will be compared.

There have been mixed results from other studies concerning students' attitudes. A few studies (Boyd & Baker, 1987; Denton, Clark, Rossing, & O'Connor, 1984-1985; and Johnson, O'Connor, & Rossing, 1983-1984) reported positive attitudes, while Parkinson & Parkinson (1989) reported less positive attitudes with the use of interactive television. Their findings might have been due to the fact that the interactive TV class group had only one-third of the faculty contact time that the traditional class group had.

The examination scores of students in both sites will be compared to determine differences in learning. There is consensus in studies by Boyd and Baker (1987); Johnson, O'Connor, and Rossing (1983-1984), and Parkinson and Parkinson (1989), who have examined the impact of interactive television on student learning. They found no differences in student performance on examinations. Finally, success rates in the National Council Licensing Examination (NCLEX) for registered nurses will also be compared between the two groups.

Informal feedback received from faculty suggests that interactive television has motivated them to be more organized in the preparation and delivery of lectures, perhaps because the classroom or studio away from the campus precludes running back to one's office. Although occasional technical problems (e.g., microphone feedback) are an annoyance, the faculty recognize that the technician and site coordinator keep the "down time" to a minimum. They also voiced the benefits of seeing themselves on video. This experience has enhanced their teaching effectiveness. Probably the largest concern that faculty have iterated is that the studio classroom is too cramped for the size of the on-campus student group. The studio, built for a maximum of 25, held an on-campus class group of 35 students.

The on-campus student group, although troubled by the need to travel two miles off campus to the studio site, has recognized some of the new medium's potential. Some have commented that, although they had not seen their classmates face to face in the remote site, when they finally did meet with them, it was like they had known each other for a long time.

CONCLUSIONS

There have been many positive outcomes from the use of interactive television to deliver an outreach associate degree nursing program. Benefits include 1. increased enrollment of nursing students previously denied access to career mobility options, 2. access to university-level education, 3. increased sharing with the rest of the university community, 4. increased attention by faculty to the dialogue or interactive component of teaching, and 5. increased visibility and perceived public image of educational flexibility of the School of Nursing.

The uses for interactive television need not be confined to the classroom but can be effectively used for advisement of potential students, on-going feedback and communications with enrolled students at remote sites, and faculty meetings with faculty at remote sites. These expanded uses of interactive television can help decrease travel time over difficult terrain in isolated rural areas, thereby decreasing faculty workload but maintaining the "face-to-face" human interaction that is desired in most contexts.

Innovation requires change. Innovations dependent on new partnerships necessitate considerable risk taking. In this project new partnerships were forged among many organizations. Readiness to enter into a partnership and a commitment to the goals of the project were critical factors to the success of its implementation.

Students in rural areas benefit from distance education through the provision of equal access to comparable education offered on a university campus. Students who complete a course of study delivered in this manner are able to disseminate their new knowledge of nursing practice to the rural health care environment.

REFERENCES

Baath, J. (1982). Distance students' learning-empirical findings and theoretical deliberations. *Distance education, 3*(1), 6–27.

Bates, A. W. (1982). Trends in the use of audiovisual media in distance education systems. In Daniel et al. (Eds.), *Learning at a distance: A world perspective* (pp. 99–112). Edmonton: Athabasca University.

Boyd, N. J., & Baker, C. M. (1987). Using television to teach. *Nursing & Health Care, 8,* 523–527.

Delling, R. M. (1975). Distant study as an opportunity for learning. In E. L. Josa (Ed.), *The system of distance education* (pp. 55–59). Malmo: Hermods.

Delling, R. M. (1976). Telemathic teaching? Distant study. *ICCE Newsletter, 18–21.*

Denton, J. J., Clark, F. E., Rossing, R. C., & O'Connor, J. J. (1984-1985). Assessing institutional strategies and resulting student attitudes regarding two-way television instruction. *Journal of Educational Technology Systems, 13,* 281–298.

Garrison, D. R. (1989). *Understanding distance education.* London: Routledge.

Holmberg, B. (1977). *Distance education: A survey and bibliography.* London: Kogan Page.

Holmberg, B. (1981). *Status and trends of distance education.* London: Kogan Page.

Holmberg, B. (1986). *Growth and structure of distance education.* London: Croom Helm.

Johnson, G. R., O'Connor, R., & Rossing, R. C. (1983–1984). Interactive two-way television vs. in-person teaching. *Journal of Educational Technology Systems, 12,* 265–272.

Keegan, D. (1990). Theories of distance education. In D. Sewart, D. Keegan, & B. Holmberg (Eds.), *Distance education: International perspectives* (pp. 72–94). London: Croom Helm.

Lassiter, P. (1985). Education for rural health professionals—nurses. *Journal of Rural Health, 1*(1), 23–26.

Moore, M. G. (1973). Toward a theory of independent learning and teaching. *Journal of Higher Education, 44,* 666–679.

Moore, M. G. (1983). On a theory of independent study. In D. Sewart, D. Keegan, & B. Holmberg (Eds.), *Distance education: International perspectives* (pp. 112–134). London: Croom Helm.

Parkinson, C. F., & Parkinson, S. B. (1989). A comparative study between interactive television and traditional lecture course offerings for nursing students. *Nursing & Health Care, 10*(9), 499–502.

Peters, O. (1973). *Die didaktische struktur der fernunterrichts.* Weinheim & Basel: Beltz, Switzerland.

Sewart, D. (1978). *Continuity of concern for students in a system of learning at a distance.* Hagen: Fernuniversitat (Ziff).

Sewart, D. (1981). Distance education—a contradiction in terms. *Teaching at a distance, 19,* 8–18.

Sewart, D. (1987). Staff development needs in distance education and campus-based education: Are they so different? In P. Smith & M. Kelly (Eds.), *Distance education and the mainstream* (pp. 175–200). London: Croom Helm.

Stuart-Sidall, S., & Haberlin, J. (1985). Nursing role in rural health nursing. In L. Jarvis (Ed.), *Community health nursing: Keeping the public healthy* (pp. 495–511). Philadelphia: F. A. Davis.

Thompson, D. (1989a). *Vermont Interactive Television: Compressed video between multiple sites.* Northeast Distance Learning Conference, April 10, 1989. Randolph, VT: Vermont Technical College.

Thompson, D. (1989b). A user's guide to Vermont Interactive Television. Randolph, VT: Vermont Technical College.

U.S. Department of Health and Human Services (1988). The shortage of RNs in rural areas. In U.S. Department of Health and Human Services, *Secretary's commission on nursing.* Washington, D.C.: Author.

Vermont Department of Employment and Training (1987). Occupational employment projections for Vermont to 1995. Burlington, VT: Author.

Vermont Department of Health (1987). *Vermont: A health plan 1986–1990.* Waterbury, VT: Author.

Vermont State Nurses' Association (1987). *Profile of the Vermont registered nurse.* Burlington, VT: Vermont State Nurses' Association.

Vermont Student Assistance Corporation (1988). Talking points: Nursing and teaching students. Montpelier, VT: Author.

Wedemeyer, C. A. (1974). Characteristics of open learning systems. In *Open learning systems* (pp. 27–49). Washington, D.C.: National Association of Educational Broadcasters.

White, M. A. (1989). *Distance Learning: How will we know if it really works?* (videorecording). Northeast Distance Learning Conference. Boston, MA: The Duplicating Center.

17

Rural Nursing: Developing the Theory Base

Kathleen Ann Long
Clarann Weinert

A logger suffering from "heart lock" does not have a cardiovascular abnormality. He is suffering from a work-related anxiety disorder and can be assisted by an emergency room nurse who accurately assesses his needs and responds with effective communication and a supportive interpersonal relationship. A farmer who has lost his finger in a grain thresher several hours earlier does not have time during the harvesting season for a discussion of occupational safety. He will cope with his injury assisted by a clinic nurse who can adjust the timing of his antibiotic doses to fit with his work schedule in the fields.

Many health care needs of rural dwellers cannot be adequately addressed by the application of nursing models developed in urban or suburban areas but require unique approaches emphasizing the special needs of this population. While nurses are significant, and frequently the sole, health care providers for people

Reprinted from *Scholarly Inquiry to Nursing Practice: An International Journal, 3*(2). Copyright 1989, Springer Publishing Company, Inc., New York, NY 10012. Used by permission.

living in rural areas, little has been written to guide the practice of rural nursing. The literature provides vignettes and individual descriptions, but there is a need for an integrated, theoretical approach to rural nursing.

Rural nursing is defined as the provision of health care by professional nurses to persons living in sparsely populated areas. Over the past eight years, graduate students and faculty members at the Montana State University College of Nursing have worked toward developing a theory base for rural nursing. Theory development has used primarily a retroductive approach, and data have been collected and refined using a combination of qualitative and quantitative methods. The experiences of rural residents and rural nurses have guided the identification of key concepts relevant to rural nursing. The goal of the theory building process has been to identify commonalities and differences in nursing practice across all rural areas and the common and unique elements of rural nursing in relation to nursing overall. The implications of developing a theory of rural nursing for practice have been examined as a part of the ongoing process.

The theory building process was initiated in the late 1970s. At that time, literature and research related to rural health care were limited and focused primarily on the problem of retaining physicians in rural areas and providing assessments of rural health care needs and prescriptions for rural health care services based on models and experiences from urban and suburban areas (Coward, 1977; Flax, Wagenfield, Ivens, & Weiss, 1979). The unique health problems and health care needs of extremely sparsely populated states, such as Montana, had not been addressed from the perspective of the rural consumer. No organized theoretical base for guiding rural health care practice in general, or rural nursing in particular, existed.

QUALITATIVE DATA

The target population for qualitative data collection was the people of Montana. Montana, the fourth largest state in the United States, is an extremely sparsely populated state, with nearly

800,000 people and an average population density of approximately five persons per square mile. One half of the counties in Montana have three or fewer persons per square mile, with six of those counties having less than one person per square mile. There is only one metropolitan center in the state; it is a city of nearly 70,000 people, with a surrounding area that constitutes a center of approximately 100,000 (*Population Profiles,* 1985).

Qualitative data were collected through ethnographic study by Montana State University College of Nursing graduate students. These data provided the initial ideas about health and health care in Montana. Since general propositions about rural health and rural health care did not exist, the gathering of concrete data was the first step toward subsequent development of more general theoretical propositions.

Graduate students used ethnographic techniques as described by Spradley (1979) to gather information from individuals, families, and health service providers. Interview sites were selected by students on the basis of specific interest and convenience. During a six-year period, data were gathered from approximately 25 locations. In general, each student worked in depth in one community, collecting data from ten to 20 informants over a period of at least one year. Data were gathered primarily from persons in ranching and farming areas and from towns of less than 2,500 persons. In some instances, student interest led to extensive interviews with specific rural subgroups, such as men in the logging industry or elderly residents in a rural town (Weinert & Long, 1987). Open-ended interview questions were developed using Spradley's (1979) guidelines. The questions emphasized seeking the informants' views without superimposing the cultural biases of the interviewer. The opening question in the interview was, "What is health to you . . . from your viewpoint? . . . your definition?" Interviewers used standard probes and a standard format of questions regarding health beliefs and health care preferences.

Spradley (1979) indicated that the goal of ethnographic study is to "build a systematic understanding of all human cultures from the perspective of those who have learned them" (p. 10). The goal of data collection in Montana was to learn about the culture of rural Montanans from rural Montanans. Emphasis in the cultural learning process was on understanding health beliefs, values, and practices. Rigdon, Clayton, and Diamond (1987) have noted that understanding the meaning that persons attach to subjective experiences is an important aspect of nursing knowledge. The ethnographic approach captured the meanings that rural dwellers ascribe to the subjective states of health and illness and facilitated the development of a rich data base.

As the data base developed, the following definitions and assumptions were accepted as a foundation for theory development. Rural was defined as meaning sparsely populated. Within this context, states such as Montana, which are sparsely populated overall, are viewed as rural throughout, despite the existence of some population centers within them. Further, based on this definition, rural regions or areas can be identified within otherwise heavily populated states. The assumption is made that, to some degree, health care needs are different in rural areas from that of urban areas. Also, all rural areas are viewed as having some common health care needs. Finally, the assumption is made that urban models are not appropriate to, or adequate for, meeting health care needs in rural areas.

Retroductive Theory Generation

Faculty work groups were developed to examine and organize the qualitative data. The work groups involved three to five nursing faculty members, each with rural nursing experience, but with varied backgrounds and expertise. Thus, a work group included experts from various clinical areas, as well as persons with direct experience either in small rural hospitals or in larger, metropolitan centers within rural states. Standard ethnographic content analysis (Spradley, 1979) was used to sort and categorize the ethnographic data. Groups worked toward consensus about the meaning and organization of specific data. Recurring themes were identified, and these were viewed as having relevance and importance for the rural informants in relation to their views of health.

A retroductive approach, as originally described by Hanson (1958), was used to examine the initial ethnographic data and build the theory base. Specific concepts and relational statements were derived from the data, and more general propositions were induced from these statements. The new propositions were then used to develop additional specific statements which could be supported by existing data or which were categorized for later testing. The retroductive approach was literally a "back and forth" process that permitted persons familiar with the data to move between the data and beginning-level theoretical propositions. The process was orderly and consistent and required group consensus about data interpretation and the relevance of derived propositions. The retroductive process continued in work groups over several years as additional ethnographic data were gathered. Consultants participated at key points in the process, in order to raise questions, add insights, and critically evaluate the group's theory building approach. Walker and Avant (1983) have noted that the retroductive process "adds considerably to the body of theoretical knowledge. It is, in fact, the way theory develops in the 'real world'" (p. 176).

QUANTITATIVE DATA

Following several years of ethnographic study, the faculty members involved in theory development wished to enrich the qualitative data base by collecting relevant quantitative data. Kleinman (1983) stated, "Qualitative description, taken together with various quantitative measures, can be a standardized research method for assessing validity. It is especially valuable in studying social and cultural significance, e.g., illness beliefs, interaction norms, social gain, ethnic help seeking, and treatment responses" (p. 543). Hinds and Young noted (1987), "The combination of different methodologies within a single study promotes the likelihood of uncovering multiple dimensions of a phenomenon's empirical reality" (p. 195).

A survey developed by Weinert in 1983 attempted to validate some of the rural health concepts that had emerged from the ethnographic data. These concepts were: health status and health beliefs, isolation and distance, self-reliance, and informal health care systems. Survey instruments with established psychometric properties were selected to measure the specific concepts of interest. A mail questionnaire completed by the respondents included the Beck Depression Inventory (Beck, 1967) and the Trait Anxiety Scale (Spielberger, Gorsuch, & Lushene, 1970), to tap mental health status, and the General Health Perception Scale (Davies & Ware, 1981), to measure physical health status and health beliefs. A background information form assessed demographic variables, including length of residence and geographic locale. The Personal Resource Questionnaire (Brandt & Weinert, 1981) assessed use of informal systems for support and health care.

The convenience sample of survey participants was located through the Agricultural Extension Service, social groups, and informal networks. All participants lived in Montana, completed the questionnaires in their homes, and returned them by mail to the researcher. The 62 survey participants were middle-class whites, with an average of 13.5 years of education and a mean age of 61.3 years, who had lived in Montana an average of 45.6 years. The survey sample consisted of 40 women and 22 men residing in one of 13 sparsely populated Montana counties. The most populated county has a population density of 5.9 persons per square mile and one town of nearly 6,000 people. In the most sparsely populated county, there is one town of 600 people and an average population density of 0.5 persons per square mile.

Findings from the quantitative study were used throughout the theory development process to support or refute concept descriptions and relational statements derived from the ethnographic data. Survey findings are discussed in the following section as they relate to key concepts and relational statements.

REFINING THE BUILDING BLOCKS OF THEORY

To order the data and foster the formation of relational statements, an organizational scheme for theory development was adopted. Using the paradigm first described by Yura and Torres (1975) and later by Fawcett (1984), ethnographic data were categorized under the four major dimensions of nursing theory: person, health, environment, and nursing. The data were then ordered from the more general to the more specific. This process led to the identification of constructs, concepts, variables, and indicators.

An example helps to illustrate this process. Ethnographic data had been gathered from "gypo" loggers. These men are independent logging contractors from northwestern Montana who work in rugged isolated areas, usually living in trailers or tents while working. Examples of quotes from these loggers and their associates as found in the data are: A logger states, "We worry about the here and now"; a local physician says, "Loggers enter the health care system during times of crisis only"; the public health nurse in the area says, "Loggers don't want to hear about health care problems; they don't return until the next accident."

Table 17–1 shows the scheme used to organize these data. The concepts "present time" orientation and crisis orientation to health are identified. These are placed under the person dimension. In this example, the constructs are not fully developed, but are viewed as psychological and/or sociocultural. The important variables identified thus far are definitions of time and of crisis. Possible indicators are measures of time, such as hours or seasons, and measures of crisis, such as numbers of illnesses or injuries.

Key Concepts

In the process of data organization it was noted that some concepts appeared repeatedly in ethnographic data collected in several different areas of the state. In addition, aspects of several of these concepts were supported by the quantitative survey data (Weinert, 1983). Using Walker and Avant's (1983) model of concept synthesis, these concepts were identified as key concepts in relation to understanding rural health needs and rural nursing practice. These key concepts are as follows: work beliefs and health beliefs, isolation and distance, self-reliance, lack of anonymity, outsider/insider, and old timer/newcomer.

As key concepts in this theory, work beliefs and health beliefs are viewed as different for rural dwellers as contrasted with urban or suburban residents. These two sets of beliefs appear to be closely interrelated among rural persons. Work, or the fulfilling of one's usual functions, is of primary importance. Health is assessed

Table 17–1
Data Ordering Scheme

Component	Examples
Dimension	Person
Construct	Psychological/sociocultural
Concept	"Present time" orientation Crisis orientation to health
Variable	Definitions of time Definitions of crisis
Indicators	Hours, minutes, days Seasons, work seasons Number of injuries Number of illnesses

by rural people in relation to work role and work activities, and health needs are usually secondary to work needs.

The related concepts of isolation and distance are identified as important in understanding rural health and nursing. Specifically, they help in understanding health care-seeking behavior. Quantitative survey data indicated that rural informants who lived outside of towns traveled a distance of almost 23 miles, on average, for emergency health care and over 50 miles for routine health care. Despite these distances, ethnographic data indicated that rural dwellers tended to see health services as accessible and did not view themselves as isolated.

Self-reliance and independence of rural persons are also seen as key concepts. The desire to do for oneself and care for oneself was strong among the rural persons interviewed and have important ramifications in relation to the provision of health care.

Two key concept areas, lack of anonymity and outsider/ insider, have particular relevance for the practice of rural nursing. Lack of anonymity, a hallmark of small towns and surrounding sparsely populated areas, implies a limited ability for rural persons to have private areas of their lives. Rural nurses almost always reported being known to their patients as neighbors, part of a given family, members of a certain church, and so on. Similarly, these nurses usually know their patients in several different social and personal relationships beyond the nurse-patient relationship. The old timer/newcomer concept, or the related concepts of outsider/insider, is relevant in terms of the acceptance of nurses and of all health care providers in rural communities. The ethnographic data indicated that these concepts were used by rural dwellers in organizing their view of the social environment and in guiding their interactions and relationships. Survey data revealed that those who had lived in Montana over ten years, but less than 20, still considered themselves to be "newcomers" and expected to be viewed as such by those in their community (Weinert & Long, 1987).

Relational Statements

In an effort to move from a purely descriptive theory to a beginning-level explanatory one, some initial relational statements were generated from the qualitative data and were supported by the quantitative data that had been collected thus far. The statements are in the early stages of testing.

The first statement is that rural dwellers define health primarily as the ability to work, to be productive, to do usual tasks. The ethnographic data indicate that rural persons place little emphasis on the comfort, cosmetic, and life-prolonging aspects of health. One is viewed as healthy when able to function and be productive in one's work role. Specifically, rural residents indicated that pain was tolerated, often for extended periods, so long as it did not interfere with the ability to function. The General Health Perception Scale indicated that rural survey participants reported experiencing less pain than an age-comparable urban sample (Weinert & Long, 1987). Further, scores on the Beck Depression Inventory and the Trait Anxiety Scale (Weinert, 1983) revealed that they experienced less anxiety and less depression.

The second statement is that rural dwellers are self-reliant and resist accepting help or services from those seen as "outsiders" or from agencies seen as national or regional "welfare" programs. A corollary to this statement is that help, including needed health care, is usually sought through an informal rather than a formal system. Ethnographic data supported both the second statement and its corollary. Numerous references were found showing, for example, a preference for "the 'old doc' who knows us" over the new specialist who was unfamiliar. Data from the Personal Resource Questionnaire (Weinert, 1983) indicated that rural dwellers relied primarily on family, relatives, and close friends for help and support. Further, the rural survey respondents reported using health care professionals and formal human service agencies much less frequently than did comparable urban respondents in previous studies.

A third statement is that health care providers in rural areas must deal with a lack of anonymity and much greater role diffusion than providers in urban or suburban settings. This statement has marked significance for rural nursing practice. Although limited ethnographic and survey data have been collected from rural nurses thus far, some emerging themes have been identified. In addition to identifying a sense of isolation from professional peers, rural nurses emphasize their lack of anonymity and a sense of role diffusion. There is an inability to keep separate the activities and behaviors of the individual nurse's various roles. In a small town, for example, the nurse's behavior as a wife, a mother, and a church attender are all significantly related to her effectiveness as a health care professional in that community. Further, in their professional role, nurses reported experiencing role diffusion. Nurses are expected to perform a variety of diverse and unrelated tasks. On a single shift, a nurse may work in obstetrics delivering a baby, care for a dying patient on the medical-surgical unit, and initiate care of a trauma patient in the emergency room. Likewise, on evening shift or weekends, a nurse may be required to carry out tasks reserved for the pharmacist or dietician on the day shift.

RELATIONSHIP OF CONCEPTS AND STATEMENTS TO THE LARGER BODY OF NURSING KNOWLEDGE

How people define health and illness has a direct impact on how they seek and use health care services and is a key concept in understanding client behavior and in planning intervention.

Definition of Health

The rural Montana dwellers primarily define health as the ability to work and to be productive. The work of other researchers supports the finding that residents of sparsely populated areas view health in terms of ability to work and remain productive. Ross (1982), a nurse anthropologist, studied the health perceptions of women living in the Lake District along the coast of Nova Scotia. She conducted in-depth interviews with 60 women of both British and French backgrounds in small coastal fishing communities. Similar to the rural dwellers in Montana, these women described good health as being "able to do what you want to do" and to "be able to work." Lee's (1987) recent work in Montana supports earlier findings on which the rural nursing theory was built. She found that work and health practices were closely related among farmers and ranchers; health is viewed as a functional state in relation to work. Scharff's (1987) interviews with nurses practicing in small rural hospitals in eastern Washington, northern Idaho, and western Montana indicated that they viewed the health needs of rural people as overlapping those of people living in urban situations in many instances. The nurse informants, however, noted that rural people equate health with the ability to work or function in their daily activities. Rural people were viewed as delaying health care until they were very ill, thus often needing hospitalization at the point of seeking care.

Self-Reliance

The statement derived from the Montana data that "rural dwellers resist accepting help from outsiders or strangers" has been supported in data from research in rural Maryland (Salisbury State College, 1986). People living in the rural eastern shore area were described as highly resistant to care from persons viewed as outsiders, and rural shore residents often refused to go "across the bridge" to Baltimore to seek health care, even though this was a trip of less than 100 miles and would allow access to sophisticated, specialized treatment. Like the rural people in Montana, these Maryland residents sought health care information and assistance from local, and often informal, sources. The self-reliance of rural persons and their resistance to outside help were also reported by Counts and Boyle (1987) in relation to residents of the Appalachian area. Self-reliance was noted as a major feature that must be considered in planning nursing care services for this population.

The rural Nova Scotia women studied by Ross (1982) indicated informal personal networks of family, friends, and neighbors as important sources of health information who also provided the physical, financial, emotional, and social support that contributes to well-being. When these women were asked what connection there was between health and the availability of hospitals, doctors, and other medical care, 42 percent indicated that it was the individual's responsibility for health knowledge and care; 25 percent thought professionals were useful to a certain point in providing advice and services such as routine physical exams; 19 percent indicated that these services were for sick persons, not healthy persons; and 9 percent felt the formal health care system had no relationship to health (Ross, 1982, p. 311). One woman commented, "Health is not a topic to discuss with doctors and nurses" (Ross, 1982, p. 309).

Rural Nursing

The Montana data and the theory derived from it indicate that nurses and other health care providers in rural areas must deal with a lack of anonymity. Nurses are known in a variety of roles to their patients and, in turn, know their patients in a variety of roles. Most of the nurses interviewed by Scharff (1987) felt that by knowing their patients personally they could give better care. Other nurses, however, noted that providing professional care for family or friends can be a frightening experience. Nurses indicated that there was no anonymity for them in the rural community, which, at times, was reassuring and, at other times, constricting (Scharff, 1987).

The concept of role diffusion in the rural hospital setting was very apparent in Scharff's (1987) work. She reported that a rural hospital nurse must be a jack-of-all-trades who often practices within the realm of numerous other health care disciplines, including respiratory therapy, laboratory technology, dietetics, pharmacy, social work, psychology, and medicine. Examples of the intersections between rural nursing and other disciplines include doing EKGs, performing arterial punctures, running blood gas machines, drawing blood, setting up cultures, going to the pharmacy to pour drugs, going to the local drugstore to get medications for patients, ordering x-rays and medications, delivering babies, directing the actions of physicians, and cooking meals when the cook gets snowed in. As Scharff (1987) noted, some of these functions are carried out by urban nurses practicing in particular settings such as a trauma center or intensive care unit. Rural nurses, however, are usually not circumscribed by assignment to a particular unit or department and are expected to function in multiple roles, even within one work shift.

This generalist work role and the lack of anonymity of rural nurses are substantiated by findings and descriptions from several other rural areas of the United States (Biegel, 1983; St. Clair, Pickard, & Harlow, 1986). A study of nurses in rural Texas noted, "Nurses play roles as nurse, friend, neighbor, citizen, and family member" within a community; further, rural nurses in their work roles were described as needing to be "all things to all people" (St. Clair et al., 1986, p. 28).

Generalizability

The issue of a situation or locale-specific theory and its relationship to the larger body of nursing knowledge needs serious consideration. The work of Scharff (1987) indicated that the core of rural nursing is not different from urban nursing. The intersections, however, those "meeting points at which nursing extends its practice into the domains of other professions"; the dimensions, that is, the "philosophy, responsibilities, functions, roles, and skills"; and the boundaries, which "respond to new and growing needs and demands from society" (American Nurses Association, 1980), appear to be very distinct for rural nursing practice.

Questions remain as to how generalizable findings from Montana residents are to other rural populations. Clearly, there is a need for more organized and rigorous data collection in relation to rural nursing before these questions can be answered. A sound theory base for rural practice requires continued research, conducted across diverse rural settings.

IMPLICATIONS FOR NURSING PRACTICE

The findings from the Montana research about people living in sparsely populated areas have implications for nursing practice in rural areas. Since work is of major importance to rural people, health care must fit within work schedules. Health care programs or clinics which conflict with the rural economic cycle, such as haying or calving, will not be used. Since health is defined as the ability to work, health promotion must address the work issue. For example, health education related to cardiovascular disease should highlight strategies for preventing conditions that involve long-term disability, such as stroke. These aspects will be more meaningful to rural dwellers than preventive aspects that emphasize a longer, more comfortable life.

The self-reliance of rural dwellers has specific nursing implications. Rural people will often delay seeking health care until they are gravely ill or incapacitated. Nursing approaches need to address two distinct aspects: nonjudgmental intervention for those who have delayed treatment and a strong emphasis on preventive health teaching. If the nurse can provide adequate health knowledge, the rural dweller's desire for self-reliance may lead to health-promotion behaviors. With a good information base, rural people can make appropriate decisions about self-care versus the need for professional intervention.

Health care services must be tailored to suit the preferences of rural persons for family and community help during periods of illness. Nurses can provide instruction, support, and relief to family members and neighbors, who are often the primary-care providers for sick and disabled persons. The formal health care system needs to fit into the informal helping system in rural areas. A long-term community resident, such as the drugstore proprietor, can be assisted in providing accurate advice to residents through the provision of reference materials and a telephone back-up system. One can anticipate greater acceptance and use by rural residents of an updated but old and trusted health care resource, rather than a new, professional, but "outsider" service (Weinert & Long, 1987).

Nurses who enter rural communities must allow for extended periods prior to acceptance. Involvement in diverse community activities, such as civic organizations and recreational clubs, may assist the nurse in being known and accepted as a person. In rural communities acceptance as a health care professional is often tied to personal acceptance. Thus it appears that rural communities are not appropriate practice settings for nurses who prefer to maintain entirely separate professional and personal lives.

The stresses that appear to affect nurses in rural practice settings have particular importance. Rural nurses see themselves as cut off from the professional mainstream. They are often in situations where there is no collegial support to assist in defining an appropriate practice role and its boundaries. The educational preparation of those who wish to practice in rural settings needs to emphasize not only generalist skills, but also a strong base in change theory and leadership techniques. Nurses in rural practice need a sound orientation to techniques for accessing diverse sources of current information. If the closest library is several hundred miles away, for example, can an arrangement for interlibrary loan and access to material via telephone, bus, or mail be arranged? Networks that link together nurses practicing in distant rural sites are particularly useful, both for information exchange and for mutual support.

SUMMARY

It is becoming increasingly clear that rural dwellers have distinct definitions of health. Their health care needs require approaches that differ significantly from urban and suburban populations. Subcultural values, norms, and beliefs play a key role in how rural people define health and from whom they seek advice and care. These values and beliefs, combined with the realities of rural living—such as weather, distance, and isolation—markedly affect the practice of nursing in rural settings. Additional ethnographic and quantitative data are needed to further define both the common and the locale-specific conditions and characteristics of rural populations. Continued research can provide a more solid base for the nursing theory that is required to guide practice and the delivery of health care to rural populations.

REFERENCES

American Nurses Association. (1980). *Nursing: A social policy statement* (No. NP-63 20M 9/82R). Kansas City, MO: Author.

Brandt, P., & Weinert, C. (1981). The PRQ: A social support measure. *Nursing Research, 30,* 277–280.

Beck, A. (1967). *Depression: Causes and treatment.* Philadelphia: University of Pennsylvania Press.

Biegel, A. (1983). Toward a definition of rural nursing. *Home Health Care Nursing, 1,* 45–46.

Counts, M., & Boyle, J. (1987). Nursing, health and policy within a community context. *Advances in Nursing Science, 9,* 12–23.

Coward, R. (1977). Delivering social services in small towns and rural communities. In R. Coward (Ed.), *Rural families across the life span: Implications for community programming* (pp. 1–17). West Lafayette, IN: Indiana Cooperative Extension Services.

Davies, A., & Ware, J. (1981). *Measuring health perceptions in the health insurance experiment.* Santa Monica, CA: Rand.

Fawcett, J. (1984). *Analysis and evaluation of conceptual models of nursing.* Philadelphia: F. A. Davis.

Flax, J., Wagenfield, M., Ivens, R., & Weiss, R. (1979). *Mental health and rural America: An overview and annotated bibliography.* Rockville, MD: U.S. Government Printing Office.

Hanson, N. (1958). *Patterns of discovery.* Cambridge: Cambridge University Press.

Hinds, P., & Young, K. (1987). A triangulation of methods and paradigms to study nurse-given wellness care. *Nursing Research, 36,* 195–198.

Kleinman, A. (1983). The cultural meanings and social uses of illness: A role for medical anthropology and clinically oriented social science in the development of primary care theory and research. *Journal of Family Practice, 16,* 539–545.

Lee, H. (1987). *Relationship of hardiness and current life events to perceived health and rural adults.* Manuscript submitted for publication.

Population profiles of Montana counties: 1980. (1985). Bozeman, MT: Montana State University Center for Data Systems and Analysis.

Rigdon, I., Clayton, B., & Diamond, M. (1987). Toward a theory of helpfulness for the elderly bereaved: An invitation to a new life. *Advances in Nursing Science, 9,* 32–43.

Ross, H. (1982). Women and wellness: Defining, attaining, and maintaining health in Eastern Canada. *Dissertation Abstracts International, 42,* DEO 82-12624.

Salisbury State College (1986, June). *Discussion of Salisbury State College rural health findings.* Presented at the Contemporary Issues in Rural Health Conference, Salisbury, MD.

Scharff, J. (1987). *The nature and scope of rural nursing: Distinctive characteristics.* Unpublished master's thesis, Montana State University, Bozeman, MT.

Spielberger, C., Gorsuch, R., & Lushene, R. (1970). *STAI manual for the State-Trait Anxiety Questionnaire.* Palo Alto, CA: Consulting Psychologist.

Spradley, J. (1979). *The ethnographic interview.* New York: Holt, Rinehart, and Winston.

St. Clair, C., Pickard, M., & Harlow, K. (1986). Continuing education for self actualization: Building a plan for rural nurses. *Journal of Continuing Education in Nursing, 17,* 27–31.

Walker, L., & Avant, K. (1983). *Strategies for theory construction in nursing.* Norwalk, CT: Appleton-Century-Crofts.

Weinert, C. (1983). *Social support: Rural people in their "new middle years."* Unpublished raw data.

Weinert. C., & Long, K. (1987). Understanding the health care needs of rural families. *Journal of Family Relations, 36,* 450–455.

Yura, H., & Torres, G. (1975). *Today's conceptual frameworks with the baccalaureate nursing programs* (NLN Pub. No. 15-1558, pp. 17–75). New York: National League for Nursing.

Acknowledgments: Qualitative data collected and analyzed by Montana State University, College of Nursing graduate students and faculty, form the basis for a substantial portion of this paper. Ethnographic data collection and analysis was supported, in part, by a U.S. Department of Health and Human Services, Division of Nursing, Advanced Training Grant to the Montana State University, College of Nursing (#1816001649A1). The project that provided the survey data was funded by a Montana State University Faculty Research/Creativity Grant. This article is based partially on a paper presented at the Western Society for Research in Nursing Conference, Tempe, AZ, May 1987.